THE NICER YEAR BOOK 1996

Ultrasonography

ISBN 1-899066-66-7

9 781899 066667

THE NICER YEAR BOOK 1996

Ultrasonography

Edited by

Barry B. Goldberg, MD
Professor of Radiology
Jefferson Medical College
Thomas Jefferson University Hospital
Philadelphia, PA, USA

and

Holger Pettersson, MD
Professor of Radiology
University Hospital
Lund, Sweden
Educational and Scientific Director,
the NICER Institute

Series on Diagnostic Imaging
from
The NICER Institute

ISIS MEDICAL MEDIA

The NICER program and the NICER books

NICER

The NICER program is a unique approach to continuing education in diagnostic imaging, and consists of a global program provided by some of the world's leading authorities. Its goal is the provision of high-quality education, dissociated from any commercial interests or influences, to radiologists throughout the world. The teaching program is run by:

the NICER Institute

which is an educational foundation based on a collaboration between

The Department of Radiology,
Lund University, Sweden,
and
The Nycomed Imaging A/S, Oslo, Norway

The NICER program is based on two pillars:
The NICER Courses
The NICER Publications

The NICER Courses comprises a series of 2–4 courses, given in different regions of the world, each series running over a period of 2–4 years. The courses in a complete series cover the whole field of diagnostic imaging, each course dealing with one or two organ systems.

The NICER Publications embrace a wide spectrum of radiological knowledge ranging from the basic to state-of-the art. The first book series, published in 1991–1992, comprised five volumes of 300–600 pages per volume. Each multi-author volume covered one or two organ areas, different aspects of the subject matter being written by leading radiologists and edited by world authorities.

Since 1994 NICER publishes a new series on diagnostic imaging called the NICER Yearbook Series. Each year we will publish one volume devoted to a particular radiological topic, but presented in a manner that will be informative and interesting to both the general radiologist and the specialist.

The first book in this series, 1994, was devoted to interventional radiology. The NICER Yearbook 1995 – A Global Textbook of Radiology – was called "centennial" to celebrate the first century of diagnostic imaging. It was published in English, with translations to Chinese, Russian, and Spanish. It is now a pleasure for the NICER Institute to present the Yearbook 1996, "Ultrasonography".

Until now (1996) more than 6 500 course participants have attended the courses around the world, and more than 70 000 NICER books have been distributed.

The NICER Institute welcomes you, the Readers. We hope that you will enjoy the reading, and we look forward to seeing you at future courses.

Lund University
Sweden

NYCOMED
IMAGING

The NICER Institute

ISBN 82-990882-2-4

Published by: The NICER Institute, Oslo · Graphic design cover: Mons Rønning
Design, repro and printing by: Elanders Norge AS, Oslo

Reprinted papers are available from The NICER Institute
Po.Box 4462, Torshov, N-0401 Oslo, Norway

Distributed by: ISIS MEDICAL MEDIA
ISBN 1-899066-66-7

Contents

List of Authors

Archie Alexander, MD
Associate Professor of Radiology
Division of Diagnostic Ultrasound
Department of Radiology
Thomas Jefferson University Hospital and Medical College
PHILADELPHIA, PA, USA

Paul L. Allan, MD, FRCR, FRCPE
Senior Lecturer in Medical Radiology
Honorary Consultant Radiologist
Royal Infirmary
EDINBURGH, Scotland

Torbjörn Andersson, MD
Chairman
Department of Radiology
Örebro Medical Center Hospital
ÖREBRO, Sweden

Harm-Gerd Blaas, MD
National Center for Fetal Medicine
Department of Gynecology and Obstetrics
Trondheim University Hospital
TRONDHEIM, Norway

Maria Chiara Bossi, MD
Department of Radiology
European Institute of Oncology
MILAN, Italy

James D. Bowie, MD
Professor of Radiology
Assistant Professor of OB/GYN
Department of Radiology
Duke University Medical Center
DURHAM, NC, USA

Mark Brooks, FRACR
Consultant Radiologist
Department of Radiology
Austin and Repatriation

Medical Center
MELBOURNE, Australia

Terry L. Coates, MD
Assistant Professor of Radiology
Department of Radiology
UCD Medical Center
SACRAMENTO, CA, USA

Dennis L. Cochlin, MB, BCh, FRCR
Department of Radiology
Division of Diagnostic Ultrasound
University Hospital of Wales
CARDIFF, United Kingdom

Peter L. Cooperberg, MD
Professor of Radiology
Department of Radiology
University of British Columbia
VANCOUVER, Canada

David O. Cosgrove, MA, MSc, FRCR, FRCP
Consultant in Radiology
Department of Diagnostic Radiology
Hammersmith Hospital
LONDON, United Kingdom

Rose de Bruyn, MD
Consultant Pediatric Radiologist
The Hospital for Sick Children
LONDON, United Kingdom

Keith Dewbury, MD, FRCR
Consultant Radiologist
Department of Radiology
Southampton General Hospital
SOUTHAMPTON, United Kingdom

Paul Dubbins, BSc, MBBS, FRCR
Consultant Radiologist
Department of Radiology
Derriford Hospital
PLYMOUTH, United Kingdom

Sturla H. Eik-Nes, MD, PhD
Professor of Obstetrics and Gynecology
National Center for Fetal Medicine
Department of Obstetrics and Gynecology Trondheim
University Hospital
TRONDHEIM, Norway

Bruno D. Fornage, MD
Professor of Radiology
Chief, Section of Ultrasound
The University of Texas
M.D. Anderson Cancer Center
HOUSTON, TX, USA

Flemming Forsberg, PhD
Assistant Professor of Radiology
Division of Diagnostic Ultrasound
Department of Radiology

Thomas Jefferson University
Hospital and Medical College
PHILADELPHIA, PA, USA

Andrew M. Fried, MD
Professor of Diagnostic Radiology
Department of Diagnostic Radiology
College of Medicine
University of Kentucky
LEXINGTON, KY, USA

Barry B. Goldberg, MD
Professor of Radiology
Division of Diagnostic Ultrasound
Department of Radiology
Thomas Jefferson University
Hospital and Medical College
PHILADELPHIA, PA, USA

Gretchen A.W. Gooding, MD
Professor and Vice Chairman
Department of Radiology
University og California, San Francisco
Chief, Radiology Service
Veterans Administration Medical Center
SAN FRANCISCO, CA, USA

Barbara S. Hertzberg, MD
Associate Professor of Radiology
Assistant Professor of OB/GYN
Department of Radiology
Duke University Medical Center
DURHAM, NC, USA

Cheryl L. Kirby, MD
Assistant Professor of Diagnostic Imaging
Department of Radiology
Albert Einstein Medical Center
PHILADELPHIA, PA, USA

Per G. Lindgren, MD
Associate Professor of Radiology
Department of Radiology
Uppsala Academic Hospital
UPPSALA, Sweden

Ji-Bin Liu, MD
Research Assistant Professor of Radiology
Division of Diagnostic Ultrasound
Department of Radiology
Thoms Jefferson University
Hospital and Medical College
PHILADELPHIA, PA, USA

John R. Mathieson, MD
Instructor
Department of Radiology
University of British Columbia
VANCOUVER, Canada

John P. McGahan, MD
Professor of Radiology
Department of Radiology
UCD Medical Center
SACRAMENTO, CA, USA

Ellen B. Mendelson, MD
Clinical Associate Professor of Radiology
The University of Pittsburg School of Medicine
Director, Mammography and Women's Imaging Department of Radiology
The Western Pennsylvania Hospital
PITTSBURGH, PA, USA

Henrietta Kotlus Rosenberg, MD
Professor and Chairman, Diagnostic Imaging
Department of Radiology
Albert Einstein Medical Center
PHILADELPHIA, PA, USA

Glenn A. Scheske, MD
Clinical Assistant Professor
Department of Radiology
University of British Columbia
VANCOUVER, Canada

Nancy H. Sherman, MD
Assistant Professor of Radiology
Director of Ultrasound
Alfred L. DuPont Institute
WILMINGTON, DE, USA

Eva Tegnander, CNM
National Center for Fetal Medicine
Department of Gynecology and Obstetrics
Trondheim University Hospital
TRONDHEIM, Norway

Corinne E. Tobin, MD
Breast Diagnostic Imaging Center
Nassau Radiologic Group
GARDEN CITY, NY
USA

Peter N.T. Wells, DSc, FEng
Department of Medical Physics and Bioengineering
Bristol General Hospital
BRISTOL, United Kingdom

Preface

Diagnostic imaging today comprises a broad battery of imaging modalities, to be used in varying combinations depending on the level of specialisation of the diagnostic unit and the type of diagnostic problem to be solved. Of all these modalities ultrasound, together with traditional radiography (x-ray), are by far the two most commonly used techniques, irrespective of level of specialisation, economic possibilities and geographic surroundings where the examination is performed.

Ultrasonography has important implications within all organ areas and the general radiologist, as well as the specialist at any level, needs both theoretical knowledge and technical skills in its use. It is, therefore, natural that the NICER Institute has devoted one volume in the NICER Yearbook Series to ultrasound. The book is intended to be a basic overview of diagnostic ultrasound of today, to be of value both for the general radiologist and the radiologist in training. It is also intended as broad and basic information to specialised radiologists.

A basic book like this will never be able to cover all aspects within the field of ultrasound. It should provide a broad survey and an adequate update of ultrasound of today as a basic diagnostic imaging tool. It is the editors' sincere hope that the book will fulfill these goals.

Philadelphia and Lund, March 1996

Barry B. Goldberg
Holger Pettersson

CHAPTER 1

Physics and Instrumentation

Peter N.T. Wells, DSc, FEng

Nearly seventy years have passed since the pioneers of sonar first noticed that small fish were killed when they swam into their ultrasonic beams (1). Since then, medical ultrasound has evolved from being a laboratory curiosity into one of the mainstays of modern medical diagnosis.

Since the late 1950s, when ultrasonic pulse echo methods developed for the detection of flaws in metal (2, 3) first began to be applied to the solution of medical problems (4, 5), progress has been increasingly rapid and often dramatic. The application of modern electronic techniques of signal processing and display, and improvements in transducer materials, have resulted in the development of advanced ultrasonic scanners capable of producing high resolution two-dimensional images, in real time, of the soft-tissue structures of the body, together with pictorial representations of blood flow.

Although it will always be prudent to be concerned about the possibility that the exposures used in ultrasonic imaging might result in harmful biological effects, there is no evidence of this in the techniques currently used in clinical practice (6).

PROPAGATION OF ULTRASOUND IN BIOLOGICAL TISSUES

The human body is composed of "soft" and "hard" tissues. The soft tissues include organs like the liver, kidney and the heart, and materials like blood; the hard tissues are the skeleton and the teeth. Besides these broad distinctions, there are tissues with intermediate properties: these include the lung, which is composed of soft tissue and gas, and cartilage and the lens of the eye.

Ultrasonic diagnosis is generally confined to regions composed of soft tissues, which have favorable propagation properties (7). Soft tissues support longitudinal waves, in which the particles move backwards and forwards in the same direction as the ultrasonic beam as it travels through the tissue as a progression of compressions and rarefactions. (For practical purposes, soft tissues can be considered not to be able to support other kinds of wave motion, such as transverse waves in which the particles oscillate from side-to-side across the direction of propagation.) Ultrasound travels at nearly equal speeds, virtually independent of frequency, in the different soft tissues (8). The speeds (c) range from about 1480 meters per second (m s^{-1}) in fat to about 1600 m s^{-1} in muscle. The speed in water is about 1520 m s^{-1} at 37° C (normal body temperature).

In any system in which radiation is used directly to form an image, one of the factors controlling the spatial resolution is the wavelength of the radiation. This is the reason why mechanical vibrations with frequencies of millions of cycles per second (megahertz, MHz) are used in medical diagnosis. The relationship between the wavelength (λ) and frequency (f) is given by

$$\lambda = c/f.$$

The wavelength in soft tissues is about 1.5 mm at 1 MHz, and proportionally shorter at higher frequencies.

It is, however, necessary to compromise between resolution and attenuation, because both increase with frequency. Thus, other things being equal, the amount of energy which reaches any given depth in the tissue, for a given input energy, is reduced with increasing frequency. In soft tissues, the half-power distance is about 5 mm at a frequency of 1 MHz. Usually, it is more convenient to describe attenuation not in terms of half-power distance, but in logarithmic units known as decibels. Mathematically, it is the ratio of the powers P_1 and P_2 carried by waves of different amplitudes which is expressed in decibels; thus:

$$[dB] = 10 \log P_1/P_2.$$

Two advantages result from the use of the decibel scale. First, the ratios of powers differing by many orders of magnitude (such as are commonly experienced in ultrasonic diagnosis) can be expressed in terms of quite small numbers; and second, the processes of amplification and attenuation (which occur at the various steps in the signal processing chain of an ultrasonic imaging system) can be described simply by adding or subtracting signal levels expressed in decibels, instead of needing to carry out multiplications and divisions of the actual signal levels themselves.

As explained in the following section, pulse-echo ultrasonic diagnosis (7) depends on the detection of ultrasound reflected or scattered within the examined tissues. When an ultrasonic wave, travelling in one medium, encounters the interface with another medium, two distinct phenomena occur. First, the wave is refracted from the first medium into the second. In the case of a plane interface, the angle of refraction depends on the angle of incidence and the speeds of ultrasound in the media on each side of the interface. If these speeds are equal, which, for soft tissues, can be assumed to be the case for the purpose of this discussion, the direction of the wave is not changed as it travels across the interface. The second phenomenon is that of reflection, or scattering. The amount of energy reflected at the interface, or scattered by small structures, depends on the difference between the characteristic impedances of the media on each side of the interface. The characteristic impedance (Z) of a medium is equal to the product of its density (ρ) and the speed of sound in it. Although the different soft tissues have similar densities and speeds of sound, in practice these two quantities do differ by sufficient amounts to cause reflection or scattering strong enough to allow echoes to be detected and images to be formed. Again, expressed mathematically, and for normal incidence on a flat interface,

$$R = [(Z_2 - Z_1)/(Z_2 + Z_1)]^2,$$

where R is the ratio of the power of the reflected wave to that of the incident wave and Z_1 and Z_2 are the characteristic impedances of the media on the incident and other sides of the interface, respectively. Note that if the characteristic impedances of the media on each side of the interface are equal, no reflection or scattering occurs. The greater the difference between the characteristic impedances, however, the larger the fraction of the incident wave that is reflected; thus, ultrasound is strongly reflected or scattered at the interfaces between soft tissue and, for example, gas or bone.

It is now easy to understand why attenuation controls the frequency that can be used for ultrasonic imaging and, consequently, the resolution of the imaging system. The strength of the echo reflected or scattered from a structure within the tissue at any given depth depends not only on the power of ultrasound transmitted into the body and the reflectivity of the interface, but also on the attenuation of the ultrasound as it travels in both directions through the overlying tissue. An average value for attenuation in tissue (8) is 0.5 dB cm^{-1} MHz^{-1}; thus, for example, a wave with a frequency of 3 MHz travelling through 10 cm (20 cm of go-and-return path length) in tissue experiences attenuation of about 30 dB. (To help to grasp what this means, a 50 per cent loss of power is equal to a loss of 3 dB so that the tissue path in this example corresponds to 10 half-power thicknesses. Thus, after travelling through the 20 cm of tissue, the remaining power of the wave is a little less than 0.1 per cent of that of the wave originally entering the tissue.) Thus, it is now obvious that the strength of the echo is reduced, other things being equal, as the frequency of the ultrasound is increased at any given penetration. As explained later, the detectability of the echo depends on its strength in relation to the ”noise” of the ultrasonic signal processing chain; when the echo amplitude falls below the level of the noise, it ceases to be detectable. This is the reason why, in the search for better resolution, there is a limit to the maximum frequency that can be used in any particular anatomical situation.

GENERATION AND DETECTION OF ULTRASOUND

In medical ultrasonics, a transducer is required to convert electrical energy to mechanical vibrations and vice versa. Piezoelectric ceramics are generally used for this purpose, although piezoelectric plastics and composites, which have advantage in some aspects of performance, are beginning to become available (9).

Except in simple A-scan and Doppler instruments, which are described later, the ultrasonic beam has to be scanned to form an image. A two-dimensional image is formed by scanning the beam in a plane, usually in a format which is a rectangle, parallelogram or sector, or in some variant of these. This can be accomplished either mechanically or electronically.

The shape of the ultrasonic beam is fundamentally determined by the size of the aperture from which it originates (7). For mechanical scanning, the transducer is usually disk-shaped. The beam can be focused, either with a lens or by means of an annular array. Transducer arrays, of which the annular array is an example, make it possible for the beam profile to be controlled by the introduction of small time differences in the signal paths associated with each of the elements in the array. Thus, an annular array can be used to simulate the lens. That both operate in the same way can be understood by considering a focal point at some particular position on the central axis of the ultrasonic beam. For this point to be the focus of the beam, the requirement is that the same time should elapse for ultrasound to travel from any point on the transducer surface to the focus, and vice versa for focusing on reception. A lens functions by including appropriate thicknesses of material in which ultrasound travels at a different speed from that in tissue, to correct for the different path lengths at different transducer radii. With a focused annular array, these different time delays are introduced electronically. With lens focusing, the focal length is fixed and the same for both transmission and reception. With an annular array, the position of the transmitted focus can be preselected to any desired depth along the beam axis. Since received signals are delayed with time according to depth, as explained later, however, the position of the focus during reception can be swept continuously along the ultrasonic beam axis: this means that the entire image can be kept sharply in focus.

Electronic beam control depends on the use of transducer arrays such as those shown in Figure 1. In principle, the linear array (Figure 1 A) is the simplest. A typical array consists of 100 transducer elements, distributed uniformly along an assembly 50 mm long and 10 mm wide. Since the beam shape depends on the size of the aperture, in this example it is typical for the aperture to be formed from 20 elements, thus having a 10 mm-square shape. Operated in this way, such an array is able to scan in a rectangular

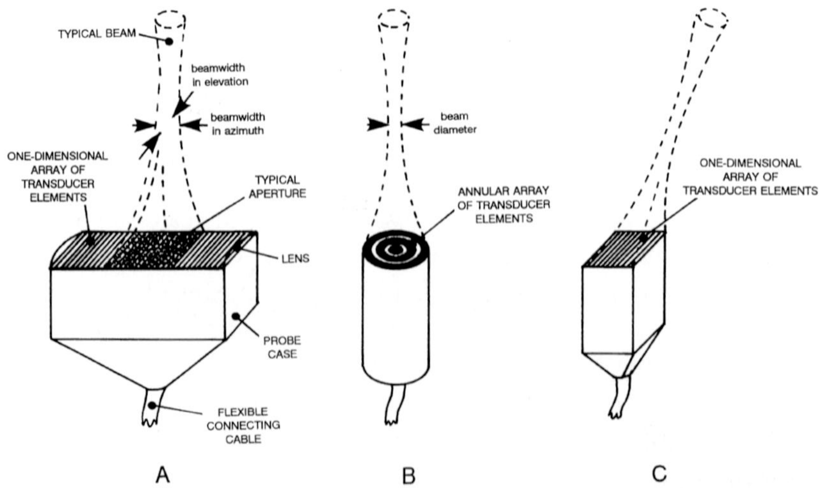

Figure 1 *Some examples of transducer arrays for electronic beam control. (A) Linear array, producing rectangular format scans with fixed lens focusing in elevation and dynamically swept electronically controlled focusing in azimuth on reception. (B) Annular array, producing a beam with circular cross-section and dynamically swept electronically controlled focusing on reception. (C) Phased array, producing a scan with a sector format.*

format with 81 separate beam positions, each separated from its neighbor by a distance of 0.5 mm. Each beam can be electronically focused within the scan plane – in azimuth – at any chosen fixed depth on transmission and dynamically throughout the scanned depth on reception. Focusing in the scan plane thickness – the beam width in elevation – can be achieved with a lens but, of course, only at a fixed depth equal to the focal length. Even this limitation can be overcome, however, by the use of a two-dimensional array. As shown in Figure 1 B, this allows simultaneously swept beam focusing in both azimuth and elevation.

One-dimensional arrays, known as "phased arrays", can also be used to steer the beam off-axis. This is illustrated in Figure 1 C. The principle is the same as that for focusing, but the time delays are graded continuously across the width of the aperture. This is the electronic simulation of a prism, which simply deflects a beam rather than focusing it. By combining the time delays for beam steering and focusing, however, the beam can be completely controlled in the plane of the scan.

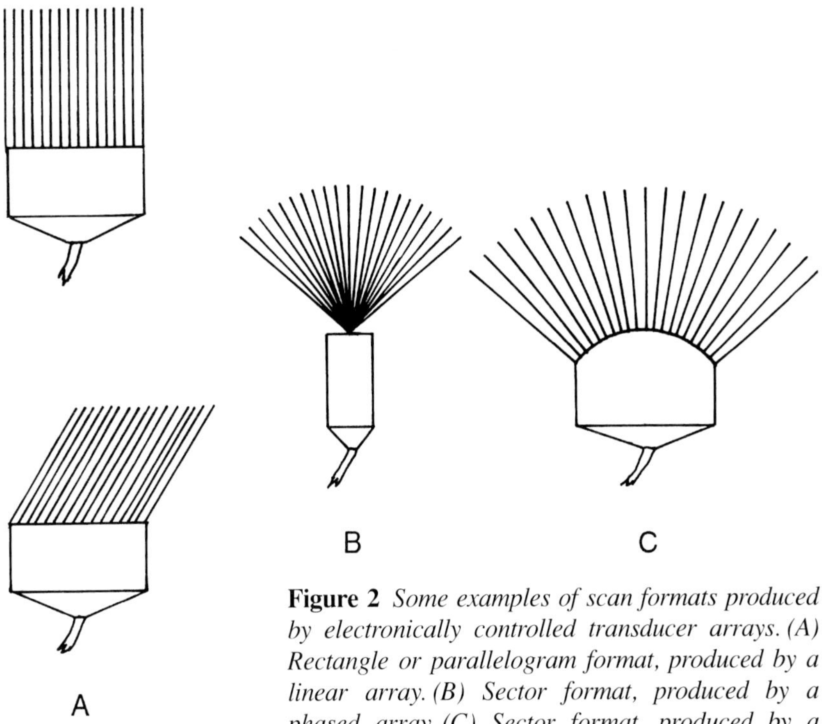

Figure 2 *Some examples of scan formats produced by electronically controlled transducer arrays. (A) Rectangle or parallelogram format, produced by a linear array. (B) Sector format, produced by a phased array. (C) Sector format, produced by a curved array.*

As shown in Figure 2 A, linear array transducers can be used to scan in formats which are rectangles or parallelograms. Phased arrays produce scans with sector formats (Figure 2 B). Sector scan formats can also be produced by curved linear arrays (Figure 2 C). This approach requires less complicated electronic circuits in the scanning instrument and the size of the transducer is very convenient for many clinical applications. Phased array scanners are suitable when the skin contact area has to be as small as possible. Linear arrays are suitable both for general purpose and specialised clinical applications.

PULSE-ECHO TECHNIQUES

General Principles

The ultrasonic pulse-echo method depends on three pieces of information (7). First, the measurement of the times that elapse between the transmission of an ultrasonic pulse into the patient and the reception of its echoes gives information about the positions of reflecting and scattering interfaces in depth along the ultrasonic beam. Second, the amplitudes of the echoes give information about some of the physical properties of the interfaces. Third, either by inference or as part of the image-forming process, account is taken of the direction of the ultrasonic beam; this gives information about the positions of the reflecting or scattering interfaces, both in elevation and in azimuth.

In a pulse-echo system, the "resolution cell" is the volume of material within which the physical interaction that provides the echo signal actually takes place. The dimensions of the resolution cell depend on its position along the ultrasonic beam, the ultrasonic beam profile and the "dynamic range" of the receiving system. The dynamic range is the range within which the echo amplitude must lie for changes in echo amplitude to produce changes in the appearance of the image. In a typical scanning situation, the dynamic range of the echoes received by the transducer is set at about 100 dB (corresponding to a ratio of 100 000 to 1 between the amplitudes of the smallest and largest signals) by limitations imposed by noise and by the maximum acceptable ultrasonic intensity. Noise in ultrasonic imaging is of various kinds and arises from several sources. Although in some respects the ultrasonic scattering process itself produces echo signals which resemble noise in that they are randomly distributed in amplitude and time, it actually gives rise to the texture which is such an important aspect of the final image. It is the noise that originates in the electrical circuitry of the receiving amplifier that in practice sets the lower limit on the amplitude of detectable signals. Fundamentally, this is "resistive noise", the origin of which lies in the physical behavior of any component which has electrical resistance; ultimately, it is unavoidable. Another source of noise is in the initial amplifying circuit elements in the receiver; it can be minimized, but not eliminated, by good circuit design. It is also pertinent that the total power of the noise signals is proportional, other things being equal, to the frequency bandwidth of the receiving amplifier. Modern scanners often feature large frequency bandwidths which, as explained later, are necessary for short pulse operation and, consequently, for high spatial resolution. Again, it is a challenge to the circuit designer to minimise the associated noise disadvantage.

There are two considerations which set upper limits on the ultrasonic power that can be transmitted into the patient. The first is the obviously increasing risk of producing untoward biological effects; this is discussed in more detail later. The second is that ultrasonic waves are increasingly distorted in tissue and other media as the power carried by the wave is increased (10). This nonlinearity is seldom a practical problem with the ultrasonic powers (or intensities) used in contemporary clinical applications. It is worth noting, however, that the presence of gas-containing structures – such as the microbubbles of some ultrasonic contrast agents – does significantly increase nonlinearity to the extent that the scattered ultrasound is rich in harmonic frequencies. The detection of the scattered second harmonic ultrasound is the basis of a potentially important and novel application of contrast agents; it is discussed in detail in Chapter 24.

The A-scope

Figure 3 shows the signal processing path of a typical ultrasonic pulse-echo system (7). The transmitter is excited by brief electrical impulses, delivered at a rate determined by the system clock; the limit on the maximum pulse repetition frequency is discussed later. The output from the transmitter causes the transducer in the probe to emit a series of ultrasonic pulses which travel along the beam into the patient, as already explained. Simultaneously with the transmission of each ultrasonic pulse, the timebase generator is triggered to produce a voltage which changes with time to drive the luminous spot on the screen of the cathode-ray-tube horizontally at constant speed across the display. Echoes returning from within the patient are amplified by the receiver, the output from which controls the vertical deflection of the spot as it is driven across the display by the timebase generator. This results in a display in which vertical deflections of the trace occur at horizontal positions corresponding to the positions of the echo-producing targets along the ultrasonic beam. Because of the attenuation of ultrasound in the overlying tissues, echoes from deeper structures

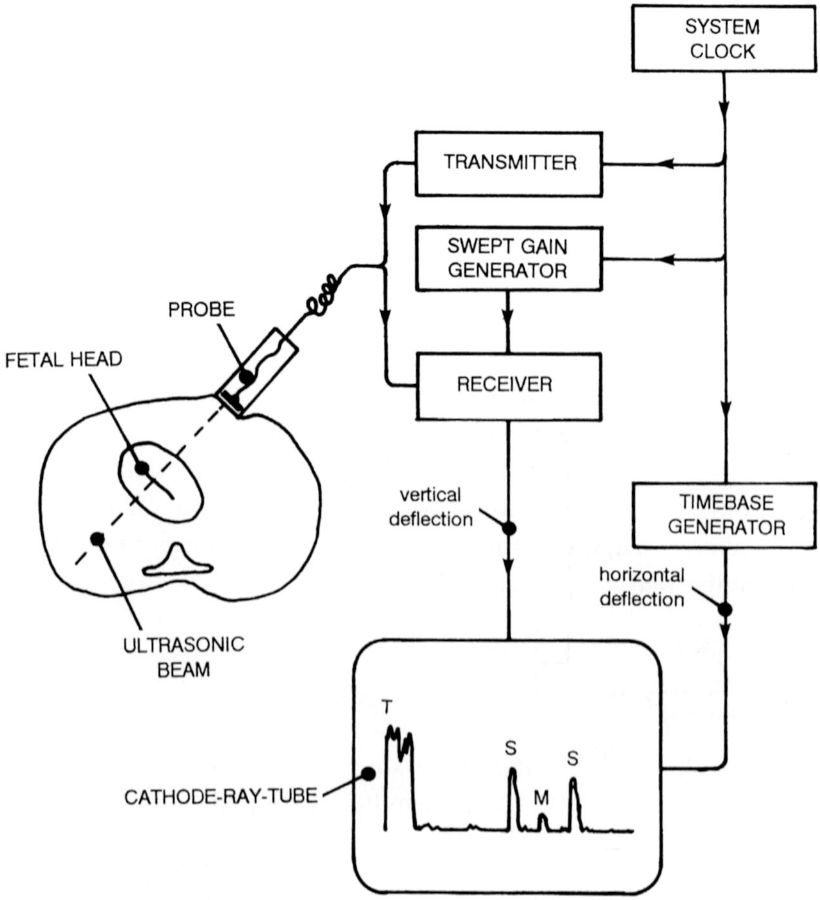

Figure 3 *Block diagram of an ultrasonic A-scope system, primarily for pulse-echo measurements of distance. In this example, the system is being used to measure the diameter of a fetal head. On the display,* T *corresponds to the transmission of the ultrasonic pulse into the patient;* S *are the echoes from the parietal bones of the fetal skull and* M*, the echo from the midline structures of the fetal brain.*

are weaker than those from similar structures located more superficially. The swept gain generator compensates for this attenuation by increasing the gain of the receiver with time following the transmission of each pulse, so that the echoes from deeper structures are amplified more than those from superficial structures.

This is the simplest kind of instrument based on the ultrasonic pulse-echo principle. It is called an "A-scope", using the terminology of radar and sonar. It was used in some of the earliest work on medical diagnostic ultrasound. Nowadays, however, its principal application is as an adjunct to other displays, particularly when accurate measurements of distance or echo amplitude are required.

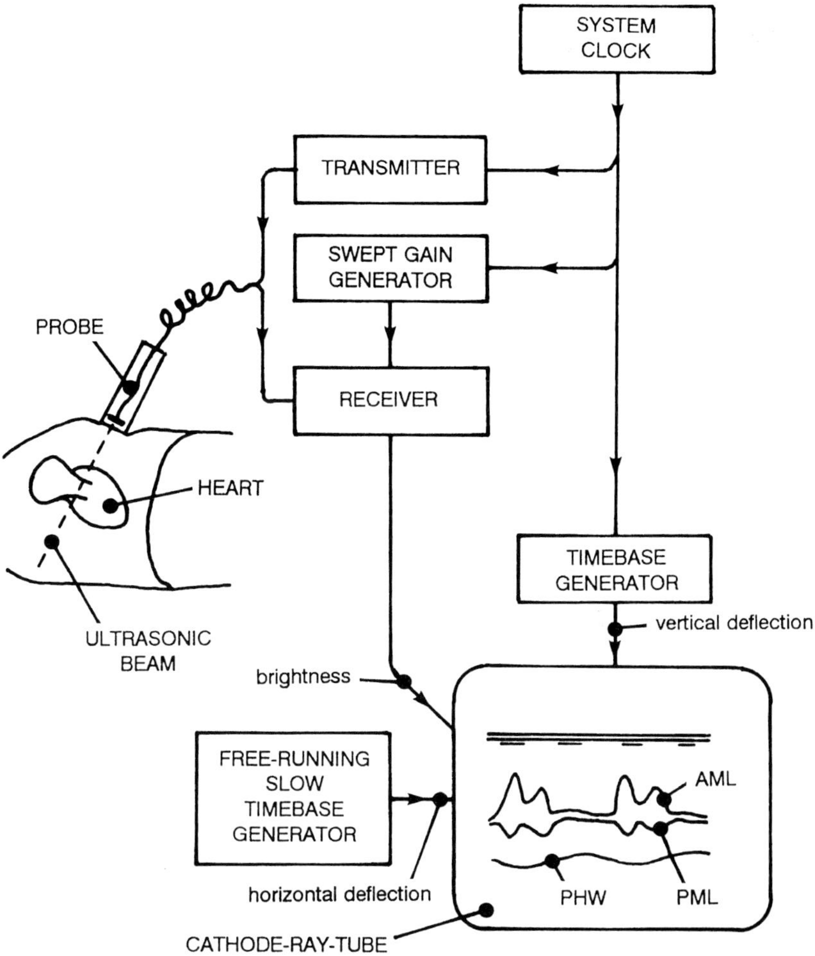

Figure 4 *Block diagram of an ultrasonic M-mode system, for the display of structure motion. In this example, the system is being used to study the motion of the mitral valve. On the display,* CW *is the chest wall;* AML *and* PML *are respectively the anterior and posterior leaflets of the mitral valve;* PHW *is the posterior heart wall.*

M-mode (Time-Position) Display

Instruments designed for time-position studies display the positions of echoes from structures lying along the ultrasonic beam as a function of time (7). This is called an "M-mode" display. Figure 4 shows a common arrangement for producing this kind of display. Actually, it quite closely resembles an A-scope, except that the timebase of the A-scope is connected to the vertical deflection circuit of the cathode-ray-tube and the output from the receiver controls the brightness, rather than the deflection, of the spot on the display. The other difference is that there is a second timebase generator, connected to the horizontal deflection circuit, which drives the spot across the display at a constant but relatively slow velocity. The result is a time-position display which allows the positions of echo-producing structures along the ultrasonic beam to be studied over a period of time. The period of time chosen depends on the particular clinical application. For example, a horizontal sweep time of a few seconds allows the behavior of the heart to be studied over a small number of cardiac cycles: this is a particularly useful clinical application of the M-mode technique.

Two-dimensional Scanning

The principles of two-dimensional ultrasonic scanning (7) are illustrated in Figure 5. The essential elements are an arrangement to sweep the ultrasonic beam across a plane which cuts through the anatomical structures to be imaged, a means to measure the instantaneous position and direction of the ultrasonic beam and to use this to control the position and direction of the timebase on the display, and electronic circuitry to form the signal processing path so that the local brightness of the display is determined by the amplitudes of the echoes from the spatially-corresponding structures in the scan plane.

Nowadays, two-dimensional scanning is almost always a real-time process. This is only mentioned here because, until about a decade ago, it was the "static B-scanner" that was in common use (7), with manual operation of the movement of a transducer mounted on some kind of gantry. In that era too, water-immersion systems capable of producing excellent images were quite popular. With even the fastest of these machines, however, the scanning time was usually at least a few seconds.

In real-time scanning, the complete image appears on the display and it is refreshed rapidly enough to allow the motion of anatomical structures to be seen as it actually happens, and changes in scan plane position to be reflected immediately in the display. The rate at which pulse-echo data can be acquired is limited by the

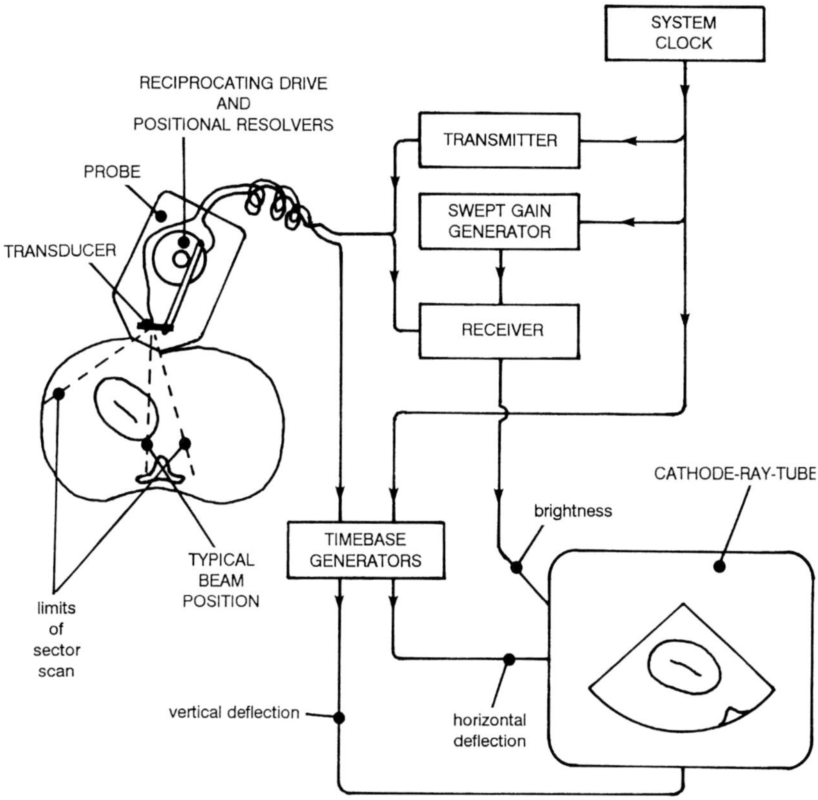

Figure 5 *Block diagram of an ultrasonic two-dimensional scanning system. In this example, a single-element disk transducer is driven mechanically to sweep the ultrasonic beam repetitively through a sector scan. Signals corresponding to the instantaneous position of the beam are provided by the probe to control the timebase generators so that the direction of the resultant timebase on the display is the same as that of the beam in the scan plane. The brightness of the display is controlled by the amplitudes of the received echoes.*

speed of ultrasound. For example, for a penetration of 150 mm into the patient, the time required for an ultrasonic pulse to traverse the 300 mm of go-and-return tissue path length is about 200 μs. This corresponds to a maximum pulse repetition frequency of 5000 per second. (If the pulse repetition frequency exceeds this, echoes resulting from the reflection of an ultrasonic pulse by superficial structures can be received at the same time as echoes from the preceding pulse being reflected by deeper structures: this causes ambiguity in the image.) Provided that the ultrasonic beam is being swept sufficiently rapidly across the scan plane, so that it passes through different tissue paths during the transmission of each pulse and the reception of the resulting echoes, a new line of image information is obtained with each pulse. Since the image frame rate is equal to the pulse repetition frequency divided by the number of lines in each image frame, this means that, in the example given here, each frame can be composed of 100 lines at a frame rate of 50 per second, and so on. Images with frame rates in excess of about 15 per second are free from flicker, because of the persistence of vision. It is worth noting that, when a less rapid frame rate is clinically useful, flicker can be avoided by image storage.

The ultrasonic beam of a real-time scanner may be steered through the scan plane by mechanical or electronic means, the principles of which have already been explained.

DOPPLER TECHNIQUES

The Doppler Effect

When a beam of ultrasound is reflected or scattered by a stationary target, the frequency of the reflected wave is the same as that of the incident wave. If the target is moving towards the source of ultrasound, however, the reflected wave is shifted upwards in frequency, and vice versa. The phenomenon is called the "Doppler effect" (7). Assuming that the velocity of the target is very much less than the speed of ultrasound (which is certainly so for physiological motion and flow within the body),

$f_D = 2\,v\,(\cos\theta)\,f/c$

where f_D is the difference between the frequencies of the transmitted and the received ultrasound, f is the transmitted frequency, v is the speed of the target, and θ is the angle between the direction of motion of the target and the effective direction of the combined transmitting and receiving beams. Typical values are f = 3 MHz, v = 1 m s^{-1} and c = 1500 m s^{-1}; the corresponding Doppler shift frequency f_D = 4 kHz. It is fortuitous that the Doppler shift frequency happens to be in the audible range for most medical ultrasonic diagnostic frequencies and physiological values of target velocity.

Continuous Wave Doppler Techniques

The simplest medical ultrasonic Doppler instruments employ continuous waves. Figure 6 is a block diagram of a typical system (7). The probe contains separate transducers for transmission and reception, arranged close together and angled so that there is a substantial length of beam overlap. The transmitting transducer is driven by a signal derived from an oscillator and it emits continuous wave ultrasound into the patient. The received echo signals are equal in frequency to that of the transmitter when the reflections are from stationary structures, but shifted in frequency by the Doppler effect if the corresponding reflecting structures (or ensembles of scatterers such as blood) are moving with components of velocity along the ultrasonic beam. In the receiver, these signals are mixed in a process that extracts the Doppler shift frequencies. The Doppler signals are audible and a skilled listener can derive much information from then, albeit in a qualitative way. The signals can also be examined quantitatively, however, using circuits ranging in complexity from simple ratemeters (for example, for measuring the fetal heart rate) to fast Fourier transform frequency spectrum analysers (for blood flow studies), as illustrated in Figure 6.

Much useful clinical information can be obtained with Doppler instruments which merely detect the amplitudes of the echoes and magnitudes of the frequencies of the Doppler-shifted signals. These instruments cannot distinguish between approaching and receding targets. The block diagram in Figure 7 shows, however, that this information can be obtained by the process of phase quadrature detection (11). A phase quadrature detector operates by determining whether the phase of the received signal leads or lags that of the transmitted signal, which serves as the reference.

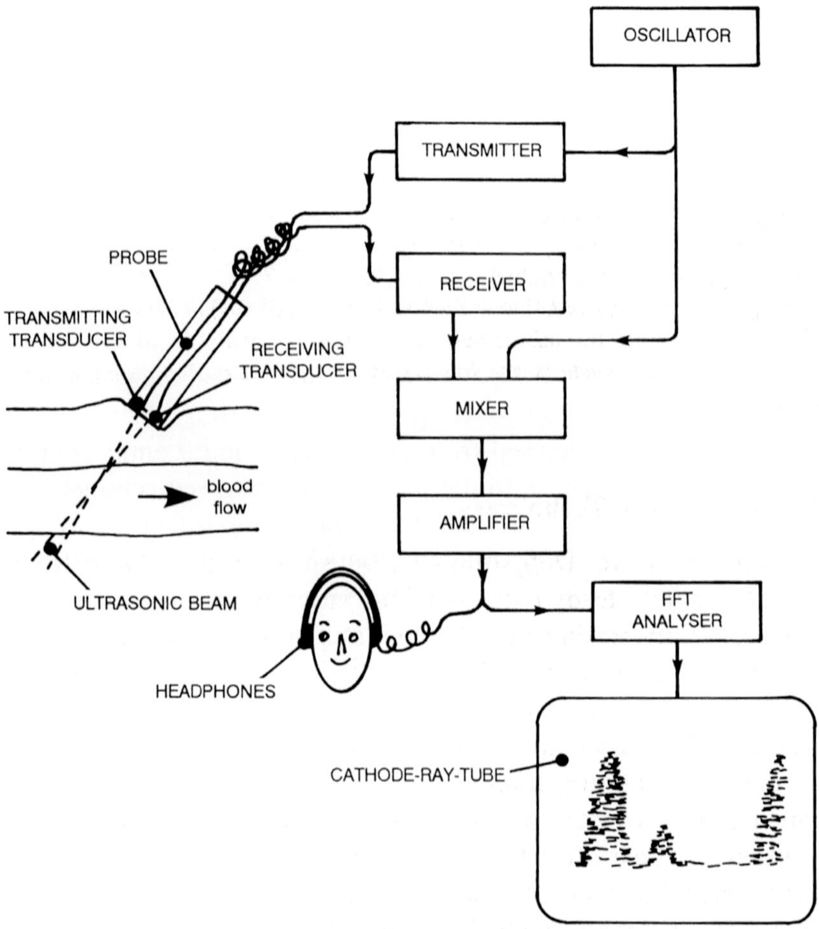

Figure 6 *Block diagram of ultrasonic continuous-wave Doppler system, with nondirectional detection. The oscillator drives the transmitter so that the transmitting transducer emits continuous wave ultrasound into the patient. Echoes, including Doppler-shifted signals, are amplified by the receiver; the output from the mixer consists of the Doppler-shifted signals. These signals can be heard directly or, after processing by the fast Fourier transform (FFT) analyser, displayed as a frequency spectrum.*

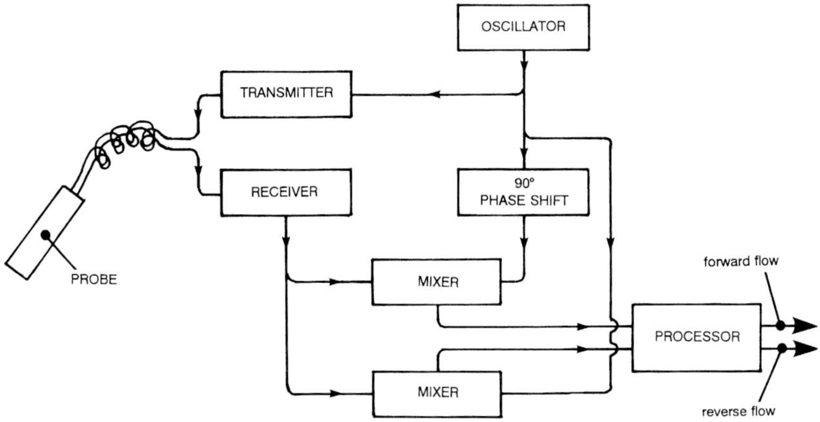

Figure 7 *Block diagram of ultrasonic continuous-wave Doppler system, with directional detection. Compared with the block diagram in Figure 6, there are two mixers; one mixer is fed with a signal derived directly from the oscillator, whilst the other mixer is fed with the same signal but shifted in phase by 90°. The outputs from the two mixers lead or lag in phase, depending on the flow direction; further arithmetic processing separates these signals according to flow direction.*

Pulsed Doppler Techniques

Continuous wave Doppler systems have no depth selectivity (apart from the steady reduction in signal strength which occurs as a result of increasing attenuation in increasing thickness of intervening tissue), unless this is provided by physical limitation of the cross-over region of the transmitting and receiving beams (12). It is possible, however, to pulse the transmitted signal so that the round-trip transit time between the transducer and the target can be selected by having an electronic gate (opened at an appropriate time after the transmission of the pulse) in the received signal path (7). As shown in Figure 8, this enables the position along the ultrasonic beam of the "Doppler sample volume" to be chosen by the operator. For simplicity, Figure 8 does not show the circuitry needed to provide directional information but this can be obtained by phase quadrature detection, as already explained.

In a pulsed Doppler system, there is an upper limit to the unambiguously-detectable Doppler shift frequency. According to the Nyquist criterion, this is equal to half the pulse repetition frequen-

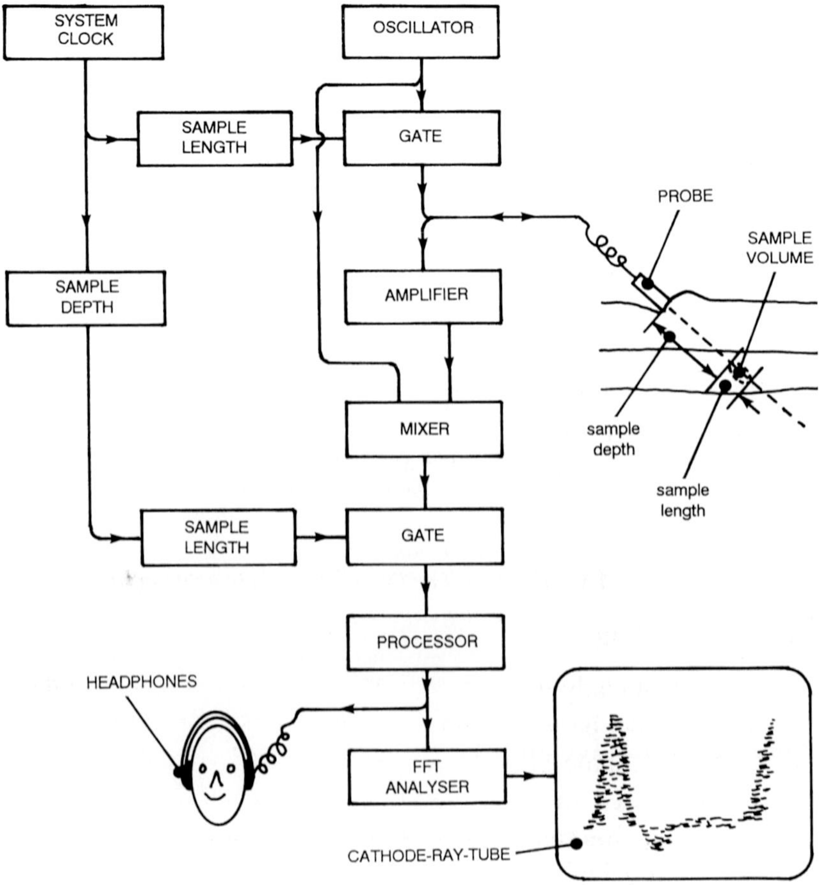

Figure 8 *Block diagram of pulsed Doppler system. Each time that the system clock produces a pulse, the first sample length generator opens the first gate to allow the oscillator to excite the transducer to emit a pulse of ultrasound of the desired length into the patient. Simultaneously, the clock triggers the sample depth generator so that the second sample length generator opens the second gate in readiness to allow the Doppler sample to be transferred to the processor. In the processor, the sample is stored until the system clock provides a fresh, updated sample. For simplicity, the circuitry necessary for directional detection is now shown.*

cy (11). Ordinarily, the pulse repetition frequency itself is limited by the required depth of penetration, as with any pulse-echo technique. This affects the choice of the ultrasonic frequency used for pulsed Doppler studies. In principle, reducing the ultrasonic frequency relaxes the constraint on the maximum unambigiously-detected target velocity, but this may be at the expense of lower signal strength (since the scattering from blood increases with frequency) and poorer resolution (since the beam becomes wider and the pulse becomes longer as the frequency falls, other things being equal).

There are some clinical applications of techniques which use pulsed Doppler for range selectivity, unsupported by imaging for target identification and localization. In many respects, these applications resemble the independent use of the A-scope; it is necessary to know the orientation of the transducer and the local anatomy in order to interpret the Doppler signals. In clinical practice, however, it turns out that the optimum pulsed Doppler ultrasonic frequency is usually somewhat lower than the optimum frequency for imaging in the same clinical situation.

COMBINED IMAGING AND BLOOD FLOW STUDIES

Duplex Scanning

Although, as already explained, a hand-held probe without imaging guidance can be used to obtain useful pulsed Doppler clinical information in some circumstances, usually it is helpful to have imaging guidance in order to provide the confidence of target identification. This can most easily be achieved by what is known as "duplex scanning" (11). The principle is illustrated in Figure 9. Real-time pulse-echo imaging is performed in the usual way; the scan plane is selected so as to locate the anatomical region for Doppler investigation. Superimposed on the real-time image is an electronically-generated overlay which shows the direction of the ultrasonic beam selected by the operator to pass through the region-of-interest and the position along the beam at which the Doppler sample volume is to be located. If a mechanically-scanned transducer is used for real-time imaging, it is usually not possible to switch instantaneously between imaging and Doppler signal acquisition; the transducer scanning motion has to be arrested with the ultrasonic beam in the desired position for Doppler signal acquisition. With transducer array scanning, however, this is not a problem because the beam position can be controlled virtually instantaneously; as far as the operator is concerned, imaging and

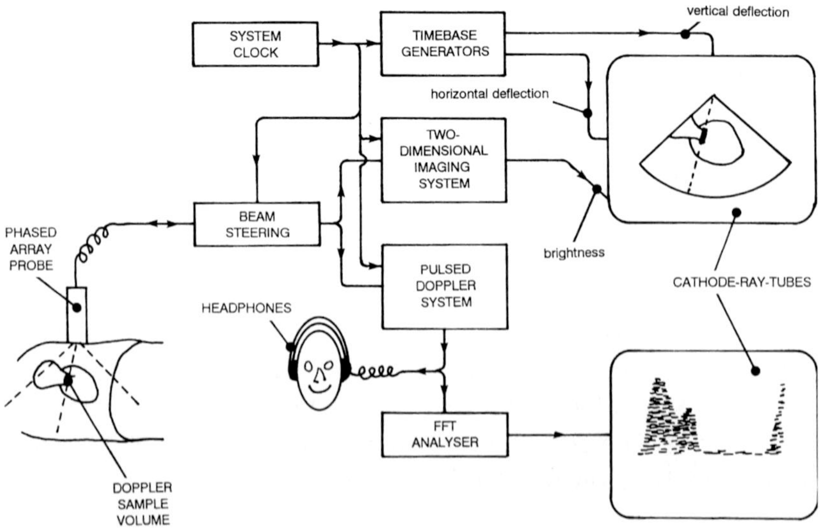

Figure 9 *Block diagram of duplex scanning system. In this example, the beam steering circuit produces a sector scan with the phased array probe. The real-time two-dimensional imaging system is used to decide the placement of the Doppler beam and sample volume; the pulsed Doppler system provides audible signals from the sample volume, which can also be displayed as a frequency spectrum after fast Fourier transform analysis.*

Doppler signal acquisition can be alternated sufficiently rapidly for both to be performed apparently simultaneously in real time.

The main clinical value of duplex scanning lies in the ability that it provides to permit a thorough investigation of the Doppler frequency spectrum acquired from an anatomical site the location of which is confirmed by two-dimensional imaging. The range of clinical applications is large; particularly important are studies of blood flow in the heart and in peripheral, cerebral and abdominal vessels.

Color Flow Imaging

In principle, duplex scanning can be used to study blood flow at every point in a two-dimensional real-time image. This is, however, a somewhat theoretical capability. Duplex scanning is clinically useful when the operator knows in advance the anatomical site at which the flow conditions are likely to be of interest. It is a slow process and, consequently, it is impracticable to explore the flow conditions throughout the entire image plane.

Figure 10 shows how blood flow information throughout the entire image plane can be acquired and displayed in real-time (11). The display consists of a real-time grey-scale two-dimensional anatomical image, acquired in the manner already explained. Superimposed on this grey-scale image is a two-dimensional image in which blood flow is represented by a color map. There are two distinct approaches to the derivation of the flow information; these are frequency and time domain processing. Moreover, the color in the image can represent either the magnitude of the flow velocity, or it can be related to some measure of the quantity of flowing blood.

Frequency Domain Processing

Frequency domain processing for color flow imaging can be regarded as a pulsed Doppler technique (13). In the block diagram in Figure 10, the "flow imaging system" is what is known as an "auto-correlation detector". Doppler signals from a phase quadrature de-

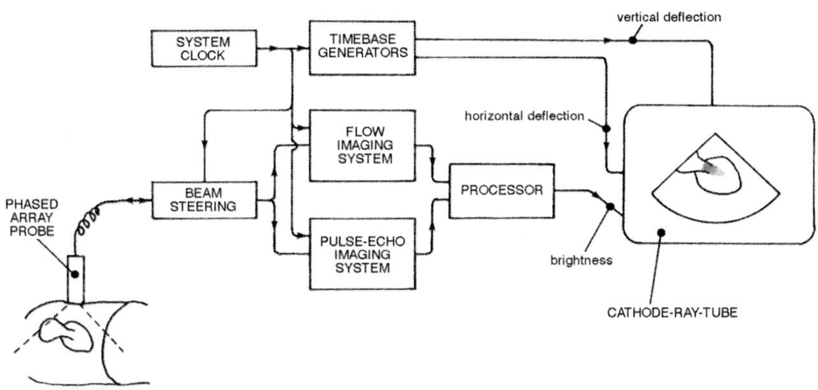

Figure 10 *Block diagram of color flow imaging system. In this example, the beam steering circuit produces a sector scan with the phased array probe. The pulse-echo imaging system operates in the usual way to produce a real-time two-dimensional scan, which is combined in the processor with the output from the flow imaging system; the resulting display is a color flow image. The flow imaging system can employ either frequency or time domain processing.*

tector are split into two paths. One path leads directly to one input to an electronic circuit which performs the process of multiplication. The other path leads to other input to the multiplier but through a time delay circuit that introduces a delay exactly equal to the interval between the transmission of consecutive ultrasonic pulses. If the echo wavetrains corresponding to consecutive pulses originate only from stationary structures, these wavetrains are identical and the output from the multiplier is a constant (i.e., non-time-varying) waveform. If there is movement anywhere along the ultrasonic beam, however, consecutive wavetrains have phase shifts due to the Doppler effect. The output from the multiplier then contains segments of wavetrain that vary in amplitude from pulse to pulse. These variations correspond to the Doppler signals along the entire length of the ultrasonic beam. It is then a simple step to scan the ultrasonic beam through a two-dimensional plane and thus to obtain a two-dimensional Doppler flow image, in real time.

Time Domain Processing

The M-mode display, as already explained, shows how the positions of echo-producing structures along the ultrasonic beam change with time. Although blood is usually thought of as not being echogenic, blood flow is occasionally seen in real-time two-dimensional scanning when the sensitivity of the scanner is high. Time domain processing for flow imaging (14) depends on the measurement of the actual distances moved by the echo-producing ensembles in blood on a line-by-line basis, with the ultrasonic beam being swept through the entire scan plane in real time. This is the function of the "flow imaging system" when this is the modus operandi in Figure 10. For this approach to be successful, the sensitivity of the pulse-echo system has to be high enough to permit the continuous detection of the echoes from blood.

Comparison between Frequency and Time Domain Processing

In comparing frequency and time domain processing for color flow imaging, the most important considerations relate to image frame rate, sensitivity and spatial resolution (14).

The maximum image frame rate (for a given number of lines per frame) is controlled by the time that it is necessary for the ultrasonic beam to remain stationary at each position in the scan plane in order to acquire sufficient information to allow the lowest blood flow velocity of interest to be estimated. This is likely to be rather longer for frequency domain than for time domain processing. In principle, with time domain processing, the target has only to move far enough along the beam for there to be a measurable change in its spatial position and this, in turn, is limited by the range resolution of the pulse-echo imaging system. Intuitively, this means that the color image frame rate is likely to be able to approach half the grey scale image frame rate. With frequency domain processing, on the other hand, it is, in effect, the Doppler shift frequency that has to be estimated. Other things being equal, the Doppler shift frequency falls as the target velocity is reduced. Again intuitively, the beam has to be stationary in each position in the scan plane for at least a substantial fraction of the time occupied by a complete cycle of the lowest Doppler shift frequency; for example, for a Doppler frequency of 400 Hz (corresponding to a flow velocity of about 10 cm s^{-1} with an ultrasonic frequency of 3 MHz and coincident beam and flow directions), the corresponding time is 2.5 ms. This means that, if there are 100 separate color lines in the image, the image frame rate is only four per second, which hardly qualifies as real time.

The sensitivity of a color flow imaging system employing frequency domain processing is likely to be similar to that of a regular pulsed Doppler system. Since the Doppler method depends on the comparison of the frequencies (or, more accurately, the phases) of the transmitted and received pulses, it is a physical requirement that the pulse duration should be quite long. This is because short pulses contain energy spread over a wide frequency spectrum and this is inappropriate for Doppler frequency comparison. One consequence of the use of a long pulse, with its narrow frequency band, is that a narrow frequency band receiving amplifier can be employed; this means that the signal-to-noise ratio is low so that the gain of the amplifier can be high with correspondingly high sensitivity. In contrast, short pulses are needed to provide the range resolution necessary for target tracking by time domain processing, particularly with low velocity targets. Short pulses have wide frequency bands: the signal-to-noise ratio is correspondingly low and so is the sensitivity. Intuitively, however, a given amount of ultrasonic energy transmitted into the patient provides an equivalent amount of information, whether frequency or time domain processing is employed. For a given average intensity, the pulse intensity with time domain processing is higher than that for frequency domain processing. To a large extent, this compensates for the inherently lower sensitivity of time domain processing and the practical result is that the sensitivities of the two methods are actually quite similar.

The spatial resolution in color flow imaging is determined by the width of the ultrasonic beam and the length of the ultrasonic pulse. The width of the beam is similar with both frequency and time domain processing. Another consequence of the narrow frequency band necessary for satisfactory operation with frequency domain processing, however, is that the pulse length has to be longer than that for optimum operation with time domain processing. This means that the range resolution with frequency domain processing is likely to be worse than that with time domain processing.

One of the most important challenges for the circuit designer, no matter whether frequency or time domain processing is adopted, is to minimize the artifactual color coding of signals from moving solid tissues within the scan plane. Solid tissues generally move at slow velocities in comparison with the velocities of blood flow, but the amplitudes of their echoes are relatively high. Circuits known as "stationary echo cancellers" are used to reduce the amplitudes of these solid tissue echoes, which otherwise would overwhelm the weak echoes from the blood. Color flow imaging instruments also usually incorporate circuits which inhibit color display in areas of the image containing echo signals exceeding a level selected by a "color write priority" control which can be adjusted by the operator. The effect of this is to prevent the color-coding of the display by echoes from moving tissues which, for some reason or another, escape effective rejection by the stationary echo canceller.

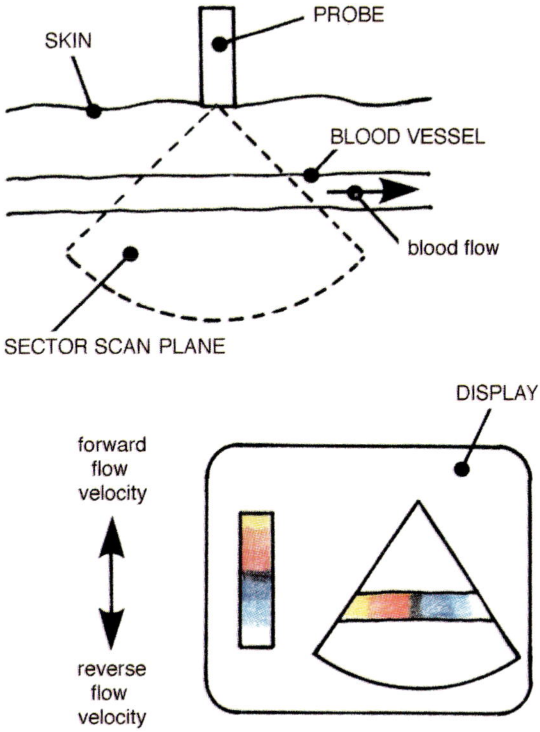

Figure 11 *The vector problem with velocity-encoded color flow imaging. In the top diagram, a phased array probe is shown scanning an idealised blood vessel in which blood is flowing at constant velocity from left to right. In the lower diagram, the color scale is represented: interpretation of the color flow image has to take account of the changing vector direction of the ultrasonic beam relative to the direction of flow.*

Color Coding Schemes

One option, and one which is a good choice in many clinical applications, is to use a coding scheme in which color is related to the velocity of blood flow (14). Increasing flow velocity towards the probe is usually coded on a red-orange-yellow scale, whereas increasing reverse flow velocity is coded in increasingly light blue. Figure 11 shows why, in interpreting color flow velocity images, it is necessary to take account of the relative directions of the ultrasonic beam and the flow: this is sometimes referred to as the ”vector problem”. Green is a color that contrasts well with both the red-yellow and the blue scales. Because of this contrast, green is sometimes used to highlight regions of equal vector velocity, or to identify regions where there is an abnormally high value of velocity variance. Velocity variance is related to flow disturbance or to the presence of turbulence and, consequently, is of clinical significance.

Another color coding option is to display flow in monochrome independent of flow direction and to increase the brightness of the color with the strength of the flow signal (14). The strength of the signal is related to the quantity of blood flowing within the corresponding region of the scan plane. "Power" or "energy" images of this kind are easy to interpret because the color is unaffected by the flow direction, so there is no vector problem. Superficially at least, they resemble x-ray contrast or magnetic resonance angiograms, and they provide a crude qualitative representation of blood perfusion.

INSTRUMENTATION AND TECHNIQUES FOR SPECIALIZED AND EMERGING APPLICATIONS

Special Purpose Probes

There are numerous specialized clinical applications of diagnostic ultrasound that depend on purpose-built probes. These probes produce real-time and color flow images in the same ways as those for traditional studies, often using the same scanning instruments. Because of their design, however, they permit unorthodox routes of access to be employed and unusual procedures to be adopted. In addition, they have long been used for guided biopsy and now applications in minimally invasive medicine are beginning to emerge.

Figure 12 shows some examples of intracavitary and intraluminal scanning probes (15). Intracavitary scanners (Figure 12 A, B, C) are designed for insertion into body cavities where skin puncture is unnecessary. Small mechanical or transducer array systems are available for scanning from the esophagus, the rectum, the urethra, and the vagina. Transverse, longitudinal and oblique scan planes may be accessible. The great advantage of intracavitary scanning is that it can avoid the long intervening tissue paths that are often inescapable with transcutaneous scanning. This also means that higher frequencies can be used to obtain high-resolution images, because of the short penetration that is needed. The probes have to be robust and easily cleaned; except for urinary tract studies, sterilization is usually unnecessary.

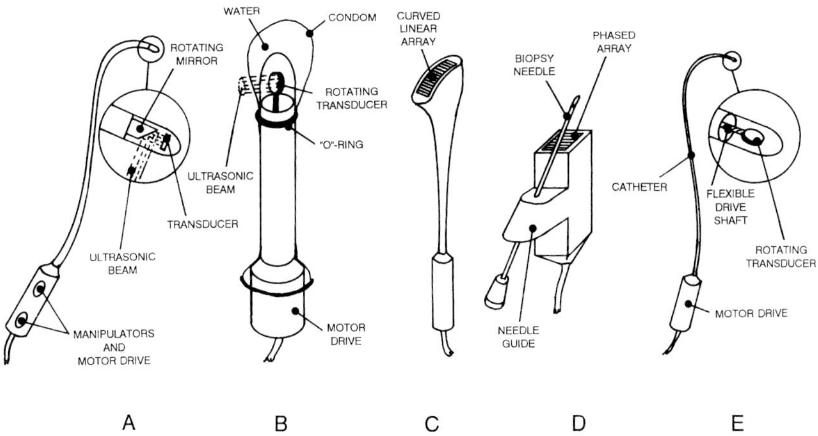

Figure 12 *Some examples of special purpose probes. (A) Esophageal probe, mounted on a flexible endoscope. (B) Rectal probe, for transverse scanning. (C) Vaginal probe, for longitudinal scanning. (D) Biopsy guidance probe. (E) Intravascular probe, mounted on a flexible catheter.*

Probes for guided procedures such as biopsy (see Figure 12 D) are designed to allow the needle track to be selected in advance of intervention. The tip of the needle can be visualized as it is advanced through the tissues.

Intraoperative scanning has already been shown to be a useful surgical aid and the range of its applications is increasing. Usually, small transducer arrays are used; what has to be inserted into the surgical field, which includes some of the probe cable, has to be sterilized or accomodated in a sterile sheath.

Endoluminal or intravascular scanning involves the use of a tiny catheter-borne transducer operating at relatively very high frequency. As shown in Figure 12 E, a typical probe consists of a small high-frequency transducer mounted at the end of a flexible catheter to obtain real-time radial scans with very high resolution. This is currently an area of active engineering and clinical research interest.

Three-dimensional Scanning

As described in Chapter 24, the development of relatively inexpensive two-dimensional image frame buffer stores and of image processing computers capable of rapid reformatting has led to a resurgence of interest in three-dimensional imaging (16). A specially-designed probe, or probe manipulator, is used to obtain a data set consisting of spatially-separated contiguous two-dimensional scans with known spatial locations. The acquisition time is necessarily protracted, because the only practicable way of increasing the rate of data acquisition is to collect several spatially separated image lines simultaneously (17) and there are limitations to the implementation of this approach. The three-dimensional information having been acquired, there are also problems in image segmentation and display. Nevertheless, promising results are being obtained and the method has great potential for novel clinical applications in the future.

Contrast Agents

Contrast agents, particularly those based on microbubbles, promise significantly to expand the clinical usefulness of ultrasonic diagnosis (18). The prospects are discussed in Chapter 24. It is already established that microbubble contrast agents can be used for "clutter rejection" (with consequential improvement in signal-to-noise ratio) by the process of second harmonic detection (19). Exploitation of this phenomenon will require the use of specially-designed ultrasonic scanning instruments.

THE SAFETY OF DIAGNOSTIC ULTRASOUND

The question of safety in the use of diagnostic ultrasound needs to be viewed in the same way as the question of safety in the use of ionising radiations in diagnosis. The risk to the patient – and to others involved in the examination and in its environment – is one component in the calculation of the cost of the test. This cost has to be balanced by the physician against the value of the benefit resulting from the test.

The physician needs to be mindful of the possibility that ultrasound as used in the examination of the individual patient might produce untoward biological effects. Also, of course, the consequences of misdiagnosis – possibly the greatest risk in contemporary ultrasonic investigations – along with hazards such as electric shock, burning and cross-infection, and the opportunity cost of the procedure, need to be taken into account; these are not considered further here.

Ultrasonic waves carry energy into the patient, which is converted into heat as it is absorbed in the tissues. In contemporary diagnostic procedures, the amount of heat produced is not large; during scanning the heat is distributed through a slice of tissue and carried away by conduction and blood flow. Nevertheless, there is at least a hypothetical risk of adverse biological effect due to thermal mechanisms. There is also the possibility of mechanical effects, due to forces resulting from streaming velocity gradients which may be amplified in the presence of cavitation bubbles of appropriate dimensions. Finally, there may be effects due to as yet unidentified interactions between ultrasound and biological tissues.

Thus, there is a scientific basis to the consideration of the safety of diagnostic ultrasound (20) and this remains a fruitful area for research. Moreover, the last two decades have witnessed a steady increase in both the time-averaged intensities and the peak pressures used in ultrasonic diagnosis (21). Consequently, both regulatory authorities and prudent physicians are right to be concerned about safety. In the USA, for example, the Center for Devices and Radiological Health has concluded that a "mechanical index" (defined in terms of the ratio of pressure to the square root of frequency) is a good predictor of the risk of particular exposure conditions. In Europe, where the use of diagnostic ultrasound is currently less vulnerable to regulation (22), there is a move towards machine classification according to potential hazard. In any event, the application of the ALARA – "as low as reasonably achievable" – principle to ultrasonic exposure is a pragmatic approach in clinical practice.

REFERENCES

1. Wood RW, Loomis AL. The physical and biological effects of high-frequency sound waves of great intensity. Phil Mag 1927;7(4):417–436.
2. Firestone FA. The supersonic reflectoscope, an instrument for inspecting the interior of solid parts by means of sound waves. J Acoust Soc Am 1946;17:287–299.

3. Desch CH, Sproule DO, Dawson WJ. The detection of cracks in steel by means of supersonic waves. J Iron Steel Inst Lond 1946;153:319–352.
4. Howry DH, Bliss WR. Ultrasonic visualization of soft tissue structures of the body. J Lab Clin Med 1952;40:579–592.
5. Wild JJ, Reid JM. Further pilot echographic studies of the histologic structure of tumors of the living intact human breast. Am J Path 1952;28:839–861.
6. Wells PNT. The prudent use of diagnostic ultrasound. Br J Radiol 1987;13:391–400.
7. Wells PNT. Biomedical ultrasonics. London: Academic Press, 1977.
8. Duck FA. Physical properties of tissue. London: Academic Press, 1990.
9. Gururaja TR, Schultze WA, Cross LE et al. Piezoelectric composite materials for ultrasonic transducer applications. IEEE Trans Sonics Ultrason 1985;32:481–499.
10. Law WK, Frizzell LA, Dunn F. Determination of the nonlinearity parameter B/A of biological media. Ultrasound Med Biol 1985;11:307–318.
11. Wells PNT. Doppler ultrasound in medical diangosis. Br J Radiol 1989;62:399–420.
12. McHugh R, McDicken WN, Thompson P, Boddy K. Blood flow detection by an intersecting zone ultrasonic Doppler unit. Ultrasound Med Biol 1981;7:371–375.
13. Kasai C, Namekawa K, Koyano A, Omoto R. Real-time two-dimensional blood flow imaging using an autocorrelation technique. IEEE Trans Sonics Ultrason 1985;32:458–464.
14. Wells PNT. Ultrasonic colour flow imaging. Phys Med Biol 1994;39:2113–2145.
15. Wells PNT. Physics and instrumentation: non-Doppler. In: Goldberg BB (ed): Textbook of Abdominal Ultrasound. Baltimore: Williams & Wilkins, 1993: 3–23.
16. Ofili EO, Nanda NC. Three-dimensional and four-dimensional echocardiography. Ultrasound Med Biol 1994;20:669–675.
17. Shattock DP, Weinshenker MD, Smith SW, von Ramm OT. Explososcan: a parallel processing technique for high speed imaging with linear phased arrays. J Acoust Soc Am 1984;75:1273–1282.
18. Goldberg BB, Liu J-B, Forsberg F. Ultrasound contrast agents: a review. Ultrasound Med Biol 1994;20:319–333.
19. Schrope BA, Newhouse VL. Second harmonic blood perfusion measurements. Ultrasound Med Biol 1993;19:567–579.
20. Docker MF, Duck FA. The safe use of diagnostic ultrasound. London: British Medical Ultrasound Society/British Institute of Radiology, 1991.
21. Duck FA, Martin K. Trends in diagnostic ultrasound exposure. Phys Med Biol 1991;16:1423–1432.
22. Whittingham TA. The safety of ultrasound. Imaging 1994;6:33–51.

CHAPTER 2

Ultrasound Artefacts

David O. Cosgrove, MA, MSc, FRCR, FRCP

Unwanted or scanner-generated signals in ultrasound are commonly referred to as artefacts, though, strictly, this term is meaningless in this context since all of the information in ultrasound scans (and all other diagnostic imaging modes) is man made. Nevertheless, the term is hallowed by usage and will be retained in this clinical sense here. In ultrasound imaging, artefacts arise whenever the assumptions underlying the pulse echo technique are broken. These are that:

1. the beam is narrow and uniform in width
2. attenuation is uniform
3. the beam travels directly to and from the echo producing interfaces, and
4. the speed of sound in soft tissues is constant.

For Doppler, additional artefacts arise from the frequency shift analysis and the calculations of velocity made from it.

Understanding artefacts is important to avoid interpretative errors, but they are often of interest in their own right because the underlying mechanisms give insight into the complex processes of ultrasound image and Doppler formation (1–3).

B-MODE IMAGING

A useful way to illustrate the artefacts produced by deviations from these "rules", first described by Fred Sample (4), is to imagine a test phantom which contains a series of objects (Figure 1).

Study of the images produced when this is scanned by a linear array demonstrates a variety of important effects.

Beam width (Figure 1 a)

The real ultrasound beam differs markedly from the uniform laser-thin ideal (Figure 2). Its pattern is complex close to the transducer face and then is narrowed by electronic and lens focusing down to its focal zone before fanning out in the far field. Sound intensity at any location reduces progressively away from the centre axis of the beam in a bell shape and this is true both within and across the scan planes.

The effect of beam width in the image is lateral smearing of discrete reflectors so that a point is depicted as a smear (Figure 3) (5). The width of the beam spread is proportional to the beam width and also to the echogenicity of the target because a strong reflector will give an echo that is above the scanner's threshold when it is further off axis than a weak reflector. Considered from the point of view of spatial resolution, the wider the

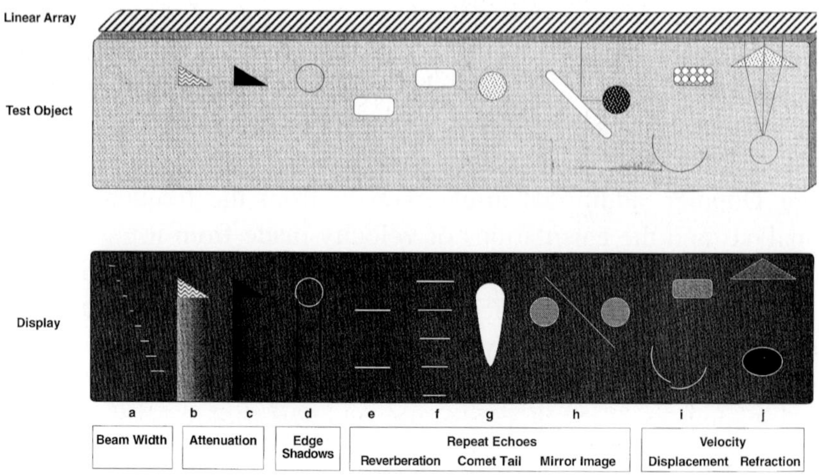

Figure 1 ***The Phantom Phantom***
An imaginary phantom or test object is depicted in the upper part of the figure with a linear array to scan it; the resultant screen display is illustrated below. Within the test object are a number of interesting targets (a-j) and the artefacts they generate are seen on the "screen".

Figure 2 ***Complexity of the Ultrasound Field*** *Visualization of the ultrasound field (using light diffraction in a transparant medium, a development of the Schlieren tank) reveals the complexity of the beam pattern. The ultrasound field from a highly focused linear array at the left in (a) shows the interference patterns and the beam spread away from the focal zone in two dimensions. There is also a marked side-lobe (arrow). The fact that this complexity is actually a three dimensional phenomenon is better revealed in the 3-D rendered version from multiple images (b) which presents a view as though looking almost directly along the beam. (Images kindly supplied by Dr. Mehboob Kadiri, Intek Research Company, Sunnyvale, CA)*

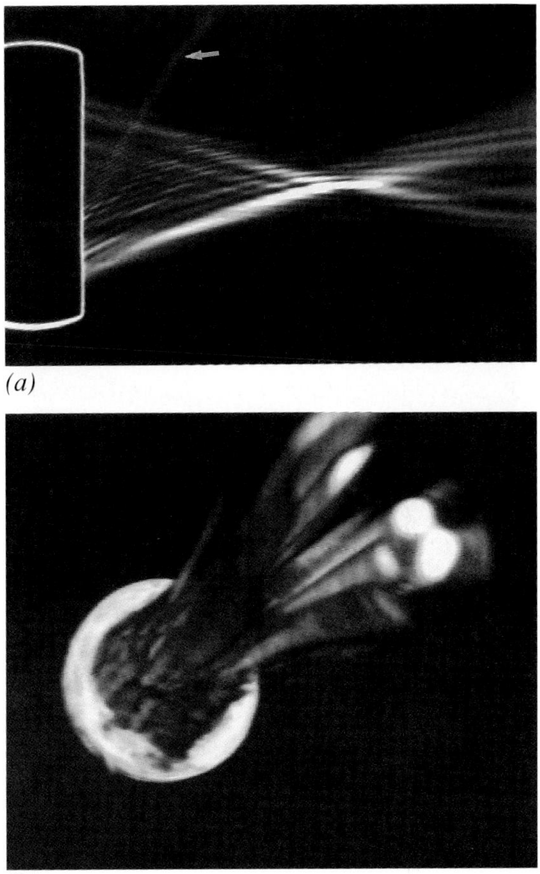

(a) *(b)*

beam the poorer the resolution because two adjacent targets will blur into one signal if they lie closer together than the beam width.

The actual beam width is difficult to define. Manufacturers quote the half-power (–3 dB) envelope at the optimum focus and this gives a figure of approximately 2 mm for a 7 MHz probe, falling to 5 mm for a 3 MHz probe. It is obvious from inspecting ultrasound images that these are best case figures and lateral resolution falls off markedly away from the focal zone and for stronger reflectors. This is why correct positioning of the focal zone is important in clinical practice and why multiple foci (multizone) are pre-

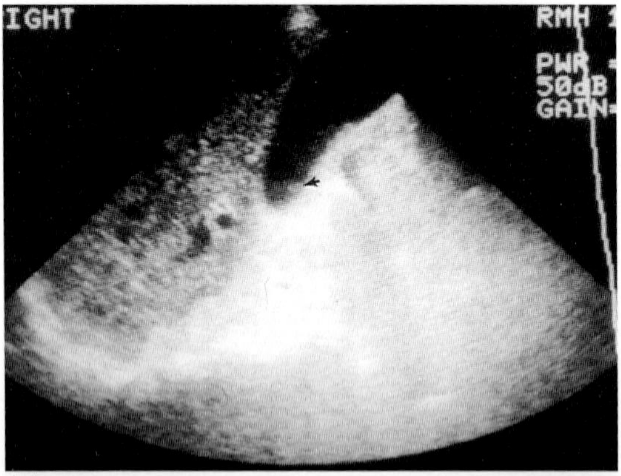

(a)

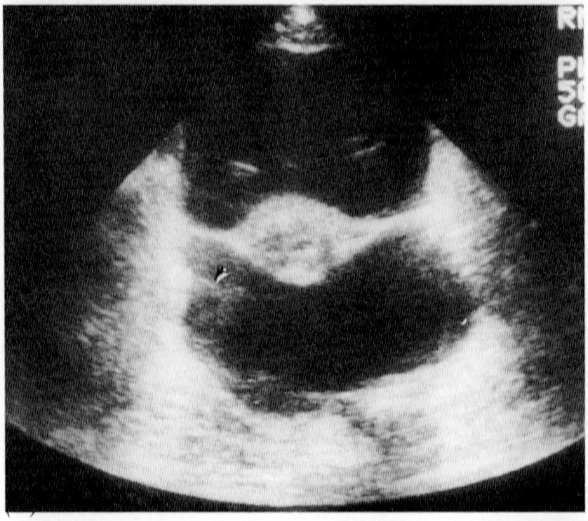

Figure 3 ***Beam Width Artefact***

Strong reflectors produce a streak on the image; they are most obvious against an anechoic background as in the gallbladder (arrowhead in a) or in the pelvis in ascites (arrowhead in b). When the offending reflector lies in the orthogonal plane the resulting slice thickness artefact is harder to recognise (arrowhead in c. – a pleural effusion) until the probe is swivelled through 90° (arrowhead in d – an aerated portion of lung).

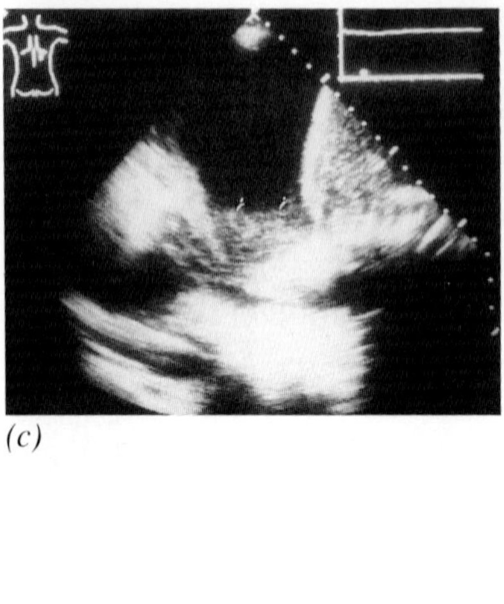

(c)

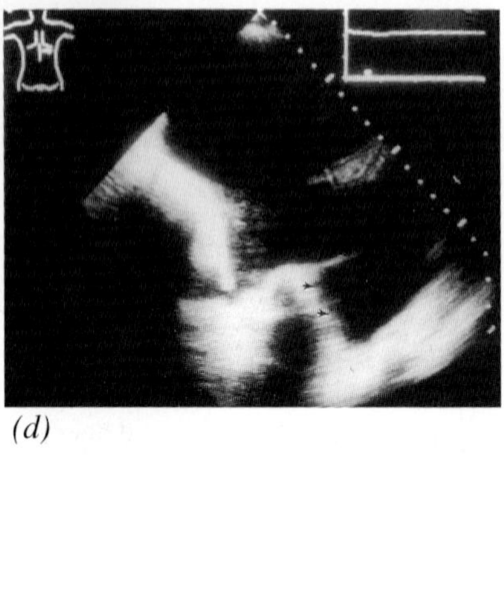

(d)

ferred whenever the loss in frame rate that this produces is acceptable. As if this non-uniformity of the beam width were not complex enough, there are also side lobes (and, for electronic arrays, grating lobes), sound beams emitted at angles from the main beam (Figures 3, 4) (6). Side and grating lobes are usually of much lower intensity than the main beam, so that only very echogenic interfaces produce discrete artefacts and generally, their effect is to introduce a wash of noice across the scan so that contrast is reduced.

The beam width sets the limit to lateral resolution while it is the pulse length that limits range resolution. Not only is the pulse length smaller but it also varies less with depth; this is why the most precise measurements in ultrasound should be made along the ultrasound beam rather than across it (e.g. biparietal diameter of the fetal head, thickness of the intima-media layer of the carotid artery).

Attenuation effects (Figure 1 b, c, d)

The ultrasound beam is attenuated as it is conducted through tissue; the main mechanism in soft tissues is absorption which occurs when the coherent vibration of tissue particles – which is sound – is disturbed and becomes random – i.e. turns into heat. Attenuation is proportional to the ultrasound frequency and it occurs at approximately 1 dB for each centimetre of tissue depth (go-and-return path) for each megahertz. If uncorrected, atten-

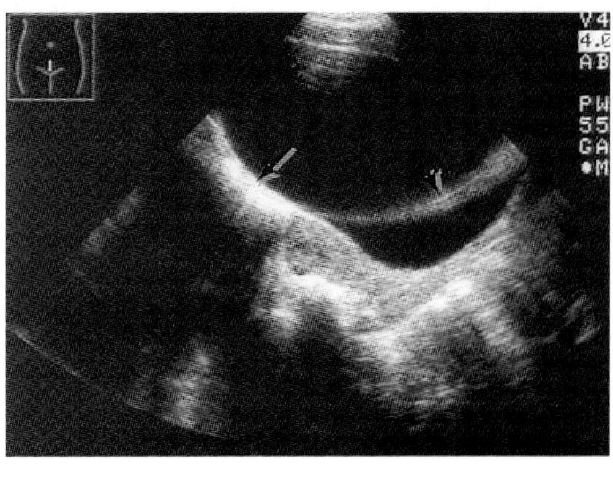

Figure 4 ***Side/Grating Lobe***
An extreme form of beam spread is occasionally seen when a very strong reflector, in this case bowel gas (arrow) is detected by the side lobe when the main beam is directed over an echofree space, here the urinary bladder. A curved artefactual line is produced (arrowhead).

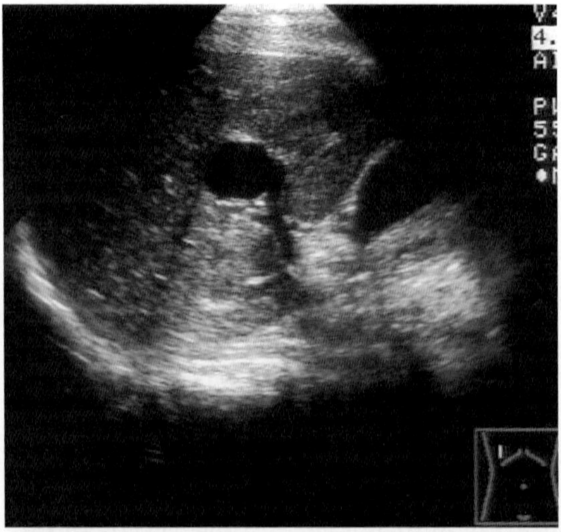

Figure 5
Enhancement
The "bright up" deep to this liver cyst indicates the lower than average attenuation of its fluid contents. This is an example of a "friendly" artefact that gives useful information.

uation would produce a scan that darkened progressively with depth and this is compensated for by the TGC (time gain compensation) amplifier which progressively boosts the signals from deeper interfaces. The setting operates across the whole image and so it is only possible to set the best average TGC for each scan.

When attenuation is lower than average for a region in the scan, e.g. in a cystic space, the TGC continues inappropriately to boost the signals deep to it (7). This over-compensates the deeper echoes and produces a bright band of increased through transmission or "acoustic enhancement" deep to the cyst (Figure 5). (Enhancing lesions are sometimes misleadingly referred to as "transonic", an unhelpful term which is better avoided). Increased through transmission is typical of fluid spaces, both normal (e.g. the gallbladder) and pathological, and may be present even when the fluid contains reflectors such as cholesterol or crystals that make it echogenic because, apart from air and bone to tissue interfaces, reflection accounts for only a small part of the ultrasound attenuation. Some solid lesions also attenuate less than average and may show increased through transmission. An example is lymphoma nodules in the liver, where the through transmission is often exaggerated by the high TGC levels required to balance the increased attenuation of the fatty liver that often coexists. Mistaking such deposits for simple cysts is a serious diagnostic error.

The exact reverse occurs for the commonest type of shadowing: a region of higher than average attenuation is undercorrected by the TGC and a dark band results. This commonly occurs with fibrosis and fat and is seen, for example, deep to the ligamentum teres in the liver and to schirrous carcinomas in the breast (Figure 6).

Shadowing can also occur deep to very echogenic interfaces where a significant proportion of the ultrasound beam is reflected. Obviously, if 90 % of the incident beam is reflected, as occurs with a tissue gas surface, there will be distal shadowing (Figure 7). In this case there is often also reverberation artefact that partly fills in the shadowed band, so called "dirty shadowing", which has a different appearance from the clean black band of

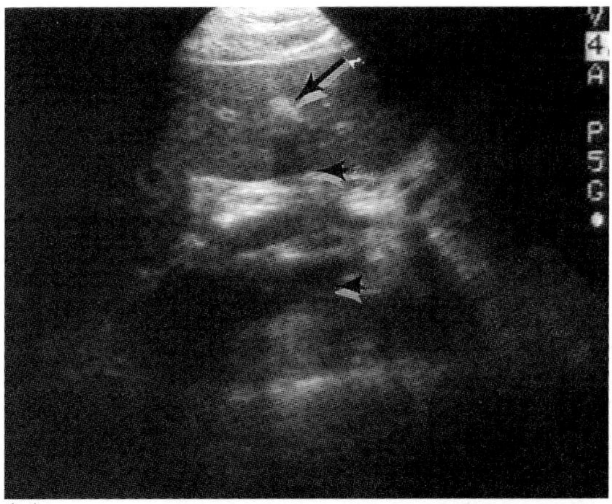

(a)

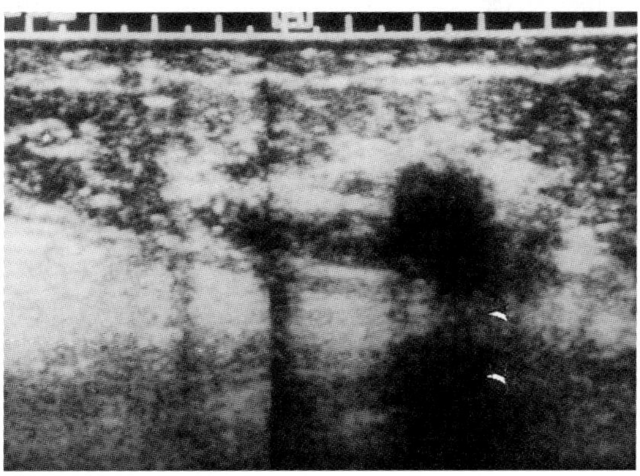

(b)

Figure 6 ***Shadowing Deep to Fibrous Tissue*** *The ligamentum teres (arrowhead) absorbs ultrasound more strongly than the surrounding soft tissues and so generates a shadow (arrow) which partly obscures deeper lying structures, here part of the pancreas. Attenuation shadowing also occurs deep to pathological fibrosis, as in this schirrous carcinoma (arrowhead in b).*

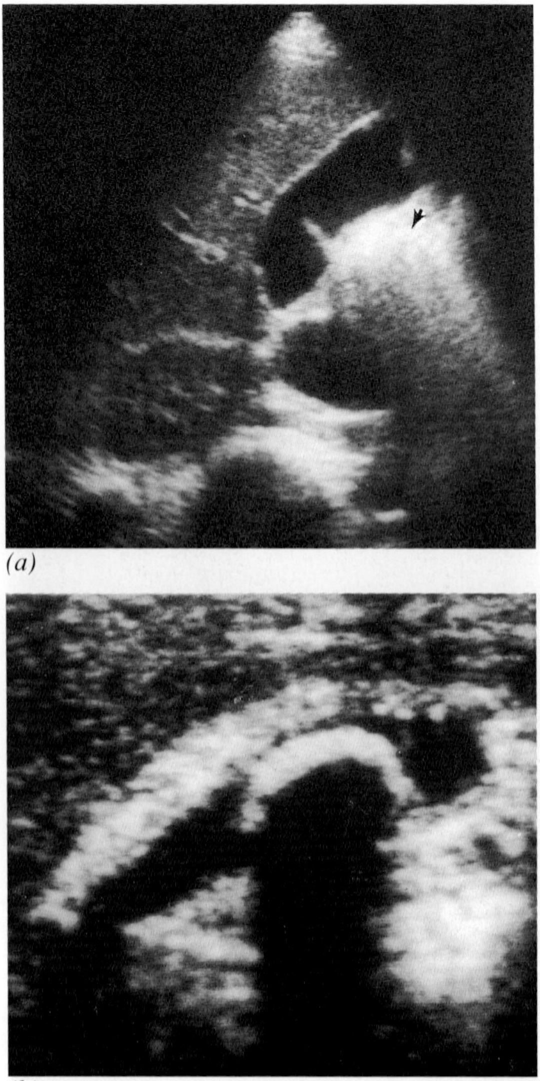

(a)

(b)

Figure 7
Reflective Shadowing
The total reflection that occurs at a gas surface such as it often found in the duodenal cap (arrowhead in a) causes reflective shadowing which is often partly filled in with echoes arising from coexisting reverberation artefacts. This appearance is different from the clean shadowing deep to a gallstone (b).

shadowing that is typical of stones where the mechanism is a combination of absorption and reflection (8).

A third and less important form of shadowing, edge shadowing, forms fine dark lines behind the edges of strongly curved structures such as the fetal skull and the walls of the cysts (Figure 8). It is not quite clear whether they are caused by absorption in the thicker band of tissue constituting the walls of these structures or

Figure 8 ***Edge Shadows***
The fine dark lines deep to the edges of the portal vein and the ivc (a) or a Cooper's ligament in the breast (b) (arrowheads) do not carry the same diagnostic significance as attenuative shadowing.

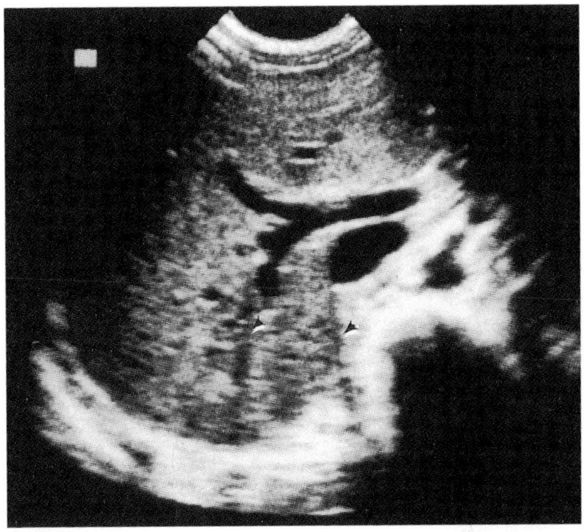

(a)

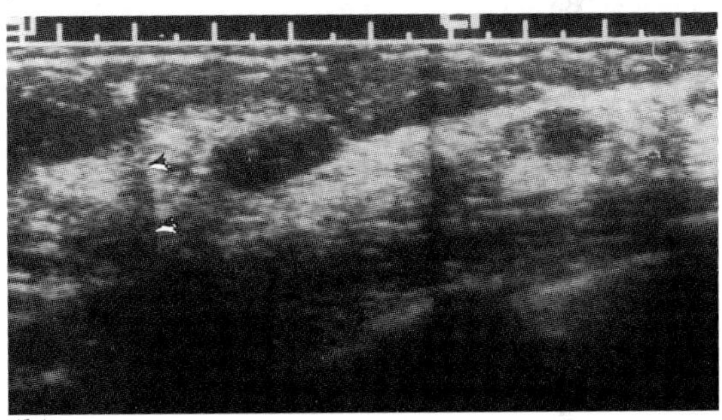

(b)

whether they are a form of refraction. The important diagnostic point is not to confuse them with the other types of shadowing, which are clinically significant. A common example occurs in the breast: edge shadows from Cooper's ligaments must not be mistaken from the attenuative shadowing of a schirrous carcinoma. Similarly, shadowing from a stone in the neck of the gallbladder, must be distinguished from the edge shadow often caused by the folds at the beginning of the cystic duct.

Multiple echoes (Figure 1 e, f, g, h)

In the pulse-echo method, which is the basis of ultrasound imaging, signals are plotted along the line of the ultrasound beam at a depth proportional to the delay in their receipt (9). Artefacts occur

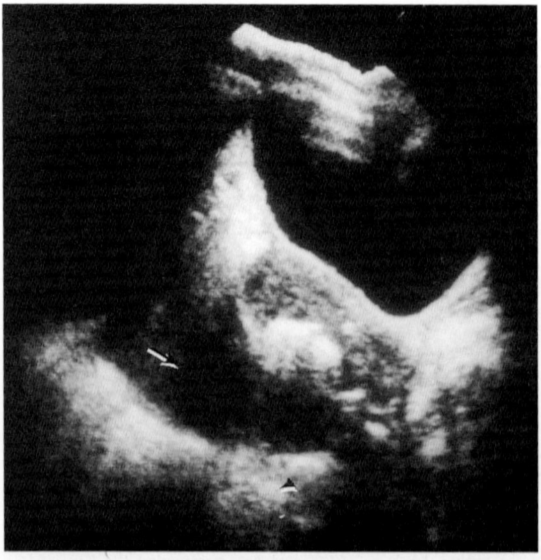

Figure 9
False Pelvic Mass
The echopoor mass deep in the pelvis (arrows) is actually formed by a repeat echo from the far wall of the bladder. It even contains recognisable structures (the calcific fibroid, arrowhead) further adding to the potential confusion.

when the transmitted pulse or its echoes follow a more complex path. A common example occurs when the strong echoes from a flat interface that lies parallel to the transducer face are reflected from the transducer back into the tissues a second time. Then a repeat echo from the interface gives a spurious signal which is indicated on the image at twice the depth of the true surface. This "second time around" artefact can give confusing pseudo lesions, for example in the pelvis, where gas in the rectosigmoid colon is

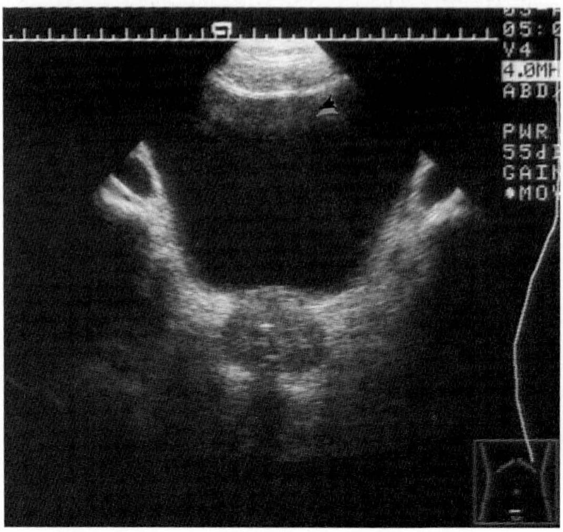

Figure 10
Reverberation Artefact
The echoes in the superficial portion of the filled bladder (arrowhead) are spurious signals arising from multiple internal reflections within the soft tissues of the anterior abdominal wall and between them and the transducer face.

the reflecting surface: the whole bladder appears as an echopoor "mass" deep in the pelvis (Figure 9). When the reflective layer is close to the skin, multiple repeat echoes can occur and this gives rise to parallel stripes in the image that extend deep to the real surface (Figure 10). These "reverberations" are easily recognised when they fall over a fluid space such as the gallbladder or amniotic fluid but, where they fall over soft tissue, they may be more difficult to recognise and they add to the general noise background so that contrast is reduced. The reflections from the transducer face can be minimised by applying matching coatings to the front of the crystal; they work in much the same way as the coatings of an optical lens by improving transmission into the crystal so that reflections are reduced.

Reverberations may also be produced by any two parallel tissue layers: the effect is commonly seen as blurring of the superficial

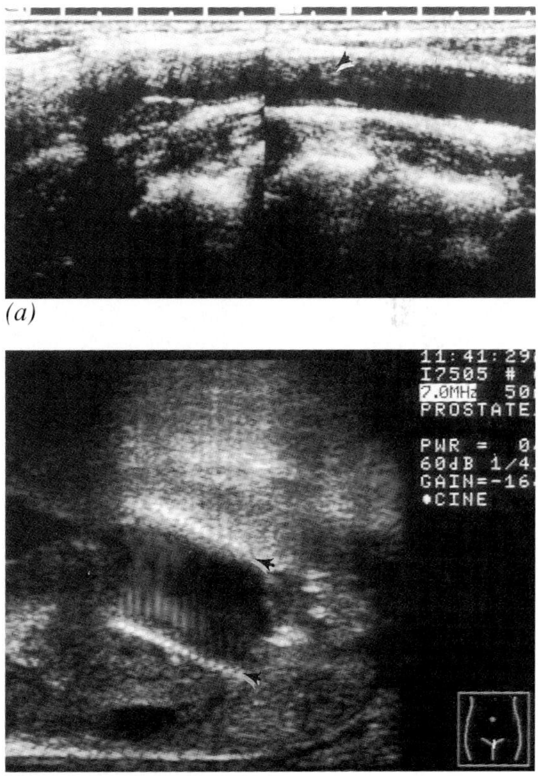

(a)

(b)

Figure 11
Reverberation Artefact
The blurring of the superficial intima-media layer of the carotid artery (arrowhead in a) is caused by reverberations. Sometimes known as "ring down artefact" it means that the IML thickness is usually better measured at the deep surface of the artery where it is clearer. The multiple parallel signals deep to the prostatic stent (arrowhead in b) in this transrectal scan are a striking example of multiple reverberations.

intima-media layer of the carotid artery and deep to metal or plastic prostheses (Figure 11) – this is why the deep intima-media layer should be selected for measurements. Bowel gas is a very strong reflector so that reverberations almost always fill what would otherwise be an echo free shadow deep to bowel; it is known as "dirty shadowing" (Figure 7 a) by comparison with the absence of signals in the shadowing from stones (Figure 7 b). The same effect occurs at the lung surface. Some of the apparent bright echoes in the parenchyma of the liver are probably also reverberations.

An interesting form of reverberation where a narrow and very echogenic streak extends deep to bowel gas has been termed the "comet tail" artefact (Figure 12). It is commonly seen in the duodenum and is probably caused by a foamy aggregate of air bubbles, each of which acts as a very efficient reflector of sound. Echoes bounce repeatedly between adjacent bubbles in random directions and from time to time some echoes escape and return to the transducer to produce a train of signals that fades gradually as the ultrasound energy is dissipated.

When a flat strong reflector lies at an angle to the ultrasound beam, the echoes are directed back into the overlying tissue at an oblique angle (10). Ordinarily, they would not be detected by the transducer but, if the reflected beam strikes interfaces, these

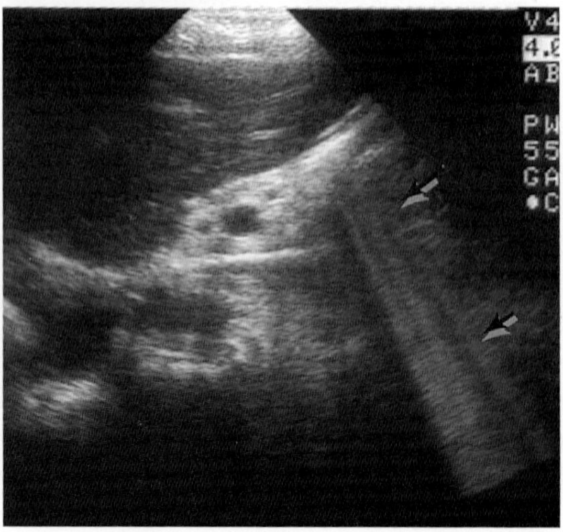

Figure 12 ***The Comet Tail Artefact***
A band of intense signals (arrows) is seen extending deep to this pocket of gas in the stomach. It probably arises from multiple reflections from the numerous gas surfaces in a foamy gas pocket.

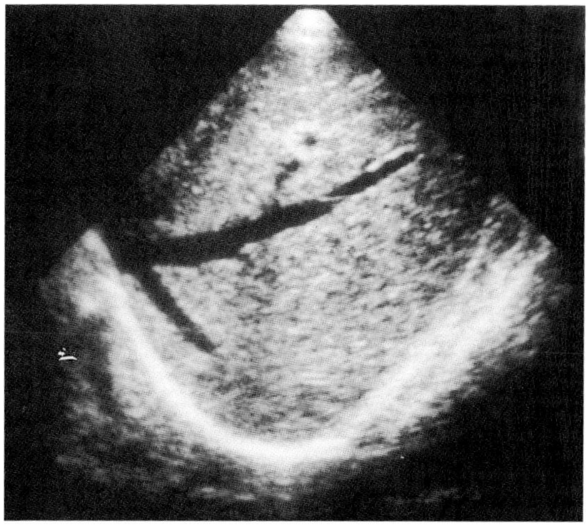

Figure 13 ***Mirror Image Artefact***
The echoes above the diaphragm are actually a mirror image of the subdiaphragmatic structures, often liver. Sometimes anatomical detail can be recognised, in this case, part of the right hepatic vein (arrowhead) (cf. Figure 16).

echoes retrace the original path and return to the transducer indirectly. This produces the "mirror image artefact" in which a structure or lesion is seen twice: one is correctly positioned and the other is depicted behind the mirror exactly as with an optical mirror. A common site where this occurs is at the parietal pleura over the diaphragm (Figure 13). The air surface here is a good reflector and so hepatic or splenic tissue, as well as lesions within them, can be depicted in the position of the lower zones of the lung. If a pleural effusion is present, the mirror is destroyed and then true information about the chest is obtained.

Velocity artefacts (Figure 1 i, j)

Generally, the assumption that the velocity of ultrasound in soft tissue is constant at 1540 m/sec is true but some tissues, notably fat (1450 m/s) and silicone implants (600 m/sec) conduct more slowly. An echo from within or beyond these materials takes longer to reach the transducer and so is indicated on the image as lying deeper than it really is (11). The difference in velocity with fat is so slight than only subtle distortions are seen even from larger regions of fatty tissue but occasionally a notch where the diaphragm seems to be displaced posteriorly behind a lipoma in the liver or an angiomyolipoma in the kidney is seen. This is a signature of fatty tissue. The velocity difference with silicone is much greater and makes

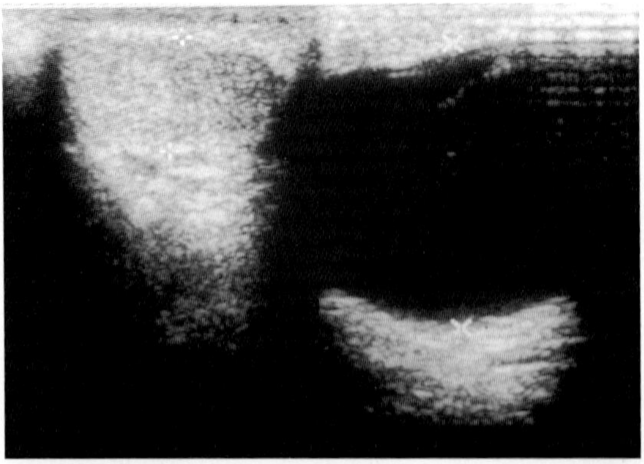

Figure 14 ***Testicular Prosthesis***
The prosthetic left testis seems to be about twice as deep as the natural right testis. This artefact is produced by the slow speed of sound in the silicone.

prostheses (e.g. in the breast and scrotum) seem approximately twice as thick as they actually are (Figure 14). The chest wall deep to a breast prosthesis often appears as a U-shaped valley.

Unless it is normal to the interface, the ultrasound beam is refracted when it crosses between tissues of different velocities, exactly as with a light beam. This beam bending can result in side-by-side double images in the same way that a fish in an aquarium can be seen twice when it is viewed through the corner of its tank (12). The commonest situation where this occurs is in the abdomen where the fat occupying the spaces between the rectus abdominus muscles has a wedge shape in transverse sections. Thus it behaves like an optimal prism, so that a midline structure in the pelvis is imaged both directly in the midline and again by the refracted beam from slightly to one side (Figure 15). This second image is placed on screen as though originating from the straight line path of the beam. Overlapping or sometimes even completely separate images are produced, for example, of the prostate, a catheter bulb, or most importantly, of the gestational sac. This artefact is more pronounced for deeper structures (because the same refraction angle produces a greater lateral distortion when the path is longer) and in the lower abdomen (because there is more fat here) but occasionally a double superior mesenteric artery can be seen. Moving the transducer away from the midline or imaging in the longitudinal plane to avoid traversing the wedges of fat removes the artefact and often greatly improves the general image quality. This same effect occurs in a less dramatic way at every interface between fatty and watery tissue and it disperses the beam

Figure 15 ***The Split Image Artefact***
The double wall appearance of a catheter bulb (arrowheads in a) and the duplicated superior mesenteric artery in b are the result of the ultrasound beam being refracted by the wedge shaped layers of the anterior abdominal wall (c).

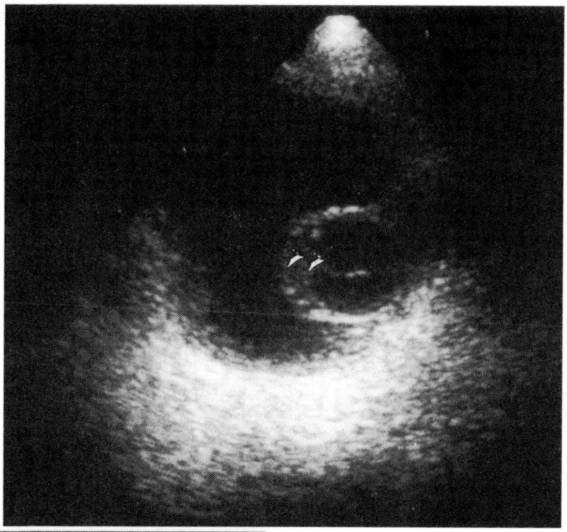

(a)

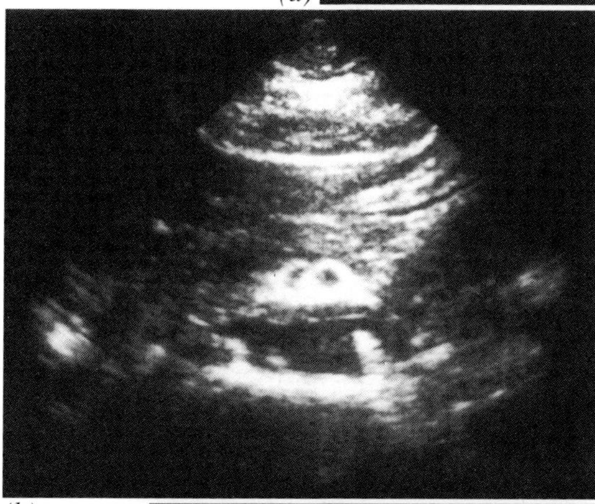

(b)

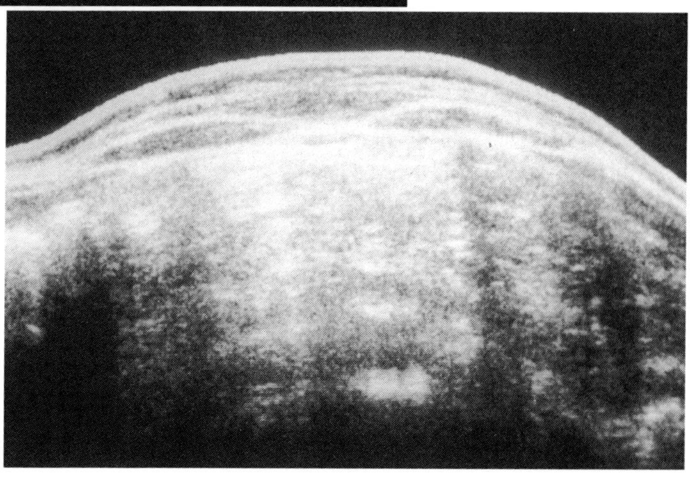

(c)

so that it broadens resulting in loss of resolution and also, importantly, in an increase in background signal So that contrast as well as spatial resolution are compromised. These refraction effects probably account for the great range in ultrasound image quality between different subjects. Overcoming this would be a great advance for ultrasound imaging.

DOPPLER

Because the ultrasound beam used for Doppler is determined by exactly the same physical principles as that used for imaging, all the artefacts that affect imaging also occur with Doppler. Particularly important are attenuation, beam-width, refraction effects and mirror image phenomenona (Figure 16).

In addition, artefacts that are unique to Doppler need to be considered (13). Some concern Doppler calculations, others the frequency analysis system. An example of the latter is the pervasive problem with pulsed Doppler (i.e. both spectral and colour Doppler) of aliasing which occurs when the pulsed repetition frequency is too low to sample the Doppler shift frequency adequately. This undersampling leads to erroneous estimations of the Doppler shift that is depicted as fast reversed flow and displayed as though the trace had gone off scale and wrapped around the back to conti-

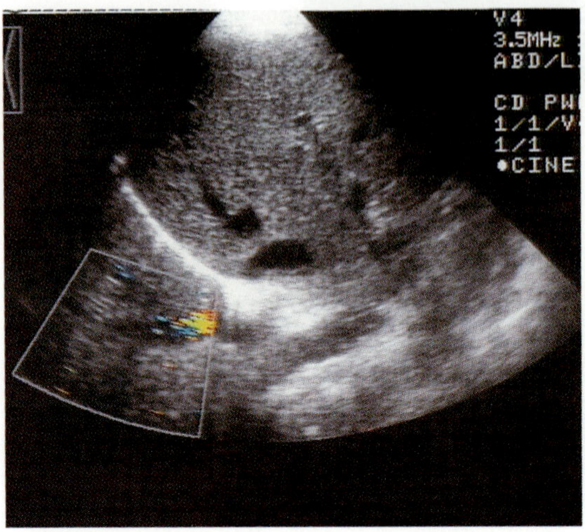

Figure 16 ***Mirror Image Artefact – B-mode and Doppler*** *The air surface at the pleura has produced a mirror image artefact of the structures in the liver. Here an hepatic vein is projected across the diaphragm and colour Doppler signals are obtained from it.*

Figure 17 ***Aliasing in Spectral Doppler***
The frequency shift in (a) is too large to be adequately sampled by the pulse repetition rate chosen; the Doppler signals from the faster flowing blood at each systole is falsely positioned as fast reverse flow as though the display had wrapped around the back of the screen (arrow). Increasing the PRF (by increasing the scale) (b) corrects the artefact.

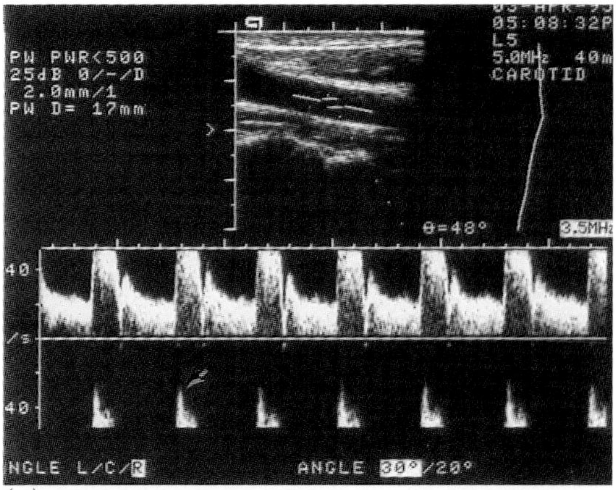

(a)

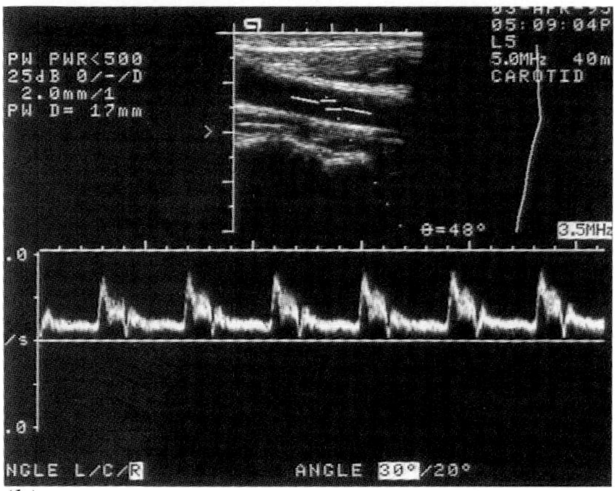

(b)

nue in the reverse channel (Figure 17). In extreme cases it may cross the baseline and even wrap around twice so that the Doppler signals are difficult even to recognise. In colour Doppler, a mosaic of colours is seen with colours at opposite ends of the colour bar adjacent to each other (Figure 18). This continuity of colours helps to distinguish aliasing from true flow reversal where the transient phase of stationary blood is shown as a black band around each colour block.

Aliasing can be corrected by increasing the PRF (usually labelled "scale" on the display panel) but with the penalty of reduced sensitivity to slow flow. Shifting the baseline adjusts the display and may be all that is needed in many cases. Other techniques that may suffice are reducing the Doppler frequency and

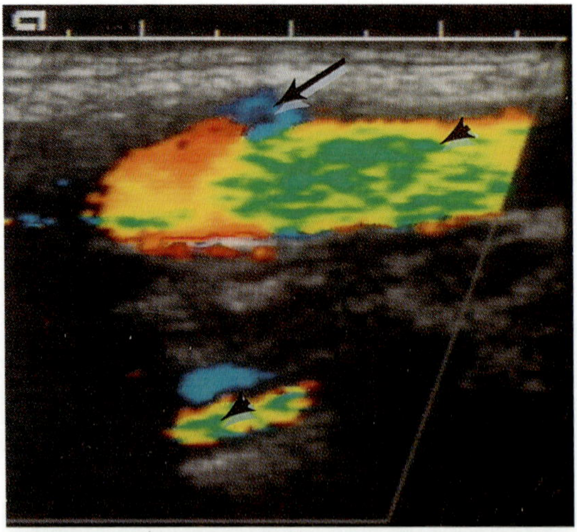

Figure 18 ***The Mosaic Effect Produced by Aliasing in Colour Doppler***
In this carotid Doppler a mosaic of colours from opposite ends of the colour bar indicate that flow is changing instantaneously from fast forward to fast reverse (arrowheads) in the hall mark of aliasing. In true flow reversal, such as at the boundary layer separation in the carotid bulb (arrow) the colours are separated by a black band representing the stationary layer of blood.

increasing the beam to vessel angle towards 60°, all directed towards reducing the numerator in the "Doppler equation". In some situations, for example when the question is simply whether there is flow or not, aliasing can be ignored; where flow direction is important, moderate aliasing can be tolerated with due care to avoid misinterpreting double aliasing. However, aliasing precludes measurements of peak or mean velocity and must be eliminated where these need to be measured.

A key practical aspect of Doppler techniques is the beam to vessel (strictly "flow") angle. Not only does the Doppler frequency shift reduce as the angle increases towards 90° (so that poorer signals are obtained), but also the accuracy with which the angle can be measured reduces sharply. In practice, angles of less than 60° should be aimed at and, while one may be obliged to override this rule in some situations, especially for deep Doppler in the abdomen, measurements based on traces obtained with larger angles are unreliable.

The siting and sizing of the sampling volume in spectral Doppler is critical to obtaining meaningful readings. Obviously, flow outside the Doppler gate is not registered and if this misses the fast jet of

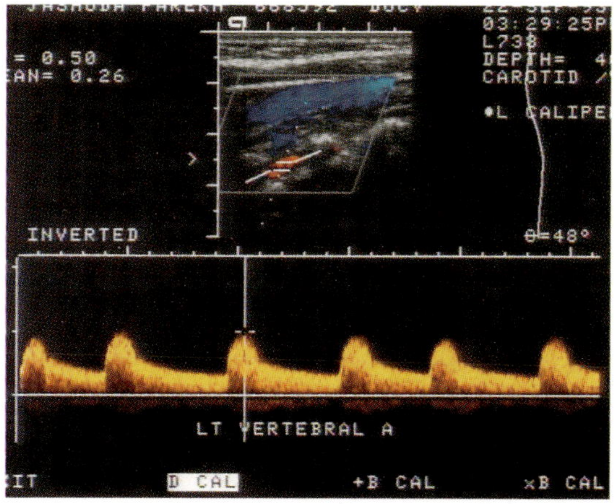

Figure 19 ***Use of Colour Doppler for Gate Placement***
The spectral gate has been positioned accurately over the vertebral artery and the angle correction cursor aligned using the colour Doppler scan as a map. (The vessel showing in blue superficial to the vertebral artery is the internal jugular vein.)

flow at a tight stenosis for example, the diagnosis will be wrong. Use of colour Doppler to guide placement of the spectral gate or use of a wide gate and meticulous scanning across the vessel minimize the problems (Figure 19). If the slow flow of the vessel margins needs to be measured, for example in calculating volume flow, then the gate must span the whole vessel lumen (Figure 20).

Calculating volume flow is a seductively simple process (vessel area × averaged mean flow velocity) but in practice both measurements are fraught with errors that multiply in the calculation to the extent that an accuracy of ± 50 % is the best achievable (14). Even

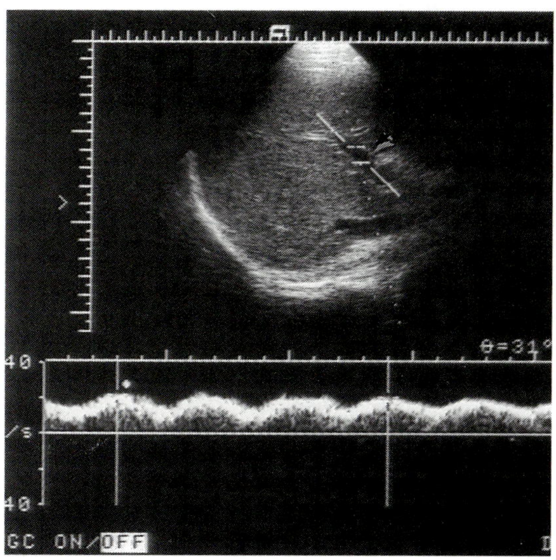

Figure 20 ***Wide Spectral Gate for Volume Flow Measurement***
In order to collect signals from as much as possible of the vessel for a volume flow estimate, as in this portal vein (arrowhead), a wide spectral gate is required otherwise flow streams outside the sample volume will be omitted. Angle correction of the frequency shift in this case gave a mean flow velocity of 13 cm/sec.

given a good beam to vessel angle, estimating the mean flow velocity depends on the scanner's calculation package and not all systems use the optimum method in which the measured values for all Doppler shift components in each sampled interval are used for the calculation (some systems merely halve the peak velocity, assuming that the flow profile is parabolic). Other factors that influence the mean value are the wall filter (which removes low velocity signals), the spread of transmitted frequencies and their change with depth (the assumed reference frequency is often wrong) and the imprecise determination of the Doppler angle, even when this is accurately measured by the operator. Measurement of the area of the vessel is also fraught: a true diameter must be obtained and, ideally, some correction for its cyclical variation, both cardiac and respiratory, should be applied. In practice, caution is needed in the clinical application of volume flow measurements because of these errors and the most useful are serial stud-

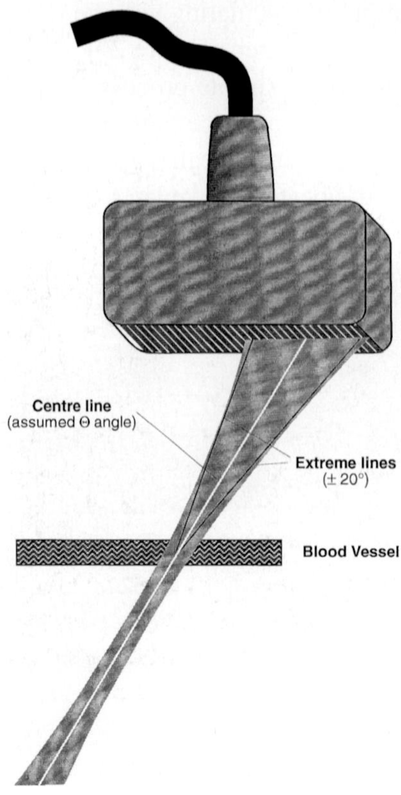

Figure 21
Beam-to-vessel Angle Uncertainty
When a wide aperture transducer is used for Doppler measurements, the angle spans a range of values for which may amount to ± 20°; this effect broadens the Doppler spectrum because some parts of the transducer have a steep angle while others have a shallow angle.

ies within a given patient. In converting the measured Doppler frequency shift to velocity, the scanner not only accepts the beam to vessel angle entered by the operator but assumes that this is a discrete value. Because the surface of the transducer has a length and is not a point, as would be ideal, in practice, there is a range of angles (Figure 21). It also assumes a single value for the frequency of the transmitted signal; in pulsed Doppler a spread of frequencies is used and this is changed by attenuation which selectively removes the higher frequencies throughout the depth of the tissue.

With colour Doppler, only the mean velocity is depicted, optionally together with the spread of velocities (variance) so the maixmum readings are lower than with spectral Doppler which is always preferred for haemodynamic measurements.

In duplex Doppler, i.e. when the scanner provides simultaneous Doppler and B-mode imaging, the time sharing necessitates compromises, notably a reduced frame rate for both B-mode and colour Doppler and a lower spectral Doppler sampling rate, so that the tracing becomes intermittent. While generally the time sharing is acceptable for small parts scanning, with deep Doppler the frame rate may become unacceptably low. The essence of the lim-

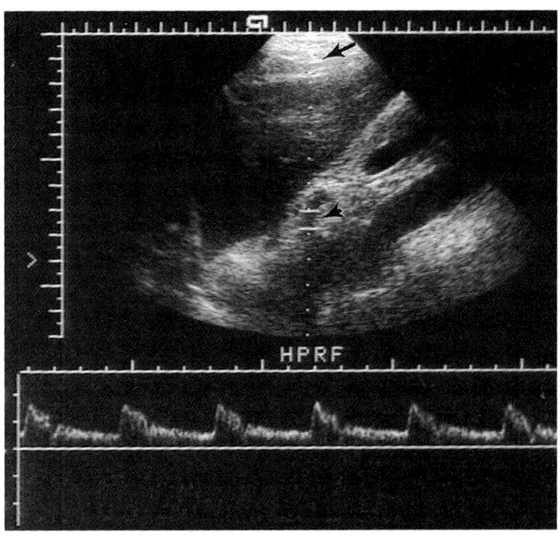

Figure 22 ***High PRF*** *An additional Doppler gate is indicated (arrow) when the PRF is increased above the nominally permitted maximum (the Nyquist limit), as may be required to obtain an alias-free tracing from the fast flow in a deep artery, here the coeliac axis (arrhowhead). As long as the HPRF gate can be seen to fall outside a second unwanted vessel, as is usually the case in practice, the faster sampling rate achieved is useful.*

itation is the need to delay sequential pulses long enough to allow the previous pulses to have decayed to background level because overlapping echoes are erroneously depicted as lying closer to the transducer than they actually are. In some spectral Doppler systems, this rule is deliberately broken to allow a higher pulse repetition frequency to be used and the regions that cause confusion are indicated on screen, as "ghost" sample volumes (Figure 22); as long as the operator ensures that no vessel lies in these overlap regions, this device allows an increase in the PRF and thus reduces aliasing.

An interesting artefact that resembles a coloured version of the comet tail artefact is sometimes seen when small calcifications lie in the colour box – it may result from physical vibrations of the calcific particles by the ultrasound beam.

A special group of Doppler artefacts arises when microbubble echo enhancing ("contrast") agents are used. Despite the fact that these agents do not change the flow characteristics at all, the spectrum shows apparent broadening with both lower and higher velocity components. This is probably caused by signals that were too weak to register with the Doppler circuitry pre-enhancement now being strong enough to be Doppler-detected; it will necessitate re-establishing the normal ranges for absolute values, though ratios can be expected to remain unchanged. "Bubble noise" is seen as transient high strength peaks on the Doppler spectrum – they are probably caused by collapse of bubbles that have been set in resonance by the Doppler beam. This effect may also contribute to the "blooming artefact" seen on colour Doppler as distal smearing of colour signals outside the positions of known vessels but multipath reverberations of the same type that cause the comet tail artefact may also be responsible.

REFERENCES

1. Cosgrove DO. Ultrasound Artefacts. In: Meire HB, Cosgrove DO, Dewbury KC (eds): Clinical Ultrasound; volume 2 (chapter 4); 1993:47–63. London: Churchill Livingstone.
2. Laing FC. Commonly encountered artifacts in clinical ultrasound. Semin Ultrasound 1983;4:1–25.

3. Kremkau FW, Taylow KJW. Artifacts in ultrasound imaging. JUM 1986;5:227–237.
4. Sarti DA, Sample WF. Diagnostic Ultrasound: Text and Cases. (chapter 1) 1980: 18. Boston: GK Hall.
5. Goldstein A, Madrazo BL. Slice thickness artifact in gray-scale ultrasound. JCU 1981;9:365–375.
6. Laing FC, Kurtz AB. The importance of ultrasonic side lobe artefacts. Radiology 1982;145:763–768.
7. Suramo I. Paivanslo M. Vuoria P. Shadowing and reverberation artefacts in abdominal ultrasonography. Eur J Radiol 1985;5:147–151.
8. Sommer FG, Taylor KJW. Differentiation of acoustic shadowing due tu calculi and gas collections. Radiology 1980;135:399–403.
9. Bly SH, Foster FS, Patterson US et al. Artefactual echoes in B-mode imaging due to multiple scattering. UMB 1985;11:99–111.
10. Cosgrove DO, Carbutt P, Hill CR. Echoes across the diaphragm: the mirror image artefact. UMB 1978;3:388–392.
11. Richman TS, Taylor KJW, Kremkau FW. Propagation speed artifact in a fatty tumor. JUM 1983;2:45.
12. Müller N, Cooperberg PL, Rowley VA et al. Ultrasonic refraction by the rectus abdominus muscle: the double image artefact. JUM 1984;4:29–34.
13. Johnston KW, Maruzzo BC, Cobbold RSC. Errors and artefacts of Doppler flowmeters and their solutions. Arch Surg 1977;112:1335–1341.
14. Gill RW. Measurement of blood flow by ultrasound: accuracy and sources of error. UMB 1985;11:625–641.

CHAPTER 3

The Liver

Mark Brooks, FRACR

THE NORMAL LIVER

The normal liver volume is approximately 1500 ± 100 cc in adult males and 1300 ± 100 cc in adult females. Accurate ultrasound measurement of liver volume is technically difficult. CT and MRI are better suited to this task. However, an ultrasound estimate of liver size can be made based on the craniocaudal extent of the right lobe and antero-posterior extent of the left lobe. When measured in the midclavicular line the right lobe normally measures up to 13 cm and is considered enlarged if more than 15 cm. The left lobe does not normally exceed 6 cm measured antero-posteriorly in the midline. Accurate positioning of the probe is important as the right lobe may measure more than 15 cm in length when measured more laterally.

Liver anatomy

Current surgical techniques of liver resection dictate a lobar and segmental approach to liver anatomy which differs from the classical description of liver anatomy. The eight liver segments (Figure 1) as described by Couinaud can be demonstrated with ultrasound and other imaging modalities (1).

The left and right lobes, roughly equal in size, are separated by a plane through the middle hepatic vein and the gallbladder bed. The right lobe is further divided into anterior and posterior sectors by the right hepatic vein. The posterior sector of the right lobe consists of segment 6 inferiorly and segment 7 superiorly each of

Figure 2 ***Normal Doppler waveforms.***
a. Hepatic artery
b. Portal vein
c. Hepatic vein

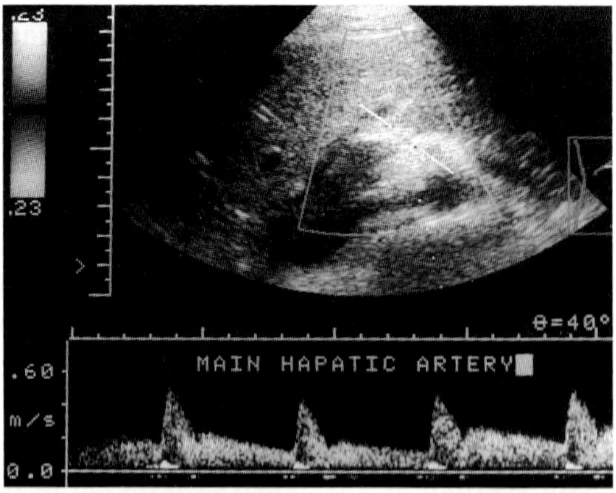

(a)

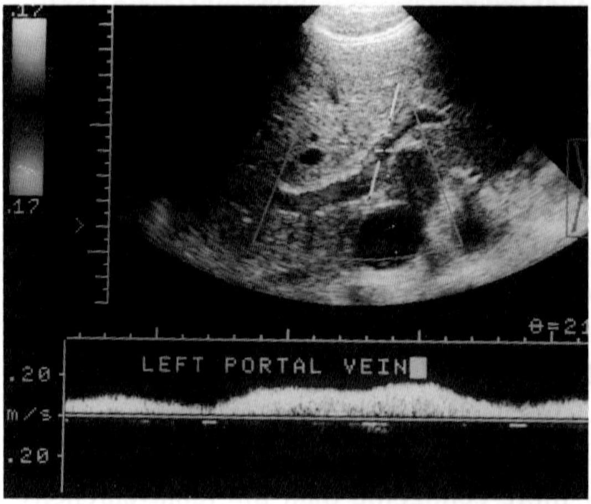

(b)

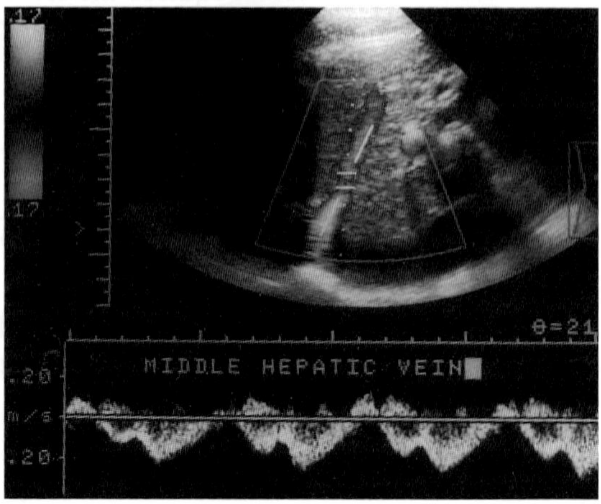

(c)

tion. Portal flow remains antegrade throughout the normal cardiac and respiratory cycle (Figure 2 b).

Hepatic vein traces have a characteristic biphasic or triphasic waveform showing hepatofugal flow during most of the cardiac cycle but transient hepatopetal flow during atrial systole corresponding with the venous "a" wave. There is also a transient slowing of flow at the end of ventricular systole which corresponds to left atrial filling in the face of a closed tricuspid valve. If this "v" wave is large enough it may also cause flow reversal resulting in a triphasic waveform. The hepatic veins also show a respiratory variation as changes in intrathoracic pressure affect venous return (Figure 2 c).

Doppler traces from hepatic vessels are best obtained either during quiet respiration or with the patient in suspended respiration at the end of a non-forced expiration.

DIFFUSE LIVER DISEASE WITH INCREASED PARENCHYMAL ECHOGENICITY

Fatty infiltration

The commonest cause of an echogenic liver is diffuse fatty infiltration. The common causes of fatty infiltration are listed in Table I. Intracellular fat globules result in an increased number of highly reflective small interfaces throughout the liver parenchyma causing a diffusely echogenic parenchyma as well as reduced

Table I ***Common causes of fatty infiltration of the liver***

NUTRITIONAL
- Obesity
- Intestinal bypass
- Parenteral nutrition

METABOLIC
- Diabetes mellitus
- Glycogen storage disease
- Hyperlipidaemias

DRUG RELATED
- Alcohol
- Corticosteroids
- Cytotoxic agents

IDIOPATHIC

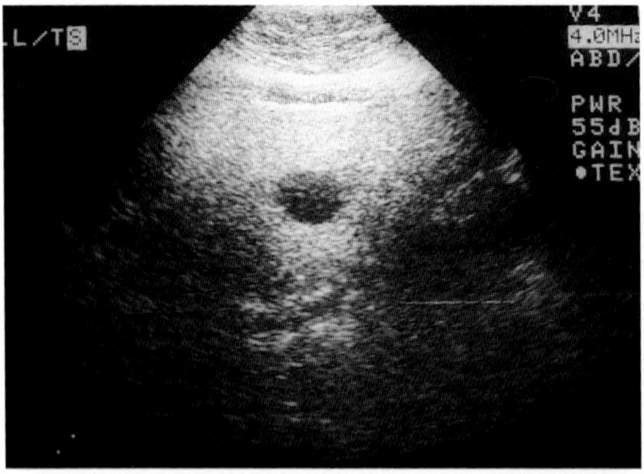

Figure 3
Diffuse fatty infiltration with an echopoor metsatasis from breast carcinoma.

through transmission (Figure 3). Increased TGC is required to image the deeper parts of the liver. Portal veins no longer stand out because the echogenicity of the liver parenchyma is similar to that of the periportal connective tissue. The liver is usually enlarged with a rounded inferior margin.

Doppler ultrasound of hepatic veins may show reduced pulsatility with loss of the normal transient flow reversal. This indicates reduced liver compliance.

Fatty infiltration does not always involve the liver uniformly. Focal fatty infiltration usually affects large areas of the liver with a geographical or wedge-shaped outline and a subcapsular distribution. Normal vessels can be seen coursing through these areas indicating preservation of hepatic architecture. Focal sparing in diffuse fatty infiltration frequently involves the gallbladder bed or the region around the falciform ligament (Figure 4) (2). As in fo-

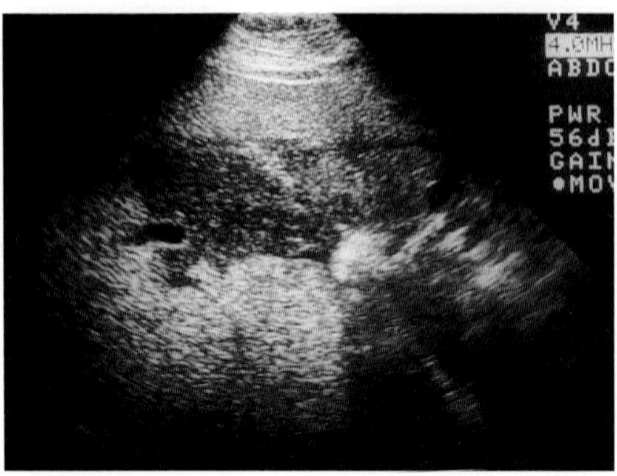

Figure 4
Fatty infiltration with focal sparing in the gallbladder bed.

cal fatty change there is no mass effect, and the lesions tend to be wedge shaped rather than round. If the ultrasound features are not typical, biopsy may be required to distinguish focal sparing from a pathological lesion.

Another potential problem in the presence of diffuse fatty infiltration is the misdiagnosis of a hypoechoic solid lesion as a simple cyst. Because the overall gain is turned down to compensate for a bright liver, low level echoes within a solid lesion may be missed. With the TGC turned up to compensate for reduced through transmission, the hypoechoic solid lesion may have posterior enhancement (Figure 3). However, the solid lesion will lack the specular reflection seen in the posterior wall of a cyst as it does not have a fluid tissue interface. Fine-needle aspiration may be necessary if the ultrasound findings are equivocal.

Fibrosis and cirrhosis

Hepatic fibrosis and cirrhosis are non-specific responses to hepatocyte injury. Their causes are listed in Table II. Collagen deposition following hepatocyte destruction is common to both conditions, but in simple fibrosis the normal architecture of the liver is preserved. In cirrhosis, fibrous bridging from central veins to por-

Table II ***Causes of fibrosis and cirrhosis***

VIRAL HEPATITIS (B and C)
ALCOHOL
METABOLIC
Haemochromatosis
Wilson's disease
Alpha-1-antitrypsin deficiency
CHOLESTASIS
Primary biliary cirrhosis
Secondary biliary cirrhosis
IMPAIRED VENOUS OUTFLOW
Budd-Chiari syndrome
Chronic cardiac failure
DRUGS
Methotrexate
Amidarone
CRYPTOGENIC

tal tracts and the presence of regenerating nodules causes distortion of the normal lobular architecture. This distortion affects drainage of blood from the portal to hepatic veins – an important factor in the pathogenesis of portal hypertension. While the progression of simple hepatic fibrosis may be arrested or even reversed by removal of the causative agent, once cirrhosis is established it is irreversible and progressive deterioration occurs.

Fibrosis is frequently accompanied by fatty infiltration. This results in an echogenic liver with reduced through transmission. In the absence of fatty change the fibrotic liver is close to normal echogenicity (3), but its texture may be slightly coarse. The liver size is normal or reduced. The liver surface is relatively smooth but fine nodularity may be visible on scanning with a 7.5 MHz probe.

Schistosomiasis causes hepatic fibrosis which is confined to portal tracts. It results in broad echogenic bands surrounding the portal tracts. Although it does not lead to cirrhosis, it is an important cause of portal hypertension. The causative organisms are S. Japonicum, prevalent in Japan, China, Indonesia and the Philippines, and S. Mansonii in Africa, South America, the Carribean and the Middle East. Cercaria enter the skin on contact with infected water and spread through the bloodstream. Adult worms produce ova which obstruct intrahepatic portal radicles and incite a granulomatous and fibrous reaction.

In advanced cirrhosis a combination of ultrasound findings strongly suggests the diagnosis.

Changes in the liver are:

1. Reduced liver size with caudate enlargement: a caudate to right lobe transverse diameter ratio of 0.65 is said to be highly specific and moderately sensitive in the diagnosis of cirrhosis (4). Caudate to left lobe antero-posterior diameter ratio of 0.5 is more easily measured (Figure 5).
2. A coarse liver texture with a mild increase in echogenicity.
3. A nodular liver surface (Figure 6).

Changes outside the liver mainly result from portal hypertension and include:

1. Splenomegaly (spleen larger than 13 cm).

Figure 5
Caudate lobe enlargement in cirrhosis.

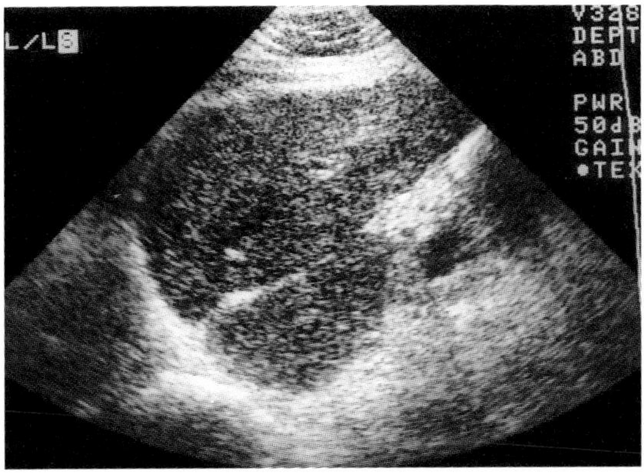

2. Portal vein enlargement > 13 mm.
3. Splenic vein enlargement > 10 mm. There is also loss of respiratory variation in the diameter of the portal and splenic vein.
4. Portosystemic shunts – short gastric, coronary vein, lienorenal and paraumbilical. These are more easily detected with the aid of colour Doppler.
5. Ascites – this results from a combination of portal hypertension and hypoalbuminemia. Ascites makes surface nodularity of the liver more easily visible.

Flow changes in the portal and hepatic veins may be demonstrated with Doppler. The main portal vein velocity is reduced or even reversed. It may be thrombosed or demonstrate cavernous transformation. When a patent paraumbilical vein is present, portal

Figure 6
Cirrhosis: a small nodular liver with ascites.

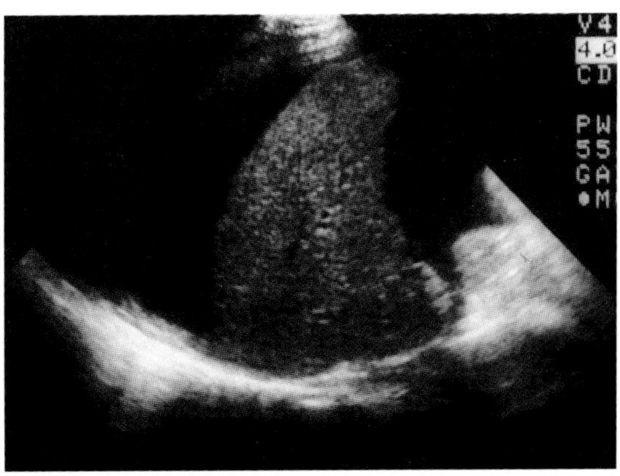

flow remains antegrade. Hepatic vein traces show a loss of normal flow reversal, reflecting the loss of compliance in liver tissue.

Early in the course of cirrhosis ultrasound changes may be subtle and many of these features may be absent. The liver size may be normal and the liver texture may appear slightly coarse or even normal.

Surface nodularity of the liver may be subtle, especially in alcoholic cirrhosis which is typically micronodular in its early stages. Dedicated scanning of the liver surface using a 7.5 MHz probe for generalized nodularity may be helpful with sensitivity and specificity above 80 % in patients presenting for investigation of abnormal liver function tests (5). This high sensitivity is associated with an increase in false positive results: Budd-Chiari syndrome, hepatic fibrosis and diffuse metastatic disease can also cause surface nodularity of the liver visible with a 7.5 MHz probe.

Alteration in the Doppler waveform of hepatic veins, with loss of normal flow reversal may be the earliest ultrasound abnormality in cirrhosis. Approximately 75 % of patients with well compensated cirrhosis (Childs Pugh class A, no clinical stigmata of liver disease and mild elevation of LFT's) show abnormal hepatic vein waveforms with loss of normal flow reversal (6). However, this finding is non-specific and is also seen in fatty infiltration and fibrosis in the absence of cirrhosis.

Because cirrhosis carries such important prognostic significance, and ultrasound findings are often non-specific, confirmation by liver biopsy is needed. Histologic evidence of the cause of the cirrhosis may also be present.

Despite the presence of regenerating nodules throughout the cirrhotic liver surprisingly few focal nodules are visible. Regenerating nodules are usually isoechoic and vary in size from a few millimetres to a centimetre or more, and are partly responsible for the coarse liver texture.

Cirrhosis is a major risk factor for the development of hepatoma. Ultrasound can be used to screen patients for hepatoma and is able to demonstrate lesions before they become clinically apparent and before they are large enough to be detected by serum alpha fetoprotein assay. Screening for hepatoma is made more difficult in cirrhotics by the coarse liver texture.

The lesion in the cirrhotic liver which more commonly mimics hepatoma is the adenomatous hyperplastic nodule. This is typically echo poor, like most small hepatomas, but is less likely to have vascularity visible on Doppler ultrasound. Serial screening of these lesions is useful to demonstrate change in size. Biopsy may also be of some use but distinction from a well differentiated hepatoma can be difficult. It seems they are part of a spectrum ranging from adenomatous hyperplasia to atypical adenomatous nodule to hepatoma. Because of their malignant potential, some authors have advocated prophylactic treatment of adenomatous hyperplastic nodules by percutaneous alcohol injection (7).

Granulomatous diseases

Granulomatous diseases of the liver include tuberculosis and sarcoidosis and also primary biliary cirrhosis.

Tuberculosis

Extrapulmonary tuberculosis and non tuberculous mycobacterial infection has increased with the spread of AIDS. In addition to intraabdominal lymphadenopathy, ultrasound may show evidence of liver involvement. Miliary lesions have been reported as causing multiple echogenic foci or even a diffusely echogenic liver (8). Larger confluent granulomata present as echo poor or echogenic lesions one to two centimetres in diameter (9). Healed granulomata may calcify (Figure 7). In AIDS patients the picture is frequently complicated by fatty infiltration.

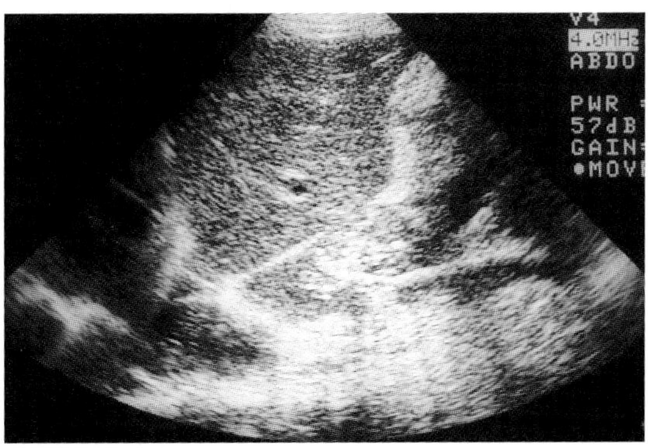

Figure 7 *Healed tuberculosis: calcified granulomata in the caudate lobe.*

Sarcoidosis

Hepatic involvement is common in sarcoidosis. Common ultrasound findings include hepatomegaly sometimes with an increase in echogenicity which may be diffuse or inhomogenous causing a coarse liver texture. The coarse texture is associated with nodularity of the liver surface (10).

Primary biliary cirrhosis

Primary biliary cirrhosis is an uncommon disorder typically presenting with pruritis and jaundice in middle aged women. Its pathology is of progressive granulomatous cholangitis of small intrahepatic bile ducts. At presentation the liver typically appears normal on ultrasound. The spleen is usually enlarged and other signs of portal hypertension develop as the disease progresses. A coarse liver texture and nodular surface are late changes reflecting progression to fibrosis and cirrhosis.

DISEASES CAUSING A DIFFUSE REDUCTION IN PARENCHYMAL ECHOGENICITY

Hepatitis most often produces an enlarged liver with normal echogenicity. A generalized reduction in echogenicity is occasionally seen reflecting increased tissue fluid and inflammatory cell infiltration (3). This results in a dark liver with relatively bright portal tracts. Marked thickening of the gallbladder wall is frequently present.

Serial measurement of liver size is useful in fulminant hepatitis as a rapidly shrinking liver carries a poor prognosis. Otherwise ultrasound has little role in hepatitis but can be useful to exclude other causes of jaundice.

Leukaemia and lymphoma may also produce the dark liver pattern with hepatomegaly, as may liver congestion associated with right heart failure. Occasionally, a dark liver is seen in a normal patient, in which case liver size and liver function tests are normal.

OTHER DIFFUSE LIVER DISEASES

Budd-Chiari syndrome

Budd-Chiari syndrome is a complex of hepatomegaly, abdominal pain and ascites resulting from occlusion of the hepatic veins. Causes include venous webs in IVC or hepatic veins and hypercoagulable states such as polycythemia rubra vera and venous invasion by tumours especially hepatoma but frequently the condition is idiopathic.

On grey scale ultrasound there is usually evidence of caudate and/or left lobe hypertrophy and sometimes a heterogenous echo texture. Ascites may be present. The hepatic veins appear abnormal and may be absent, thrombosed or small and irregular in calibre. Caudate lobe veins may be enlarged as they drain separately from the other hepatic veins directly into the IVC and are frequently spared from obstruction.

Colour Doppler and spectral Doppler may demonstrate abnormalities specific to Budd-Chiari syndrome including hepatic vein to hepatic vein collaterals (Figure 8) (10). The ultrasound changes of portal hypertension are often present. There is loss of the normal triphasic hepatic vein waveform – this may reflect loss of liver compliance or obstruction between the hepatic vein and right atrium.

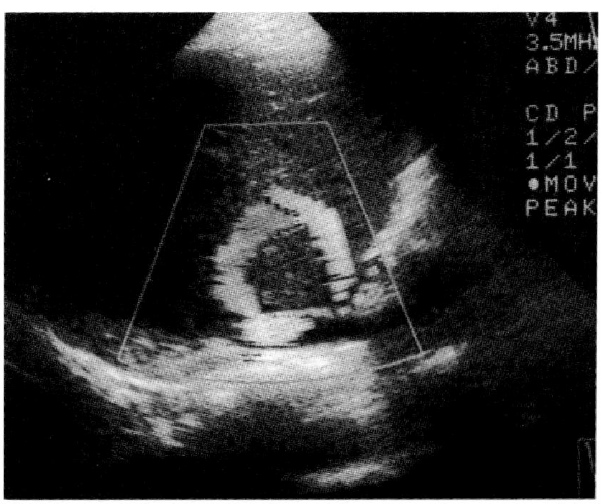

Figure 8 *Hepatic vein to hepatic vein collateral flow in Budd-Chiari syndrome.*

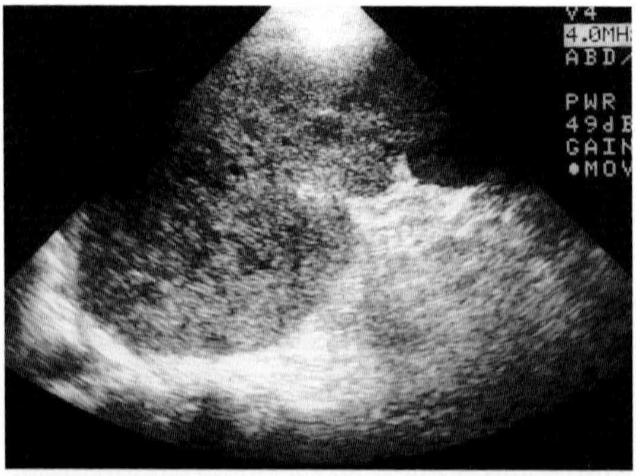

Figure 9 *Diffuse metastatic disease from primary breast carcinoma.*

Metastases

While metastatic disease is usually seen on ultrasound as one or more focal lesions, the presence of a large number of small focal lesions may produce the appearance of diffuse disease with a coarse liver texture (Figure 9). The presence of hepatomegaly and the absence of other signs of chronic liver disease helps distinguish these cases from cirrhosis. Multifocal hepatoma may also produce this appearance.

FOCAL LIVER LESIONS

Liver cysts

The simple cyst is the commonest cystic liver lesion encountered except in regions where hydatid disease is endemic. They usually arise from developmental abnormalities of the bile ducts but do not communicate with the biliary tree. They range from 1 mm in size to 10 cm or even larger, and are frequently multiple. Their characteristics are the same as those of simple cysts elsewhere – sharply defined walls with no definable thickness, anechoic contents and posterior acoustic enhancement. Occasional thin septa may be present. Hepatic cysts are not necessarily spherical.

A cystic metastasis or a hydatid cyst may mimic a simple cyst. Any deviation from the typical ultrasound findings should increase suspicion. Cysts increase in number with age and are rarely found below the age of 20. The presence of cysts in children should arouse suspicion of hydatid disease, polycystic disorders or cystic metastasis. Caroli's disease causing congenital intrahepatic duct dilatation may mimic intrahepatic cysts. Simple liver cysts occasionally casue pain or bile duct compression. Therapeutic aspiration under ultrasound guidance is a simple procedure but cysts generally recur unless a sclerosant is introduced. Communication with the biliary tree should be excluded by iodinated contrast injection prior to sclerosis of a cyst by alcohol injection.

Multiple liver cysts may be a manifestation of polycystic liver disease or von Hippel-Lindau syndrome. Approximately 30 % of patients with adult polycystic kidney disease have hepatic cysts and some 50 % of patients with polycystic liver disease have renal cystic disease. Pancreatic cysts may also be present.

Haemangioma

Haemangioma is the commonest benign liver tumour, being present in about 5 % of livers at autopsy. It is rarely symptomatic but is frequently seen as an incidental finding on abdominal ultrasound.

The typical ultrasound features are of a solitary, uniformally hyperechoic lesion which is round or ovoid and usually lies in a subcapsular location in the right lobe. The lesion usually measures up to 4 cm in diameter but larger and multiple lesions also occur. The margins are moderately well defined, but no capsule is present and no halo is seen around the lesion (Figure 10).

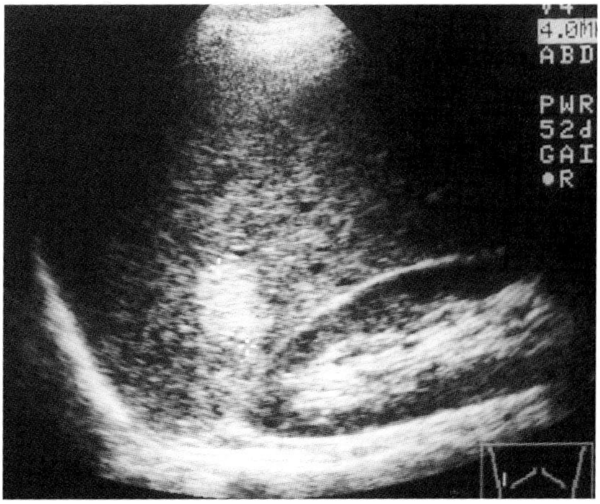

Figure 10 *Haemangioma.*

The echogenicity results from multiple reflections from the walls of the tiny vascular spaces throughout the lesion. However, because the vascular spaces contain blood, there is good through transmission and larger lesions show posterior enhancement. There is no evidence of flow on colour Doppler as blood flow within the lesions is too slow to detect.

When the appearance of the lesion is typical and there is not a high suspicion of other liver pathology, follow-up ultrasound in 3 to 6 months is sufficient to confirm the diagnosis. If there is a high clinical suspicion of metastatic disease then confirmation of the diagnosis is best performed by further imaging, either dynamic CT, MRI or labelled red cell scanning.

Around 20 % of haemangiomas have an atypical ultrasound appearance. While occasionally they are completely echo free, most of these have a partial or a complete echogenic rim and an echo poor centre (11). These changes result from thrombosis, fibrosis or myxomatous degeneration within the haemangioma.

Fatty change

Focal fatty infiltration and focal sparing in diffuse fatty infiltration have been discussed under the heading of fatty infiltration in diffuse liver disease. These conditions must be kept in mind when considering the differential diagnosis of focal liver lesions. Occasionally, focal sparing results in a round lesion which can only be distinguished from sinister liver pathology by biopsy.

Metastases

There are two distinct aims in imaging of the liver for suspected metastatic tumour. The aim in patients with an extraintestinal primary tumour such as breast carcinoma, is to demonstrate the presence or absence of liver metastases. The presence of metastases in such cases is generally an indicator of disseminated disease not amenable to local therapy.

In patients with colonic carcinoma, metastatic seeding to the liver via the portal system means that the liver may be the only site of spread. The aim in these patients is to accurately demonstrate the size, number and location of metastases. This is necessary to determine whether curative local therapy is possible and to determine the extent of resection and/or percutaneous therapy required.

The ultrasound appearance of metastases is variable but they are generally round lesions with well defined margins with mass effects, causing displacement or compression of adjacent vessels or bulging of the overlying capsule. Usually they are solid lesions and may be echo poor or echogenic. An echo poor halo is a common feature of metastases and should be carefully sought as it may be helpful in distinguishing echogenic metastases from haemangiomas (Figure 11). The halo itself is usually a result of a highly cellular tumour margin with few stromal elements (12), but may occasionally represent compression of surrounding liver tissue.

Purely cystic liver metastases are rare but should be considered with mucous secreting primary tumours or with necrotic metastases. A careful search for echogenic debris or nodular wall thickening may be rewarding but aspiration cytology may also be required.

Hepatoma

Hepatoma (or hepatocellular carcinoma) accounts for over 80 % of primary malignant liver tumours. In western countries it usually

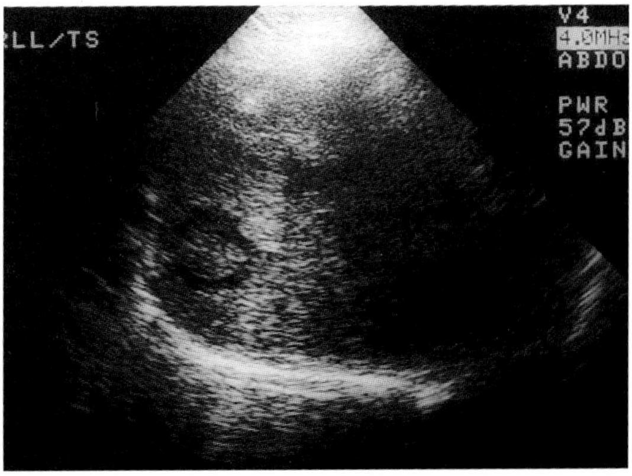

Figure 11 *Metastasis: colonic carcinoma.*

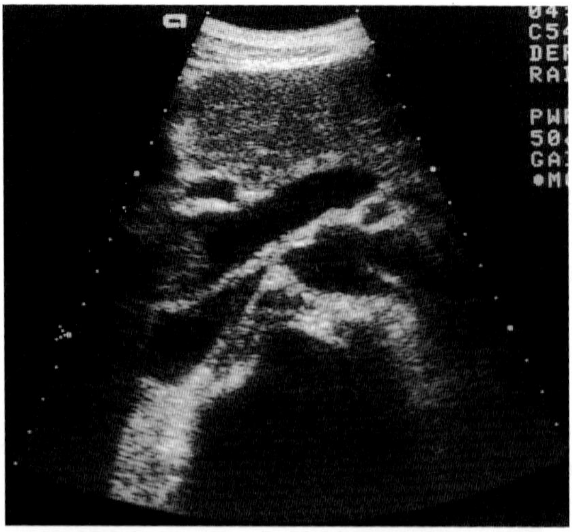

Figure 14 *Hepatoma invading the portal vein.*

The fibrolamellar variant has a central echogenic scar with radiating bands of fibrosis. It is otherwise homogeneous with no necrosis or haemorrhage.

Around 10 % of hepatomas have a complete fibrous capsule which show on ultrasound as an echogenic rim 3–15 mm in thickness. This is reported with a higher frequency in Japanese series but is also seen in non Asian patients.

Because of developments in treatment of hepatoma, including segmental resection chemoembolization and percutaneous ethanol injection, accurate demonstration of the site, size and number of hepatoma lesions in each patient is important. Invasive methods which have been shown to be highly sensitive include CT arterial portography and operative ultrasound, but more sensitive non-invasive screening is required. The advent of intravenous ultrasound contrast media should provide more sensitive imaging of smaller lesions and those which are poorly visualized because of their depth within the liver or the heterogenicity of surrounding cirrhotic or fatty liver.

Focal nodular hyperplasia (FNH)

FNH is an uncommon benign tumour-like condition usually seen in young adult women. Clinically it presents as an incidental finding on imaging or with swelling or vague upper abdominal pain and is rarely complicated by haemorrhage or rupture.

Up to 20 % of cases show multiple lesions. The lesion is typically subcapsular, measures 1 to 20 cm in diameter and is usually homogeneous and slightly echogenic or echo poor. This is not surprising as it contains all the cellular elements of normal liver but lacks the normal lobular architecture. A central scar may be present but is only occasionally seen on ultrasound as a stellate echogenic focus. The diagnosis may be confirmed by radionuclide scanning since 70 % of the lesions contain sufficient Kupffer cell activity to make them hyperintense or at least isointense. The remaining lesions require confirmation by further imaging techniques and/or biopsy.

Adenoma

Hepatic adenoma is less common than FNH. It is strongly associated with oral contraceptive pill use. Rare cases in male patients have been linked with anabolic steroid use. A 40 % incidence of hepatic adenoma is seen in type I glycogen storage disease.

Hepatic adenoma is usually a solitary well circumscribed lesion, measuring up to 15 cm in size. Like FNH it is usually slightly echogenic or echo poor but may become heterogeneous as a result of haemorrhage or necrosis.

Because of the risks of catastrophic haemorrhage and malignant transformation hepatic adenoma is treated by surgical resection.

Abscess

Liver abscesses can result from ascending cholangitis, portal pyemia or septic portal emboli, direct innoculation through trauma or biopsy, or by haematogenous seeding during generalized bacteraemia.

As well as demonstrating the liver abscess, ultrasound may show evidence of the cause such as bile duct obstruction by stone or tumour, or thrombus in the portal vein.

Usually an abscess is visible as a round, fluid filled structure, sometimes with a thickened wall (Figure 15). Its contents are va-

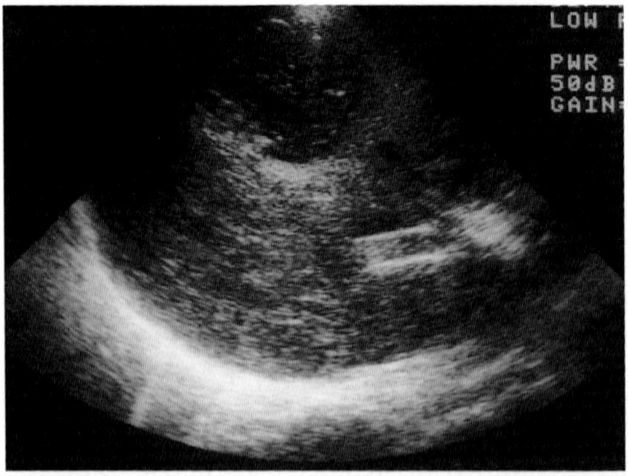

Figure 15 *Liver abscess in a patient with cholangiocarcinoma.*

riably echogenic and may even be more echogenic than surrounding liver, but posterior acoustic enhancement is usually present indicating its fluid nature.

The size and number of lesions varies with the cause of the abscess. An idiopathic abscess in an elderly patient is typically large and solitary. It has usually been present for some weeks before the diagnosis is made and therefore is well developed with a well defined wall (which may be visibly thickened) and echo poor contents. Cholangitic abscesses and those associated with portal pyemia are usually multiple.

Candida abscesses seen in immunosuppressed patients are typically small (< 1 cm) and numerous. They may be difficult to see with a standard transducer but can be visualised with high frequence probes. In the neutropaenic patient they may only become visible as the neutrophil count rises enabling a host response to the organism. These microabscesses have a typical target appearance with an echogenic focus and a surrounding echo poor halo. If there is central necrosis, an echo poor centre may be present within the echogenic focus. Sometimes the lesion is completely hypoechoic.

Hydatid disease

The tapeworm Echinococcus granulosus has the dog as its definitive host. Ova shed in faeces are ingested by the intermediate hosts – sheep, cattle, or man. The organism then burrows into the intestinal wall where it is carried by the portal vein to the liver (or beyond) where it develops into an adult cyst. The disease is common in sheep raising areas of Australia, New Zealand, Africa, South America, Southern Europe and the Middle East. Cysts within the liver grow at around 1 cm per year and can reach a diameter of 20 cm or more. Symptoms result most commonly from mass effects causing distension or a dull ache in the right upper quadrant.

The classical ultrasound appearance is of one or more cysts with slightly thickened echogenic walls containing a combination of dependent debris (hydatid sand) daughter cysts and membranes. However, initially the hydatid develops as a unilocular lesion and may mimic a simple cyst. This is particularly important in endemic areas where any liver cyst has to be considered a hydatid until proven otherwise by serological testing and clinical and ultrasound follow-up.

As the cyst grows it becomes more complex in the following ways:

1. The wall becomes thicker and more echogenic as the host fibrous reaction increases. Eventually it calcifies. Complete dense calcification usually signifies a dying or dead cyst.
2. Daughter cysts bud from the germinal membrane – initially they appear as slight focal wall thickenings, but eventually grow to fill most of the parent cyst.
3. Debris is shed into the parent cyst and daughter cysts – this is comprised of scolices which are released by daughter cysts rupturing into the parent cyst.

Together with infolding and fragmentation of the germinal membrane, this results in a parent cyst full of echogenic material surrounding multiple fluid filled daughter cysts, giving rise to the spoke wheel appearance of a mature hydatid (Figure 16) (15).

The main complications of hydatid disease are rupture, secondary infection, and anaphylaxis. Rupture into the biliary tree is the most common and leads to recurrent obstructive jaundice and cholangitis. Intraperitoneal rupture causes disseminated intraabdominal cyst formation while rupture into a hepatic vein leads to pulmonary hydatid disease. Direct extension into the pleura, pericar-

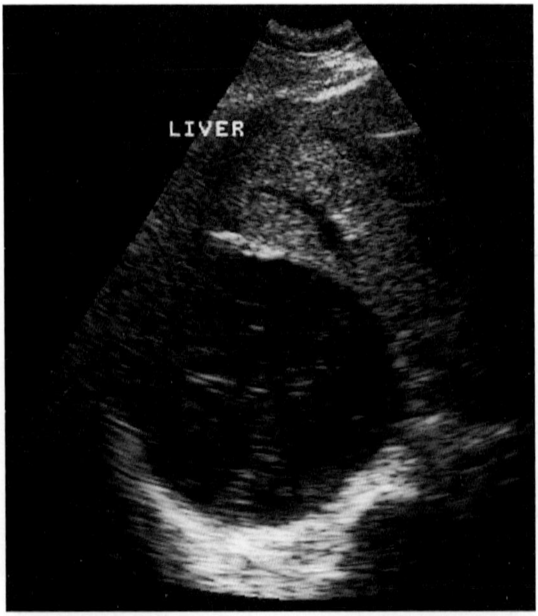

Figure 16 *Mature hydatid.*

dium and colon is less common. Fluid visible between the germinal membrane and laminated membrane, or collapse of the germinal membrane into the cyst, suggests that rupture is imminent.

With secondary infection the hydatid becomes diffusely echogenic.

Anaphylaxis occurs when there is leakage of proteinaceous fluid from the cyst into surrounding tissues. It is because of the risks of anaphylaxis and cyst rupture that percutaneous aspiration has generally been avoided. However, reports of safe and successful percutaneous diagnostic and therapeutic aspiration are increasing. Ultrasound is also useful in monitoring response to drug therapy.

Amoebic abscess

Entamoeba histolitica is endemic in Africa, South East Asia, Mexico and South America. When the cysts are ingested they pass through into the colon and change to active trophozoites. These invade the bowel wall and are carried by the portal venous system into the liver where they can produce one or more "abscesses" by a combination of infarction and proteolysis.

Amoebic abscesses are typically found anteriorly in the right lobe of the liver (possibly because the right lobe receives most of the colonic portal drainage). They have the characteristic appearance of a well defined cyst, with no visible wall, 5 to 15 cm in size containing homogeneous low level echoes, which represent the debris of lysed liver cells. Posterior enhancement is usually seen.

Around 14 % are multiple. One percent present as diffuse microabscesses (16). Extrahepatic involvement is uncommon but they may be seen in the spleen or lung. Direct extension from liver to lung occurs through the right hemidiaphragm.

Diagnosis is made by a combination of history, including travel to an endemic area, ultrasound findings and serology.

Haematoma

Liver haematoma may be seen following blunt abdominal trauma or less commonly as a result of percutaneous transhepatic cholangiography (PTC) or other invasive procedures. Early on the haematoma appears as an echogenic region within the liver. As it becomes liquified over subsequent days it forms an anechoic collection with posterior enhancement and irregular walls (Figure 17). It will usually progress to complete resolution over weeks to months but may leave a residual scar or a fluid collection with the appearance of a simple cyst.

Although ultrasound can be used to make the diagnosis of liver haematoma it is better suited to follow-up. Where available, CT is

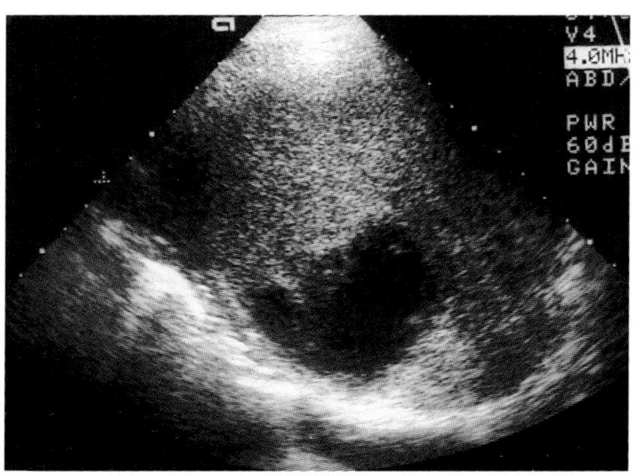

Figure 17 *Resolving haematoma.*

a more effective modality in assessing blunt abdominal trauma as it simultaneously demonstrates pathology of solid and hollow viscera, as well as musculoskeletal injury.

LIVER TRANSPLANTATION

Prior to liver transplantation it is essential to document the status of the portal venous system. Thrombosis of the portal or superior mesenteric veins makes transplantation impossible. Portal hypertension makes surgery more difficult and dangerous. Patency of the veins is well demonstrated with Doppler ultrasound, though occasionally the conglomeration of small veins present in cavernous transformation may mimic a normal portal vein. If detailed anatomy of arterial variation is required, this information is more accurately supplied by selective visceral angiography, or more elegantly by spiral CT.

In the early postoperative period Doppler ultrasound is used to document patency of the portal vein and hepatic artery anastomoses. Oedema of the transplant liver resulting in reduced compliance is a common finding and causes loss of hepatic vein flow reversal and sometimes loss of diastolic flow in the hepatic artery. These findings are non specific and do not necessarily indicate rejection.

Perihepatic fluid collections can also be documented – haematomas and serous collections are common, but if there is clinical evidence of infection, then diagnostic and therapeutic aspiration can be performed under ultrasound guidance. Bile duct strictures are common following liver transplants. These typically occur at the common duct anastomosis site or at the porta hepatis and may result in intrahepatic duct dilatation.

REFERENCES

1. Lafortune M, Madone F, Patriquis H, Breton G. Segmental anatomy of the liver: a sonographic approach to the Couinaud nomenclature. Radiology 1991;181:443–448.
2. McKenzie A, Gill G, McIntosh R et al. Computed tomographic and ultrasound appearance of focal spared areas in fatty infiltration of the liver. Australasian Radiology 1991;35:166–168.

3. Zwiebel WJ. Sonographic diagnosis of diffuse liver disease. Semin Ultrasound CT MR. 1995;16:8–15.
4. Giorgio A, Amoroso P, Lettieri G. Cirrhosis: value of caudate to right lobe ratio in diagnosis with ultrasound. Radiology 1986;161:443–445.
5. Di Lelio A, Cestari C, Lomazzi A, Beretta L. Cirrhosis: diagnosis with sonographic study of the liver surface. Radiology 1989;172:389–392.
6. Colli A, Coccicli M, Riva C et al. Abnormalities of Doppler waveform of the hepatic veins in patients with chronic liver disease: correlation with histologic findings. AJR 1994;162:833–837.
7. Livaghi T, Sangalli G, Vettori C. Adenomatous hyperplastic nodules in the cirrhotic liver, a therapeutic approach: work in progress. Radiology 1989;171:57.
8. Wetton C, McCarty M, Tomlinson D et al. Ultrasound findings in hepatic mycobacterial infection in patients with acquired immune deficiency syndrome (AIDS). Clin Radiol 1993;47:36–38.
9. Levine C. Primary macronodular hepatic tuberculosis: US and CT appearances. Gastrointest Radiol 1990;15:307–309.
10. Ralls PW, Johnson MB, Radin DR et al. Budd-Chiari syndrome: detection with color Doppler sonography. AJR 1992;159:113–116.
11. Moody A, Wilson S. Atypical haemangioma: a suggestive sonographic morphology. Radiology 1993;188:413–417.
12. Werreke K, Henke L, Varrallo P et al. Pathologic explanation for hypoechoic halo seen on sonograms of malignant liver tumours: an in vitro correlative study. AJR 1992;159:1011–1016.
13. Sachiko T, Tsugio K, Makoto F et al. Small hepatoma: differentiation from adenomatous hyperplastic nodule with colour Doppler flow imaging. Radiology 1992;182:161–165.
14. Taylor K, Ramos I, Carter D et al. Correlation of Doppler ultrasound tumour signals with neovascular morphologic features. Radiology 1988;166:57–62.
15. El-Tahin M, Omojela M, Malatani T et al. Hydatid disease of the liver: evaluation of ultrasound and computed tomography. Br J Radiol 1992;65:390–392.
16. Juimo AF, Gervez F, Angwafo F. Extraintestinal amoebiasis. Radiology 1992;182:181–185.

CHAPTER 4

The Gallbladder and Bile Ducts

Peter L. Cooperberg, MD, Glenn A. Scheske, MD and John R. Mathieson, MD

In only a relatively few short years ultrasound has evolved as the primary tool in the evaluation of the gallblader (1, 2) and bile ducts (3). In its infancy, ultrasound was mainly used for the detection of gallstones in patients with abdominal pain. However, with technological advances, and the resultant improvement in image quality, this role has expanded considerably to include the diagnosis of virtually all conditions affecting the gallbladder and biliary tree. This includes not only diagnosis, but therapy as well. Ultrasound is a valuable imaging tool in numerous interventional techniques including percutaneous cholecystostomy, biliary drainage procedures, cytological aspiration and the experimental procedure of gallblader ablation (4–14). Ultrasound has proven to be a valuable adjunct in the localization of calculi for lithotripsy (15–19) and in the intra-operative evaluation of patients with biliary obstruction. With these broader applications, the demands upon the sonographer and radiologist have also increased. Whereas in the recent past, the mere diagnosis of gallstones was considered adequate, we must now attempt to determine the size, number and in some cases, the ultrasonic characteristics of gallstones. One must also be familiar with the role of adjunctive studies such as oral cholecystography, nuclear medicine and CT.

CLINICAL CONSIDERATIONS

The overall importance and economic implicatons of gallbladder and biliary tract disease are self-evident. The fact that cholecystectomy is the second commonest abdominal operation, resulting in approximately 600,000 cholecystectomies per year in the USA alone, underlines the magnitude of the clinical problem (21). Evaluation of patients with upper abdominal pain is one of the commonest problems requiring investigation by clinicians.

Cholelithiasis is an extremely common condition in the general population and the ultrasonic diagnosis has been described in all age groups, including fetal life (22), in infancy (23), in childhood (24), and in adults up to, and including, the aged. It is commonest in females, in the obese, in patients with Crohn's disease (25), and in pregnancy (26).

The presence of gallstones in patients does not prove that this is the cause of symptoms, but this finding in the proper clinical context (patient with right upper quadrant pain, vague dyspepsia and fatty food intolerance) is usually adequate for surgical justification of cholecystectomy. Further substantiating this approach is the pathologic confirmation of changes of chronic cholecystitis in virtually all patients over the age of 40 with gallstones.

Gallbladder colic is the result of impaction of a calculus in the neck of the gallbladder. This is characterized by severe right upper quadrant pain, often after a meal containing fat. However, at the time of the ultrasound examination, the stone has usually become disimpacted, having either fallen back into the gallbladder or passed into the common bile duct.

Acute cholecystitis may ensue when the stone remains impacted. Although the full blown clinical picture of acute cholecystitis may be present (right upper quadrant pain and tenderness, positive Murphy's sign, elevated white blood count and fever) the signs and symptoms may also merge imperceptibly with those of gallbladder colic. For this reason, the term "acute gallbladder disease" is preferable to "acute cholecystitis" when considering sonographic findings. The sonographic demonstration of gallstones in a patient whose symptoms suggest acute gallbladder disease is usually considered sufficient indication for surgery. If further proof is considered necessary, a biliary isotope (IDA) scan demonstrating non-visualization of the gallbladder may be helpful in substantiating cystic duct obstruction.

ANATOMY

The location and structure of the gallbladder make it an ideal organ for sonographic evaluation. It is a tear-drop shaped structure which lies in the fossa formed by the junction of the right and left lobes of the liver. Although the location of the gallbladder fundus may be variable, the neck and body are almost invariably related to the region of the porta hepatis and the major interlobar fissure of the liver (Figure 1). The gallbladder may be folded upon itself suggesting the appearance of a septum (27). Occasionally, a fold or septum near the fundus is seen representing a Phrygian cap. There is great variability and overlap in the size of both the normal and pathological gallbladder. Large normal gallbladder and small obstructed gallbladder are not uncommon, underlining the fact that size itself is not a useful indication of pathology. Likewise, wall thickness is variable, and depends on the degree of distention and on the presence or absence of pathological changes in the tissue. Thick-walled gallbladder (greater than 3 mm) can be seen as a normal variant, but is also seen in several disease entities

Figure 1 *A diagramatic representation of the gallbladder and the biliary system. (RHD, right hepatic duct; LHD, left hepatic duct; CD, common duct; CHD, common hepatic duct; CBD, common bile duct; GB, gallbladder; DU, duodenum; PD, pancreatic duct; AV, Ampulla of Vater.)*

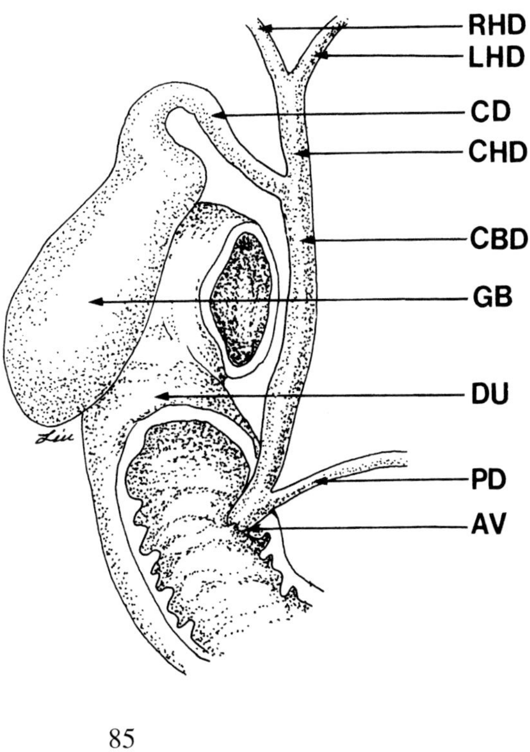

including cirrhosis, viral hepatitis, congestive heart failure, hypoalbuminemia and chronic renal failure (28).

The intrahepatic bile ducts are situated in the portal triads with the portal veins and hepatic arteries. They are normally too small to be visualized by ultrasound. The main right and left hepatic ducts accompany the main right and left portal veins into the porta hepatis. They join to form the extrahepatic common hepatic duct which passes anterior to the straight segment of the right portal vein which is just proximal to the bifurcation of the main portal vein (29). Inferiorly, the common hepatic duct continues anterior to the main portal vein in the gastrohepatic ligament, the anterior border of the foramen of Winslow (Figure 1). The cystic duct joins the common hepatic duct at a variable level to become the common bile duct. Since the cystic duct is not normally identified on ultrasound, the point at which the common hepatic duct becomes the common bile duct cannot be determined. For sonographic purposes, the more proximal portion of the extrahepatic bile duct is referred to as the common hepatic duct while the more distal portion is called the common bile duct (Figure 2). The common bile duct continues posterior to the first portion of the duodenum and directly anterior to the inferior vena cava before entering the posterolateral aspect of the head of the pancreas. It ends in the ampulla of Vater in the medial aspect of the second portion of the duodenum.

ULTRASOUND TECHNIQUE

Although conventional static ultrasound scanning was first used to visualize the gallbladder and biliary tract, this has been largely replaced with real-time techniques owing mainly to the greater versatility of this method, the involvement of the radiologist in the examination, and the technical advances in the equipment (30–34). Real-time techniques are easier to learn and are less operator dependent. The relative disadvantage of a more restricted field of view is lessened as the operator becomes more familiar with the anatomy. The relatively small field is also less critical in the examination of the gallbladder and bile ducts.

Since the cause of the patient's symptoms is usually unknown when referred for sonographic examination, we do not limit the

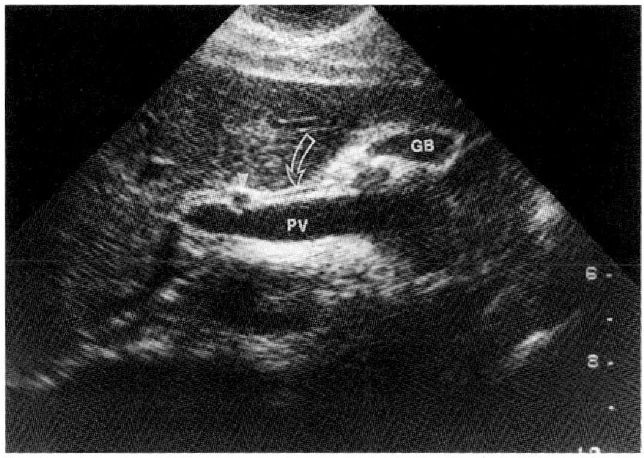

Figure 2 *Longitudinal image demonstrates a relatively empty common bile duct (arrow) located just anterior to the portal vein (PV). Note the relationship of the hepatic artery (arrow head) relative to the bile duct and the portal vein. GB, gallbladder.*

examination to a single organ. Indeed, the major advantage of ultrasound over oral cholecystography is that sonography provides an examination that is wider in scope (35). An attempt is made to visualize all upper abdominal structures in all referred patients. It has been shown that this approach results in the detection of a significant number of unsuspected abnormalities, some of which are clinically significant.

The real-time technique for gallbladder evaluation consists of examining the fasting patient in the supine or left-side down decubitus position with a 3.5 MHz transducer. Occasionally, this is supplemented with examination using a 5 MHz transducer for more superficial organs, or in cases where an attempt is being made to produce "acoustic shadows" from small calculi. Depending upon position of the gallbladder, examination is done subcostally in inspiration, or by using a lower intercostal space in expiration or shallow inspiration. After locating the gallbladder, the transducer is "swept" through the organ in its long axis. A slow sweep should be performed. If necessary, short axis views may also be obtained.

The dependent portion of the gallbladder must always be examined. Almost without exception, calculi will have a higher specific gravity than bile, and sink to the dependent portion (38). Since the definitive diagnosis of gallstones on ultrasound is dependent upon the demonstration of echogenic foci that move or roll and have distal acoustic shadows (with the exception of impacted stones), changing the patient's position is important. In addition to examining in the supine and left-side down decubitus positions, an erect or even prone view may be helpful (39).

It has been suggested that, if possible, gallbladder imaging should be performed early in the morning after overnight fasting. One study showed that, as the day progressed, about one half of subjects showed a significant decrease in bile volume, increased gallbladder wall thickness and excessive intestinal gas (40).

The common hepatic duct should then be followed more distally. This is accomplished by gently changing the obliquity and position of the transducer to maintain continuity of the duct as it passes anterior to the right portal vein. The mid-portion of the duct is frequently obscured by overlaying gas in the duodenum and colon. Occasionally, the duct can be again visualized in the head of the pancreas, especially in thin patients. It may also be hepful to follow the duct inferiorly in the transverse plane. By fixating on the small circle of the duct, the transducer is moved inferiorly, maintaining visualization of the small circle, and making it easier to differentiate the duct from the portal vein more inferiorly.

It is also important to evaluate the intrahepatic ducts. Dilatation of these structures generally occurs often in dilatation of the extrahepatic portions. Also, in cases of obstruction at the porta hepatis, intrahepatic ductal dilatation will be present in the absence of extra-hepatic dilatation.

PATHOLOGY OF THE GALLBLADDER

Cholelithiasis

Ultrasound is the investigation of choice when examining patients for gallstones. A study comparing ultrasound with oral cholecystectomy found that ultrasound was the imaging method of choice, even in patients who are morbidly obese (41).

The sonograhic appearance of an echogenic focus in the gallbladder, with an accompanying acoustic shadow, is highly specific for the diagnosis of cholelithiasis (Figure 3). This acoustic shadow is most frequently "clear", but may occasionally be "dirty" showing evidence of reverberation artifact. This has been reported in

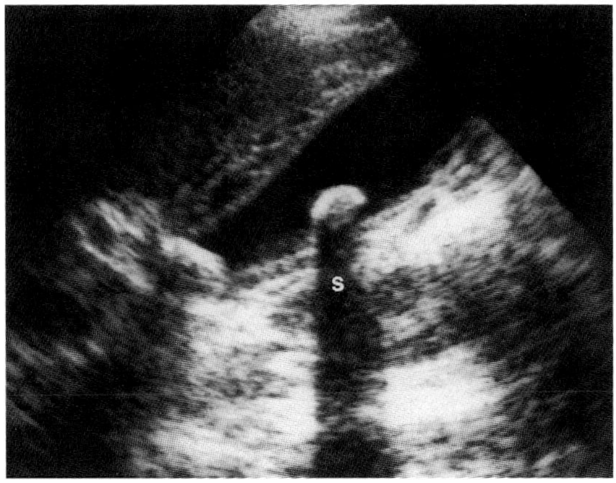

Figure 3 *Longitudinal image clearly demonstrates the presence of a gallstone as a bright curvilinear structure located within the gallbladder producing distal acoustic shadowing (S).*

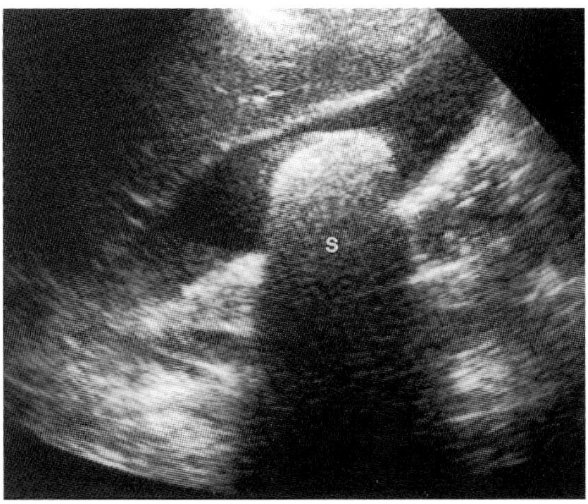

Figure 4 *Large gallstone producing "dirty" shadowing (S). The ultrasound beam has penetrated the stone because it is made up of cholesterol rather than denser calcium bilirubinate accounting for this effect. The ultrasound beam is not being totally reflected resulting in multiple echoes beyond the gallstone.*

cases where the gallstones contained calcifications or air (42, 43). In addition, pure cholesterol stones can produce "comet tail" shadowing which is also called "dirty shadowing" (Figure 4) (44, 45). False negative results are relatively rare with real-time technique and are generally the result of small calculi which are present in the gallbladder neck (Figure 5) or in a gallbladder situated deep beneath the costal cartilage. Gallstones must not be diagnosed by seeing an acoustic shadow alone, since acoustic shadows are commonly seen near the neck of the gallbladder in the absence of calculi. Other possible causes of a false negative examination include a fold in the gallbladder wall which can produce both an echo and a distal shadow. A similar possibility exists when a loop of bowel indents the gallbladder. It is much better to err on the side of a

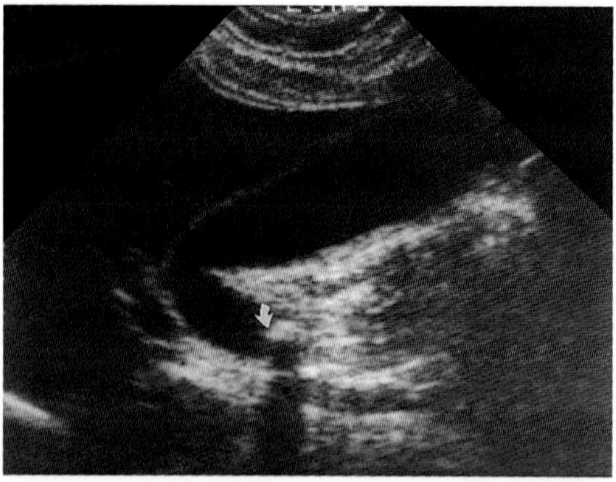

Figure 5 *Longitudinal image of the gallbladder demonstrates the presence of a small stone (arrow) in the neck. Note the distal acoustic shadowing.*

false negative diagnosis, as a false positive diagnosis usually results in surgery.

As previously mentioned, gallstones usually assume a dependent position in the gallbladder. The incidence of floating stones is rare, and although this phenomenon was formerly thought to occur only in the presence of contrast media within the gallbladder, we now know that, on occasion, stones will float in native bile (Figure 6). This is possibly due to fissuring of the stones with gas formation. The sonographic appearance of gas-containing gallstones has been described (42, 47). In patients where a thin layer of stones is suspected in the dependent position of the gallbladder but the sonographic findings are considered equivocal, the administration of

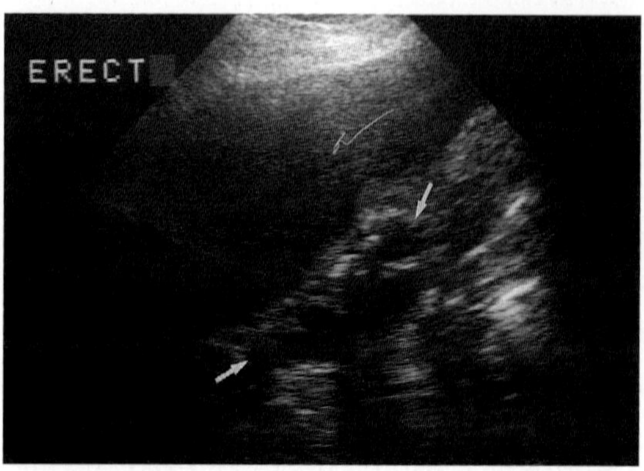

Figure 6 *Within this contracted gallbladder (arrows) can be seen several small weakly echogenic structures located predominantly anteriorly in the gallbladder, some of which are producing acoustic shadowing, consistent with a diagnosis of floating stones. This usually results when the density of the stone is lighter than the bile.*

an oral cholecystographic contrast agent has been successfully used in an attempt to produce floatation and layering of stones (48).

Although non-visualization of the gallbladder on ultrasound has been shown to be associated with an abnormal gallbladder in a very high percentage of patients, it has been demonstrated that exceptionally thick bile can produce a gallbladder which is as echogenic as the adjacent liver (sonographic "hepatization" of the gallbladder). Other causes of non-visualization of the gallbladder in a fasting patient include congenital anomalies such as ectopia (50, 51), congenital absence, conditions causing shadowing or reverberation from the near wall of the gallbladder such as porcelain gallbladder (Figure 7) (52), acute hepatic dysfunction from hepatitis of various etiologies (53), a collapsed gallbladder from

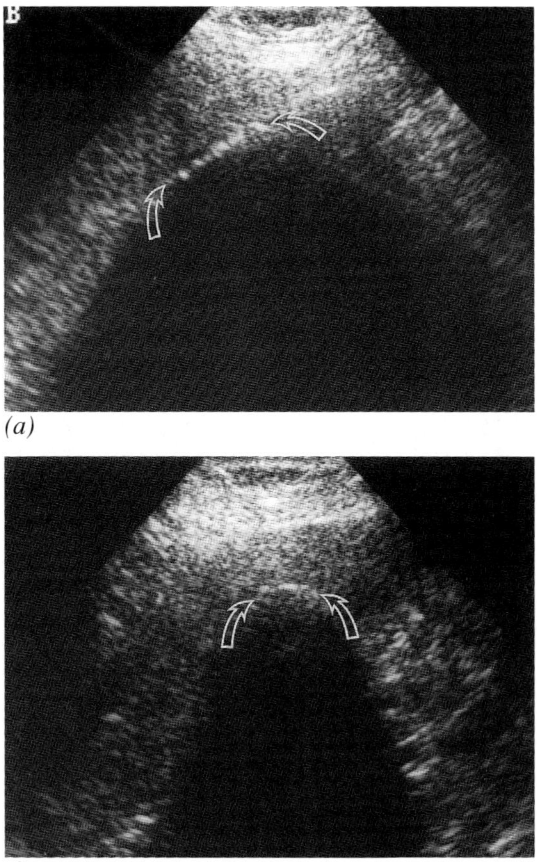

(a) (b)

Figure 7 *On the longitudinal (a) and transverse (b) images of the gallbladder bed bright reflections (arrows) represent calcifications in the anterior wall of the gallbladder (porcelain gallbladder). This may sometimes be difficult to separate from a contracted gallbladder with stones but note that the normal wall of the gallbladdder cannot be identified which would not be the case if this were a stone-filled contracted gallbladder.*

marked biliary obstruction proximal to the cystic duct, the presence of intramural or intraluminal gas as is seen in thickening of the gallbladder wall (54). All of these conditions are relatively rare and further investigation should include follow-up or repeat examinations, scintigraphy (IDA) and oral cholecystography. Cystic structures in the right upper quadrant such as an omental cyst (55) have been reported to mimic a gallbladder. Other rare cystic lesions in the right upper quadrant which must be differentiated from the gallbladder include hepatic artery aneurysm, enteric duplication cysts, abscess, and choledochal cyst (56). Occasionally, the gallbladder may be bicameral with a thick septum separating a fundus chamber from the rest of the gallbladder (57). Gallstones may only be present in the fundal chamber making diagnosis of cholelithiasis more difficult.

Cholecystitis

Although ultrasound is extremely accurate in the diagnosis of cholelithiasis, the diagnosis of cholecystitis on ultrasound can only be implied. The presence of tenderness in the region of the gallbladder from transducer pressure, in a patient with a calculus impacted in the Hartman's pouch, is highly suggestive of cholecystitis. This is the sonographic Murphy's sign, and has been reported to be present in up to 92.2% of patients with acute cholecystitis (58). However, in cases of gangrenous acute cholecystitis, the incidence of this sign has been reported to be much lower being found in only 33% of patients (59). In patients with abdominal pain and the sonographic findings of cholecystitis, the absence of a Murphy's sign increases the possibility of gangrenous cholecystitis.

Gallbladder wall thickening is also suggestive of, but not diagostic of, cholecystitis since this finding can be present in a variety of conditions including ascites, hypoproteinemia (60, 61), right heart failure and hepatitis (62–64). Other causes of a thickened gallbladder wall include adenomyomatosis (65–67), varices (68), and cirrhosis (67). Chronic cholecystitis can also be associated with a thickened gallbladder wall (Figure 8).

Hyperechoic foci in the gallbladder wall could indicate microabscess formation associated with cholecystitis, but can also be

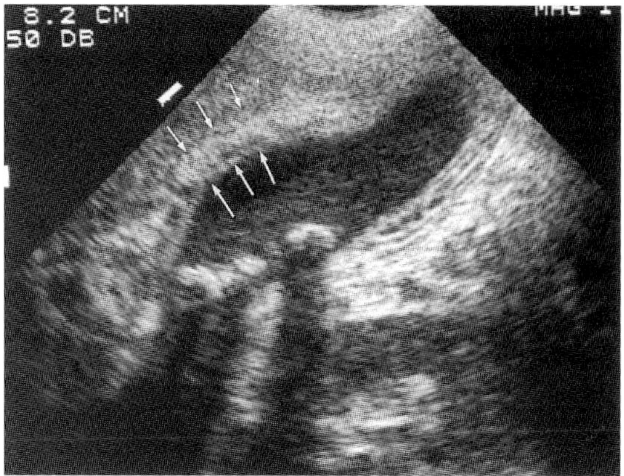

(a)

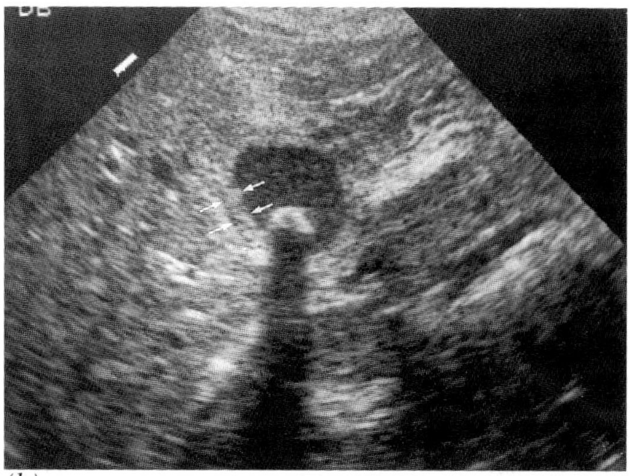

(b)

Figure 8 *Longitudinal (a) and transverse (b) views of the gallbladder show the presence of multiple small stones producing distal acoustic shadowing along with non-shadowing reflectors consistent with sludge. More importantly, note the thickened gallbladder walls (arrows). While there are many causes for such wall thickening, this proved to be chronic cholecystitis.*

the result of intramural diverticula containing inspissated bile, small stones or cholesterol crystals (69).

Other sonographic signs suggestive of acute cholecystitis include the demonstration of an intraluminal pseudomembrane within the gallbladder (70), as well as a "striated" appearance to the gallbladder wall caused by several alternating, irregular, discontinuous echo-free and echogenic bands (71). Asymmetry of the gallbladder wall and distention of the gallbladder can also be seen. While all of these sonographic signs are helpful in arriving at an accurate diagnosis, none are specific since each of them can occasionally be seen in patients without cholecystitis. Other inflammatory conditions presenting with right upper abdominal pain such as peptic ulcer disease and pancreatitis may result in similar sonographic appearances (72).

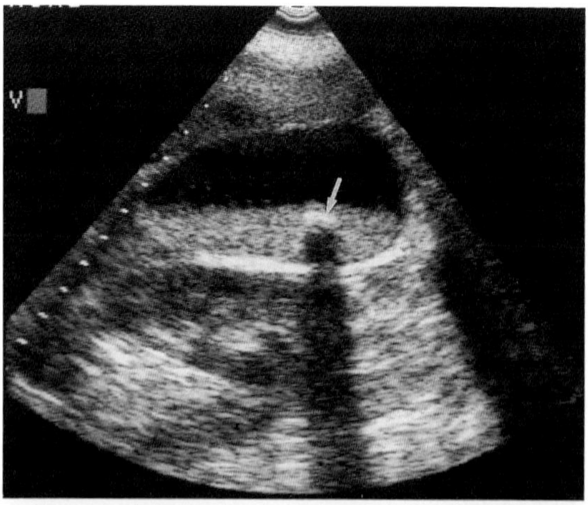

Figure 10 *Longitudinal view of the gallbladder shows multiple echogenic reflections without acoustic shadowing consistent with a diagnosis of sludge. Note the bright reflector with distal aoustic shadowing within the sludge representing a small stone (arrow).*

similar finding is seen with emphysematous cholecystitis due to gas in the gallbladder wall and in *porcelain gallbladder* because of calcium in the wall (see Figure 7). A contracted gallbladder after fasting can also be seen in cases of hepatic dysfunction such as occurs with viral hepatitis (87). A curvilinear shadow in the gallbladder bed must be differentiated from gas in the bowel. This can be accomplished by repeating the scan after a few minutes, or by rolling the patient to move the gas into a different position. A specific sonographic finding to indicate a contracted gallbladder containing calculi is the W-E-S triad. The "W" refers to the echopoor wall; the "E" refers to the echo caused by the calculi, and the "S" refers to the acoustic shadow (88).

Gallbladder sludge should not be mistaken for calculi. Sludge is echogenic bile caused by the presence of cholesterol crystals and calcium bilirubinate granules in the bile (89, 90). Sludge is due to biliary stasis secondary to prolonged fasting and is most often seen in hospital patients who have received intravenous feedings for extended periods. This is a frequent finding in neonates receiving total parenteral nutrition (91). The echogenic material generally layers out in the dependent portion of the gallbladder (Figure 10). Occasionally the gallbladder is completely filled with sludge. This appearance, which may be seen with prolonged extrahepatic biliary obstruction, can mimic a solid lesion of the gallbladder. Echogenic bile can be inhomogeneous with some brighter echo distributed through the thick bile. Tiny gallstones can be missed in these cases. Other causes of echogenic bile include hemobilia (92) and empyema (93) of the gallbladder.

Occasionally echogenic densities which do not shadow are seen in the gallbladder or biliary tree. These are referred to as "sludge balls" and should not be misinterpreted as gallstones. It has been reported that sludge balls can occasionally progress to gallstones (94).

Other abnormalities of the gallbladder

While cholelithiasis is by far the most frequent entity encountered in ultrasound evaluation of the gallbladder, the examiner must be aware of the myriad of other abnormalities, both congenital and acquired, that are seen in the gallbladder. Adenomatous polyps are frequently encountered and are visible on ultrasound as strongly echogenic foci attached to the wall. They are immobile, and without acoustic shadows (Figure 11) (95). Occasionally gallstones may be adherent to the gallbladder wall, and because of the physical characteristics of the gallstones, or for technical reasons, (stone is not in the focal zone of the transducer), there is no acoustic shadow (96). These gallstones can then simulate polyps.

Carcinomas of the gallbladder have several sonographic appearances ranging from a small density slightly larger than a polyp, to a large poorly defined mass in the right upper quadrant that has already invaded the region of the porta hepatis, liver and surrounding structures (Figure 12).

Carcinoma of the gallbladder is a difficult diagnosis to make preoperatively because of the non-specificity of the sonographic find-

Figure 11 *Longitudinal image of the gallbladder demonstrates small echogenic structures of varying size attached to the walls without evidence of acoustic shadowing consistent with the diagnosis of multiple polyps (arrows).*

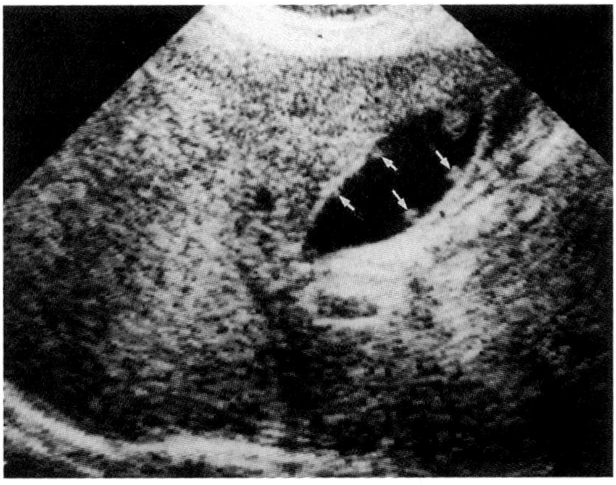

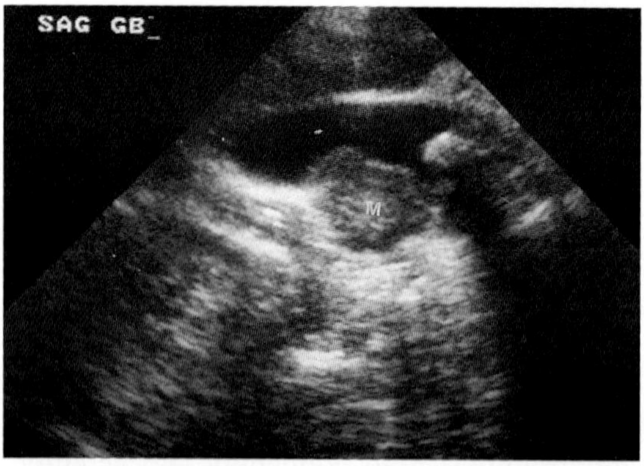

Figure 12 *Longitudinal image of the gallbladder shows a solid mass (M) involving a portion of the posterior wall of the gallbladder. This finding is consistent with a diagnosis of gallbladder carcinoma which was proven surgically. Within the gallbladder lumen inferior to this mass are several gallstones, a common finding in the presence of carcinoma.*

ings (97). The most common presentation is a large mass replacing the gallbladder (98). Other presentations include diffuse wall thickening which cannot be differentiated from inflammatory conditions, as well as fungating, polypoid masses which protrude into the lumen. The most frequent cause of a false positive diagnosis of carcinoma of the gallbladder is acute or chronic inflammation (99).

Some investigators believe that, with careful technique, early carcinoma of the gallbladder may be detected with greater frequency by cross-sectional imaging techniques (98). A large study in Finland reported a sensitivity of 25% in diagnosing gallbladder carcinoma with ultrasound (99).

It may be difficult to distinguish gallbladder carcinoma from a lesion arising in the hepatic flexure of the colon or in the liver. Gallbladder carcinoma is almost invariably associated with gallstones, and this may be helpful in the differential diagnosis. Metastases to the gallbladder while rare, do occur, especially in malignant melanoma (100). Occasionally, a mound of sludge can simulate gallbladder carcinoma, but sludge should be distinguishable by its mobility. Hyperplastic cholecystoses and adenomyomatosis can cause segmental thickening of the gallbladder which represent the Rokitansky-Aschoff sinuses (Figure 13). Polypoid masses in the gallbladder have been described sonographically in polypoid cholesterolosis (102). Primary leiomyosarcoma can occur in the gallbladder but the sonographic findings are similar to those seen in carcinoma (103).

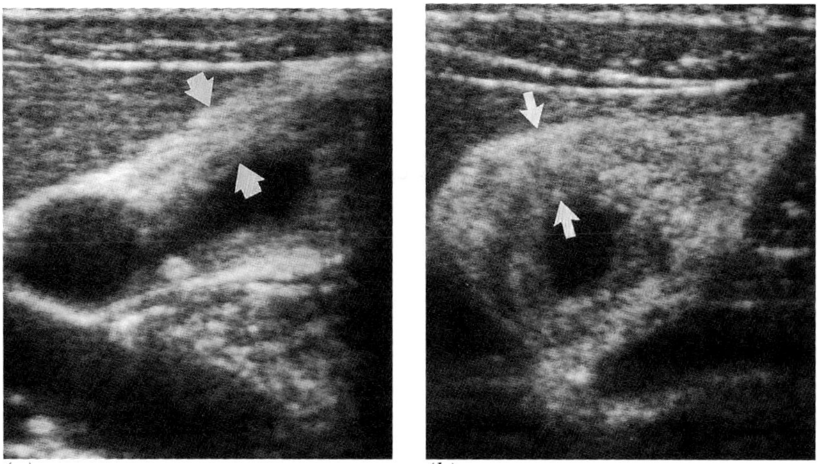

(a) *(b)*

Figure 13 *Longitudinal (a) and transverse (b) images of the gallbladder demonstrates marked thickening of the gallbladder walls (arrows) with the suggestion of some very small hypoechoic areas which may represent Rokitansky-Aschoff sinuses. These, however, may be difficult to delineate and thus differentiation from other causes for wall thickening may not be possible.*

Numerous congenital anomalies of the gallbladder may be seen sonographically. These include gallbladder duplications and multiseptate gallbladders (104). It is possible to diagnose intraluminal hematomas of the gallbladder wall in trauma patients with hemobilia (105). The sonographic features of torsion of the gallbladder have been described and include a "floating gallbladder" located below the liver but not in contact with it, a cone-shaped pedicle, and thickening of the gallbladder wall (106, 107). The sonographic diagnosis of strangulation of the gallbladder following herniation through the foramen of Winslow has also been described (108).

The combination of a calculus-containing gallbladder in an unusual location in a patient with sudden onset of severe upper abdominal pain may lead to suspicion of this entity.

PATHOLOGY OF THE BILE DUCTS

In the presence of jaundice, usually the first study ordered is an ultrasound examination (109). In almost all cases it is possible to identify the common bile duct as it courses down from the liver into the head

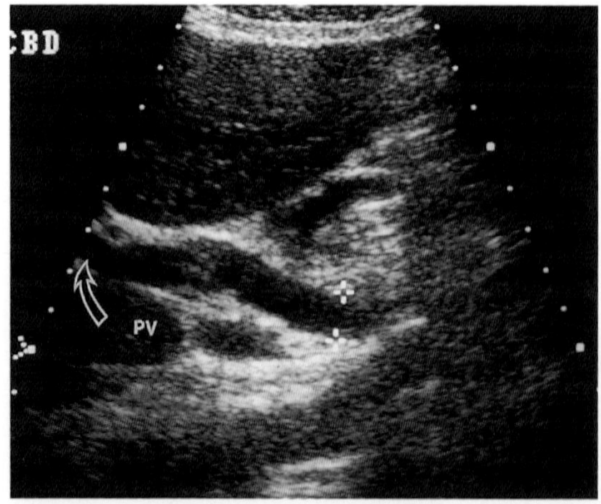

Figure 14 *Longitudinal view of the right upper quadrant shows a slightly dilated extrahepatic bile duct. Arrow delineates the region of the common hepatic duct just anterior to the portal vein (PV). It measures 9 mm in diameter which is significantly greater than the 5 mm upper normal limits expected in this region.*

of the pancreas (see Figure 1). While measurements of the common bile duct vary, normal is considered to be up to 8 mm in diameter (110). That portion of the extrahepatic bile duct located just anterior to the portal vein is usually the hepatic duct and at that point the measurement of the lumen should not exceed 5 mm (Figure 14). With increasing age, beyond the sixth decade, it is common to add 1 mm to the maximum normal measurements for each decade. In some post-cholecystectomy patients the bile duct may be slightly enlarged (110, 111). Measurement of the bile ducts after a fatty meal will often demonstrate distention and emptying of the extrahepatic biliary system. However, in cases where there is obstruction for whatever cause, this usually results in the bile duct remaining dilated. This can sometimes be helpful should there be a question in terms of bile duct size. It should, however, be noted that in cases of acute jaundice the bile ducts, although obstructed, may not yet be anatomically dilated. Thus, a follow-up examination is strongly recommended especially if the bilirubin suggests bile duct obstruction.

The intrahepatic bile ducts are located within the portal triad adjacent to the portal veins and hepatic arteries. Under normal circumstances they are not visualized except for those portions adjacent to the main right and left portal veins. However, with dilatation multiple tube-like structures can be seen adjacent to the portal veins (Figure 15). Doppler ultrasound can be used to differentiate bile ducts from blood vessels. If the obstruction is extrahepatic, it is common for the entire biliary system to dilate. It should be noted that segmental dilatations can be due to mass compression or cholangiocarcinoma (112). Intrahepatic biliary stones or strictures, the result of chronic cholangigitis, can also produce bile duct dilatation (113).

Ultrasound can often identify the cause for extrahepatic bile duct dilatation. A mass either within the head of the pancreas or Ampulla of Vater often produces bile duct dilatation (Figure 15). While it is usually possible to demonstrate the presence of such a mass, if it is small or its echogenicity blends with that of the normal pancreas it can be missed. Non-malignant masses, such as a pseudocyst can also cause bile duct obstruction. Another cause for extrahepatic bile duct obstruction is a stone (Figure 16). Careful scanning of the entire biliary system is indicated since additional stones may extend up into the major biliary branches within the liver. While an oblique longitudinal view is most commonly used to image the common bile duct, scanning transversely through the head of the

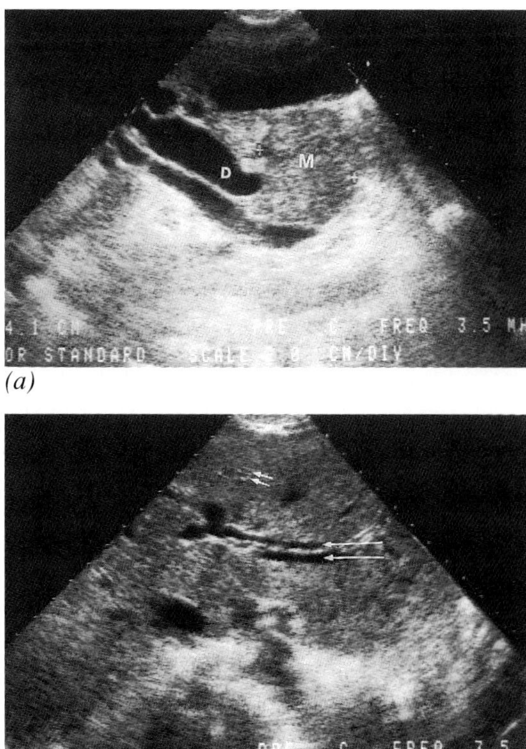

(a)

(b)

Figure 15
a. Longitudinal image of the right upper quadrant demonstrates a dilated common bile duct (D) entering the pancreas. The obstruction was caused by a clearly delineated pancreatic mass (M).
b. Transverse image of the liver clearly shows the presence of multiple tube-like structures consistent with a diagnosis of dilated bile ducts. This double tube-like appearance is quite typical for intrahepatic bile duct obstruction, with one tube representing a normal portal vein and the other the dilated bile duct (arrows).

pancreas can also be useful for identifying a stone within the distal common bile duct. If a stone is occupying the entire bile duct and there is no bile around the stone to make it stand out from the wall it may be difficult to identify. In addition, the presence of overlying bowel gas may make it impossible to fully evaluate the entire extrahepatic biliary system. Extrinsic masses, such as lymph nodes or tumor in the region of the porta hepatis or carcinoma of the gallbladder are other causes for biliary duct dilatation (Figure 17).

After passage of a stone or surgical procedures involving the biliary system, it is not uncommon for air to enter into the biliary system resulting in distinctive bright reflections along the course of the biliary tract (Figure 18).

A less common cause of bile duct obstruction is the presence of ascaris which can live within the gallbladder or bile ducts. These parasites can multiply within the biliary system and result in obstruction. When imaged, they have a typical appearance (Figure 19).

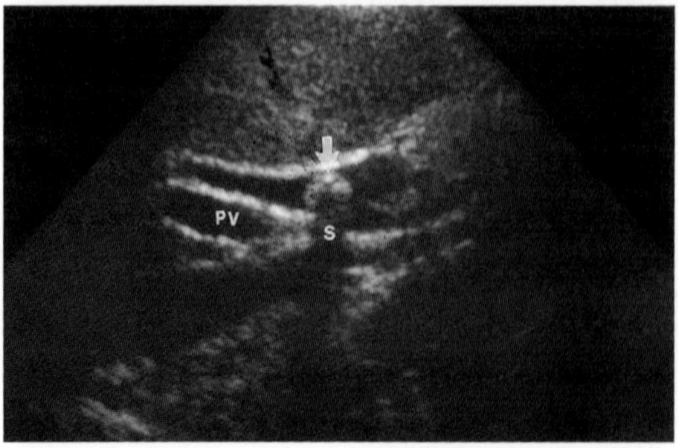

Figure 16 *Longitudinal image shows extrahepatic bile duct dilatation. Just anterior to the portal vein (PV) in the bile duct a curvilinear reflector (arrow) with distal acoustic shadowing (S) is identified consistent with a diagnosis of choledocholithiasis.*

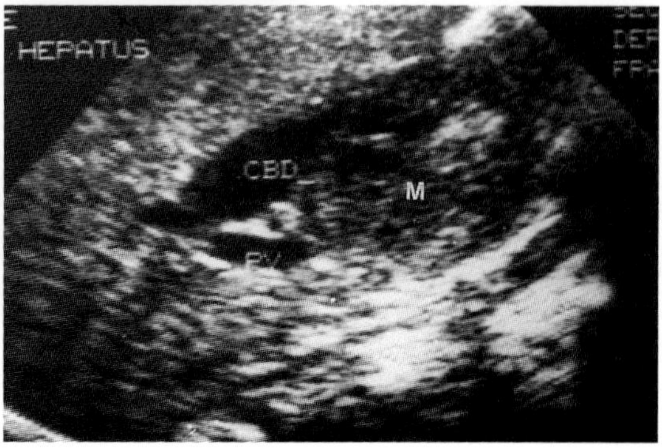

Figure 17 *Oblique image of a dilated common bile duct in a 3-year-old boy with jaundice shows the presence of a solid mass (M) in the region of porta hepatis which cannot be separated from the bile duct (CBD). This proved to be a rhabdomyosarcoma of the common bile duct.*

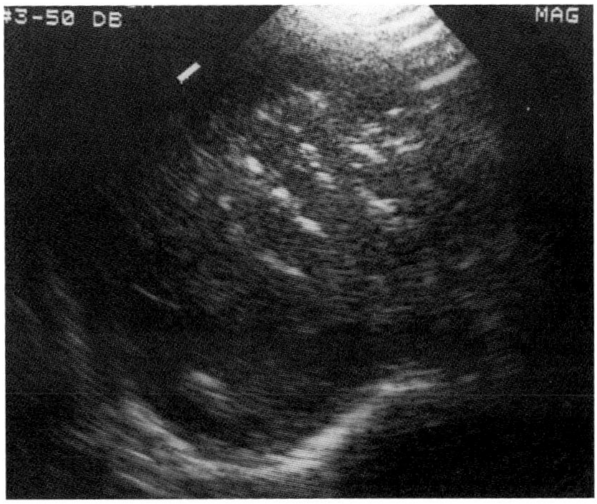

Figure 18 *Ultrasound image of the right lobe of the liver shows uniform small scattered bright reflectors predominantly throughout the upper portions of the liver following the course of the intrahepatic bile ducts. In this patient who had a previous choledochojejunostomy this pattern is characteristic of air within the biliary system.*

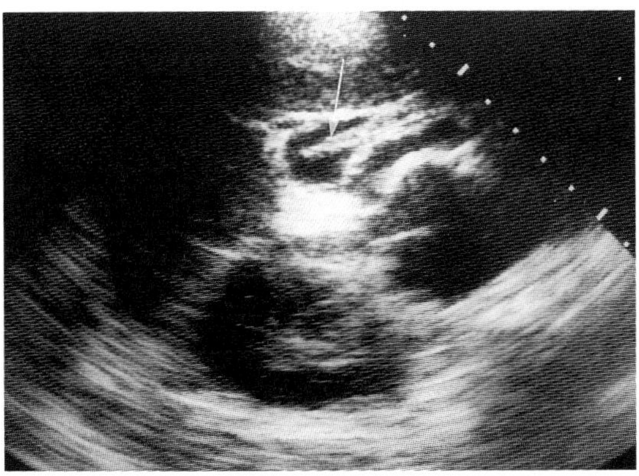

Figure 19 *Oblique ultrasound image of the right upper quadrant demonstrates a dilated common bile duct which contains tubular-like structures (arrows), which moved during real-time ultrasound examination consistent with the diagnosis of ascarias. Note the hypoechoic tube-like region within the ascaris representing its intestinal tract.*

Congenital causes of bile duct dilatation falls into two categories: extrahepatic and intrahepatic (114). By far the most common is extraheaptic where a focal dilatation can occur resulting in what is known as a choledochal cyst (Figure 20). These can occur anywhere along the length of the bile ducts, and are usually quite typical in their configuration. If they become very large they can present as a cystic mass. However, scanning in multiple planes will often demonstrate the entrance of the bile duct into the cystic area. On occasion the mass can cause bile duct obstruction. Irregular dilatations of the intrahepatic biliary system can also occur without

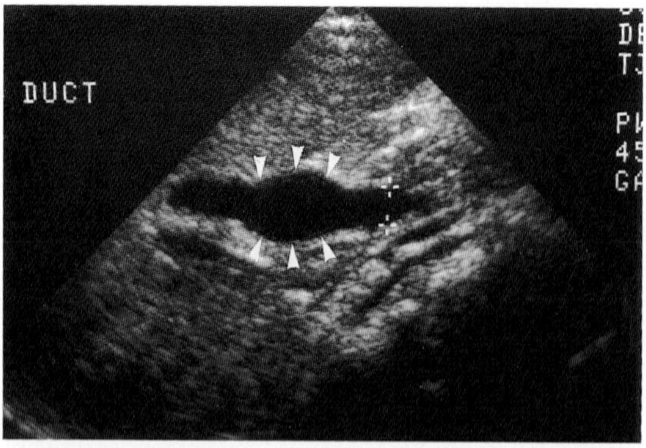

Figure 20 *Longitudinal image of focal dilatation (arrows) of the common bile duct in a 2-year-old infant consistent with the diagnosis of a choledochal cyst.*

any cause for the dilatation and is known as Caroli's disease. Atresia of the biliary system may be complete or partial. If the gallbladder is present then it is possible to drain the obstructed biliary system via the gallbladder into the adjacent bowel.

The examination of the biliary system, both extrahepatic and intrahepatic, is an important part of the ultrasound examination of the right upper quadrant. Understanding the anatomic variations, scanning techniques and pathologies will usually result in an appropriate diagnosis.

REFERENCES

1. Cooperberg PL, Burhenne HJ. Real-time ultrasonography: A diagnostic technique of choice in calculus gallbladder disease. N Engl J Med 1980;302:277–279.
2. Mogensen NB, Madsen M et al. Ultrasonography versus roentgenography in suspected instances of cholecystolithiasis. Surg Gynec Obstet 1984;159:353–356.
3. Ferrucci JT Jr, Adson MA et al. Advances in the radiology of jaundice: A symposium and review. AJR 1983;141:1–20.
4. McGahan JP, Walter JP. Diagnostic percutaneous aspiration of the gallbladder. Radiology 1985;155:619–622.
5. Teplick SK. Diagnostic and therapeutic interventional gallbladder procedures. AJR 1989;152:913–916.
6. Simeone JF, Mueller PR, Ferrucci JT. Nonsurgical therapy of gallstones: Implications for imgaing. AJR 1989;152:11–17.
7. Martin EC, Getrajdman GI. Does the gallbladder have a future? Radiology 1989;170:969–973.
8. Garel LA, Belli D et al. Percutaneous cholecystography in children. Radiology 1987;165:639–641.

9. Gibney RG, Fache JS et al. Combined surgical and radiologic intervention for complicated cholelithiasis in high-risk patients. Radiology 1987;165:715–719.
10. Lohela P, Soiva M et al. Ultrasonic guidance for percutaneous puncture and drainage in acute cholecystitis. Acta Radiol 1986;27:543–546.
11. Pearse DM, Hawkins Jr IF et al. Percutaneous cholecystostomy in acute cholecystitis and common duct obstruction. Radiology 1984;152:365–367.
12. Kerlan Jr RK, LaBerge JM et al. Percutaneous cholecystolithotomy: Preliminary experience. Radiology 1985;157:653–656.
13. Van Sonnenberg E, Wittich GR et al. Diagnostic and therapeutic percutaneous gallbladder procedures. Radiology 1986;160:23–26.
14. Becker CD, Quenville NF, Burhenne HJ. Gallbladder ablation through radiologic intervention: An experimental alternative to cholecystectomy. Radiology 1989;171:235–240.
15. Mathieson JR, So CB, Malone DE et al. Accuracy of sonography for determining the number and size of gallbladder stones before and after lithotripsy. AJR 1989;153:977–980.
16. Steinberg HV, Torres WE, Nelson RC. Gallbladder lithotripsy. Radiology 1989;172:7–11.
17. Burhenne HJ, Becker CD et al. Biliary lithotripsy: Early observations in 106 patients. Radiology 1989;171:363–367.
18. Ferrucci JT. Biliary lithotripsy: 1989. AJR 1989;153:15–22.
19. Paumgartner G. Shock-wave lithotripsy of gallstones. AJR 1989;153:235–242.
20. Rifkin MD, Mack LA et al. Intraoperative abdominal ultrasonography: Initial experience with a dedicated high-resolution operative transducer ultrasonography. J Ultrasound Med 1986;5:429–433.
21. Scholenfield IJ, Lachin JM. National co-operative study: A controlled trail of efficacy and safety of chemodiol for dissolution of gallstones. Ann Int Med 1981;95:257–282.
22. Klingensmith WC, Cioffi-Ragan DT. Fetal gallstones. Radiology 1988;167:143–144.
23. Keller MS, Markle BM et al. Spontaneous resolution of cholelithiasis in infants. Radiology 1985;157:345–348.
24. Henschke CI, Teele RL. Cholelithiasis in children: Recent observations. J Ultrasound Med 1983;2:481–484.
25. Whorwell PA, Hawkins R et al. Ultrasound survey of gallstones and other hepatobiliary disorders in patients with Crohn's disease. Dig Dis Sci 1984;29:930–933.
26. Williamson SL, Williamson MR. Cholecystosonography in pregnancy. J Ultrasound Med 1984;3:329–331.
27. Sukov RJ, Sample WF, Sarti DA et al. Cholecystosonography. The junctional fold. Radiology 1979;133:435–436.

28. Wegener M, Borsch G, Schneider J et al. Gallbladder wall thickening: A frequent finding in various nonbiliary disorders – A prospective ultrasonographic study. J Clin Ultrasound 1987;15:307–312.
29. Filly RA, Laing FC. Anatomic variation of portal venous anatomy in the porta hepatis: Ultrasonography evaluation. J Clin Ultrasound 1979;7:83–89.
30. Cooperberg PL. High-resolution real-time ultrasound in the evaluation of the normal and obstructed biliary tract. Radiology 1978;129:477–480.
31. Cooperberg PL, Li D, Wong P et al. Accuracy of common hepatic duct size in the evaluation of extrahepatic biliary obstruction. Radiology 1980;135:141–144.
32. Krook P, Allen FH, Bush Jr WH et al. Comparison of real-time cholecystosonography and oral cholecystography. Radiology 1980;135:145–148.
33. Weill F, Eisencher A, Yeltner F. Ultrasonic study of the normal and dilated biliary tree. Radiology 1978;127:221–224.
34. Cooperberg PL, Gibney RG. Imaging of the gallbladder. Radiology 1987;163:605–613.
35. Amberg JR, Leopold GR. Is oral cholecystography still useful? AJR 1978;151:73–74.
36. Field SI, Calvert-Hill MA. Clinical efficacy of screening the entire abdomen during real-time ultrasound examination. JCU 1985;13:411–413.
37. Thompson GT. Incidental findings on gallbladder sonography. J Can Assoc Radiol 1987;38:40–41.
38. Scheske GS, Cooperberg PL, Cohen MM et al. Floating gallstones: The role of contrast material. J Clin Ultrasound 1980;8:227–231.
39. Parulekar SG. Evaluation of the prone view for cholecystosonography. J Ultrasound Med 1986;5:617–624.
40. Hess ML, Cunningham JJ. Effect of examination time of day on the quality of real-time cholesonograms. AJR 1984;143:251–253.
41. Klingensmith WC, Eckhout GV. Cholelithiasis in the morbidly obese: Diagnosis by US and oral cholecystography. Radiology 1986;160:27–28.
42. Rubaltelli L, Talenti E, Rizzatto G et al. Gas-containing gallstones: Their influence on ultrasound images. J Clin Ultrasound 1984;12:279–282.
43. Parulekar SG. Ultrasonic detection of calcification in gallstones: "The reverberation shadow". J Ultrasound Med 1984;3:123–129.
44. Cover KL, Slasky S, Skolnick ML. Sonography of cholesterol in the biliary system. J Ultrasound Med 1985;4:647–653.
45. Slomic AM, Ferguson C. The ultrasonic features of an unusual cholesterol gallstone. J Canad Assoc Radiol 1988;39:155–156.
46. Sukov RJ, Sample WF, Sarti DA et al. Cholecystosonography – The junctional fold. Radiology 1979;133:435–436.

47. Mitchell DG, Needleman L, Frauenhoffer S et al. Gas-containing gallstones. The sonographic ”double echo sign”. J Ultrasound Med 1988;7:39–43.
48. Lebensart PD, Bloom RA, Meretyk S. Oral cholecystosonography: A method for facilitating the diagnosis of cholesterol gallstones. Radiology 1984;153:255–256.
49. Reinig JW, Stanley JH. Sonographic hepatization of the gallbladder: A cause of nonvisualization of the gallbladder by cholecystosonograhy. J Clin Ultrasound 1984;12:234–236.
50. Greaves FW, Nguyen KT, Sauerbrei EE. Retrohepatic gallbladder diagnosed by sonography scintigraphy. J Canad Assoc Radiol 1983;34:319–320.
51. McLoughlin MJ, Fanti JE, Kura ML. Ectopic gallbladder: Sonographic and scintigraphic diagnosis. J Clin Ultrasound 1987;15:258–261.
52. Kane RA, Jacobs R, Katz J et al. Porcelain gallbladder: Ultrasound and CT appearance. Radiology 1984;152:137–141.
53. Ferin P, Lerner RM. Contracted gallbladder: A finding in hepatic dysfunction. Radiology 1985;154:769–770.
54. Hammond DI: Unusual causes of sonographic nonvisualization or nonrecognition of the gallbladder: A review. J Clin Ultrasound 1988;16:77–85.
55. Giyanani VL, Jackson MK, Gerlock Jr AJ et al. Omental cyst mimicking the gallbladder. J Clin Ultrasound 1986;14:131–133.
56. Han BK, Babcock DS, Gelfand MH. Choledochal cyst with bile duct dilatation: Sonography and 99m Tc IDA cholescintigraphy. AJR 1981;136:1075–1079.
57. Murayama S, Mizushima A, Russell WJ et al. Sonographic diagnosis of bicameral gallbladders: A report of three cases. J Ultrasound Med 1985;4:539–542.
58. Rall PW, Colletti PM, Lapin SA et al. Real-time sonography in suspected acute cholecystitis. Radiology 1985;155:768–771.
59. Simeone JF, Brink JA, Mueller PR et al. The sonographic diagnosis of acute gangrenous cholecystitis: Importance of the Murphy sign. AJR 1989;152:2890.
60. Fiske EC, Laing FC, Brown TW. Ultrasonographic evidence of gallbladder wall thickening in association with hypoalbuminemia. Radiology 1980;135:713–716.
61. Kaftori JK, Pery M, Green J. Thickness of the gallbladder wall in patients with hypoalbuminemia: A sonographic study of patients on peritoneal dialysis. AJR 1987;148:1117–1118.
62. Saunders RC. The significance of sonographic gallbladder wall thickening. J Clin Ultrasound 1980;8:143–146.
63. Shaler WJ, Leopold GR, Scheible FW. Sonography of the thickened gallbladder wall: A nonspecific finding. AJR 1981;136:337–339.

64. Maresca G, De Gaetano AM, Mirk P et al. Sonographic patterns of the gallbladder in acute viral hepatitis. J Clin Ultrasound 1984;12:141–146.
65. Costa-Greco MA. Adenomyomatosis of the gallbladder. J Clin Ultrasound 1987;15:198–199.
66. Kidney M, Goiney R, Cooperberg PL. Adenomyomatosis of the gallbladder: A pictorial exhibit. J Ultrasound Med 1986;5:331–333.
67. Marchal GJF, Van Holsbeeck M, Tshibwabwa-Ntumba E et al. Dilatation of the cystic veins in portal hypertension: Sonographic demonstration. Radiology 1985;154:187–189.
68. Saigh J, Williams S, Cawley K. et al. Varices: A cause of focal gallbladder wall thickening. J Ultrasound Med 1985;4:371–373.
69. Graif M, Horovitz A, Itzchak Y et al. Hyperechoic foci in the gallbladder wall as a sign of microabscess formation or diverticula. Radiology 1984;152:781–784.
70. Cheong LL, Khan AN, Armstrong GR. Ultrasonic demonstration of an intraluminal pseudomembrane in the gallbladder: A definitive sign of acute cholecystitis? J Clin Ultrasound 1989;17:449–452.
71. Cohan RH, Mahony BS, Bowie JD et al. Striated intramural gallbladder lucencies on US studies: Predictors of acute cholecystitis. Radiology 1987;164:31–35.
72. Nyberg DA, Laing FC. Ultrasonographic findings in peptic ulcer disease and pancreatitis that simulate primary gallbladder disease. J Ultrasound Med 1983;2:303–307.
73. Jenkins M, Golding RH, Cooperberg PL. Sonography and computed tomography of hemorrhagic cholecystitis. AJR 1983;140:1197–1198.
74. Chinn DH, Miller EI, Piper N. Hemorrhagic cholecystitis: sonographic appearance and clinical presentation. J Ultrasound Med 1987;6:313–317.
75. Bloom RA, Libson E, Lebensart PD et al. The ultrasound spectrum of emphysematous cholecystitis. J Clin Ultrasound 1989;17:251–256.
76. Bloom RA, Fisher A, Pode D et al. Shifting intramural gas – A new ultrasound sign of emphysematous cholecystitis. J Clin Ultrasound 1984;12:40–42.
77. Nemcek AA, Gore RM, Vogelzang R et al. The effervescent gallbladder: A sonographic sign of emphysematous cholecystitis. AJR 1988;150:575–577.
78. Colletti PM, Ralls PW, Siegel ME. Acute cholecystitis: Diagnosis with radionuclide angiography. Radiology 1987;163:615–618.
79. Swayne LC, Ginsberg HN. Diagnosis of acute cholecystitis by cholescintigraphy: Significance of pericholecystic hepatic uptake. AJR 1989;152:1211–1213.
80. Smith R, Rosen JM, Gallo LN et al. Pericholecystic hepatic activity in cholescintigraphy. Radiology 1985;156:797–800.
81. Fox MS, Wilk PJ, Weissmann HS et al. Acute acalculous cholecystitis. Surg Gynec Obstet 1984;159:13–16.

82. Swayne LC. Acute acalculous cholecystitis: Sensitivity in detection using Technetium – 99m iminodiacetic acid cholescintigraphy. Radiology 1986;160:33–38.
83. Takada T, Yasuda H, Uchiyama K. et al. Pericholecystic abscess: Classification of US findings to determine the proper therapy. Radiology 1989;172:693–697.
84. Sowa M, Pamilo M, Paivansalo M et al. Ultrasonography in acute gallbladder perforation. Acta Radiol 1989;29:41–43.
85. Harbin WP, Ferrucci Jr JR, Wittenberg J et al. Nonvisualized gallbladder by cholecystosonography. AJR 1979;132:727–728.
86. Laing FC, Gooding GAW, Hergong KA. Gallstones preventing ultrasonographic visualization of the gallbladder. Gastrointest Radiol 1977;1:301–303.
87. Ferin P, Lerner RM. Contracted gallbladder: A finding in hepatic dysfunction. Radiology 1985;154:769–770.
88. Macdonald FR, Cooperberg PL, Cohen MM. The WES triad. A specific sonographic sign of gallstones in the contracted gallbladder. Gastrointest Radiol 1981;6:39–41.
89. Filly RA, Allan B, Minton MJ et al. In vitro investigation of the origin of echos within biliary sludge. J Clin Ultrasound 1980;8:193–200.
90. Thurber LA, Cooperberg PL, Clement JG et al. Echogenic fluid: A pitfall in the ultrasonographic diagnosis of cystic lesions. J Clin Ultrasound 1979; 7:273–278.
91. Matos C, Avni EF, Van Gansbeke D et al. Total parenteral nutrition (TPN) and gallbladder diseases in neonates. J Ultrasound Med 1987;6:243–248.
92. Grant EG, Smitopiotopoulos JG. Intraluminal gallbladder hematomas: Sonographic evidence of hemobilia. J Clin Ultrasound 1983;11:507–509.
93. Kane RA. Ultrasonographic diagnosis of gangrenous cholecystitis and emphysema of the gallbladder. Radiology 1980;134:191–194.
94. Britten JS, Golding RH, Cooperberg PL. Sludge balls to gallstones. J Ultrasound Med 1984;3:81–82.
95. Carter SJ, Rutledge J, Hirsch JH et al. Papillary adenoma of the gallbladder: Ultrasonic demonstration. J Clin Ultrasound 1978;6:433–435.
96. Machi J, Iwanaga D, Tanaka M et al. Gallstones simulating polyps sonographically: A report of two cases. J Ultrasound Med 1986;5:597–600.
97. Hederström E, Forsberg L. Ultrasonography in carcinoma of the gallbladder. Acta Radiol 1987;28:715–718.
98. Weiner SN, Koenigsberg M, Morehouse H et al. Sonography and computed tomography in the diagnosis of carcinoma of the gallbladder. AJR 1984;142:735–739.
99. Soiva M, Aro K, Pamilo M et al. Ultrasonography in carcinoma of the gallbladder. Acta Radiol 1987;28:711–714.

100. Stutte H, Muller PH, d'Hoedt B et al. Ultrasonographic diagnosis of melanoma metastases in liver, gallbladder and spleen. J Ultrasound Med 1989;8:541–547.
101. Anastasi B, Sutherland GR. Biliary sludge: Ultrasonic appearance simulating neoplasm. Brit J Radiol 1981;54:679.
102. Price RJ, Stewart ET, Foley WD et al. Sonography of polypoid cholesterolosis. AJR 1982;139:1197–1198.
103. Coelho JCU, Wallbach A, Kasting G et al. Ultrasonic diagnosis of primary sarcoma of the gallbladder. J Clin Ultrasound 1984;12:168–170.
104. Lef-Toaff AS, Friedman AC, Rindsberg SN et al. Multiseptate gallbladder: Incidental diagnosis of sonography. AJR 1987;148:1119–1120.
105. Kauzlarie D, Barmeir E. Sonography of intraluminal gallbladder hematoma. J Clin Ultrasound 1985;13:291–294.
106. Yeh H, Weiss MF, Gerson CD. Torsion of the gallbladder: The ultrasonographic features. J Clin Ultrasound 1989;17:123–125.
107. Quinn SF, Fazzio F, Jones. Torsion of the gallbladder: Findings on CT and sonography and role of percutaneous cholecystostomy. AJR 1987;148:881–882.
108. Bach DB, Satin R, Palayew M et al. Herniation and strangulation of the gallbladder through the foramen of Winslow. AJR 1984;142:541–542.
109. Taylor KJW, Rosenfield AT, Spiro HM. Diagnostic accuracy of gray scale ultrasonography for the jaundiced patients: A report of 275 cases. Arch Intern Med 1979;139:60–63.
110. Laing FC, Jeffrey Jr RB, Wing VW, Nyberg DA. Biliary dilatation: defining the level and cause by real-time US. Radiology 1986;160:39–42.
111. Bucceri AM, Brogna A, Ferrara R. Common bile duct caliber following cholecystectomy: a two-year sonographic survey. Abdominal Imaging 1994;19:251–252.
112. Wibulpolprasert B, Dhiensiri T. Peripheral cholangiocarcinoma: sonographic evaluation. J Clin Ultrasound 1992;20:303–314.
113. Stott MA, Farrands PA, Guyer PS et al. Ultrasound of the common bile duct in patients undergoing cholecystectomy. J Clin Ultrasound 1991;19:73–76.
114. Kim OH, Chung HJ, Choi BG. Imaging of the choledochal cyst. Radiographics 1995;15:69–88.

CHAPTER 5

The Pancreas

Andrew M. Fried, MD

Sonographic imaging of the pancreas can provide valuable information concerning size, texture, masses, ductal dilatation, and fluid collections in and about the organ as well as disease states in related organs which border or affect the pancreas. Cost, portability, and absence of ionizing radiation are distinct advantages of ultrasound whereas large amounts of bowel gas or obesity coupled with the inherent operator dependency of the technique may be considered limitations. Diagnostic and therapeutic interventional procedures under ultrasound guidance are steadily gaining favor by virtue of speed, cost and general availability of the equipment.

TECHNIQUE

The examination is generally begun with the patient supine. Curved or phased array or sector scanners are best suited to examination of the pancreas; linear arrays are generally cumbersome and do not fit well in the subcostal space. Frequencies of 3 to 5 MHz (and, more recently, the broad band transducers of 4–2 MHz for example) are suitable depending upon the patient's body habitus. Transverse scans utilize the left lobe of the liver as much as possible as a window into the pancreatic bed, covering the retroperitoneum from well above the pancreas. Visualization of the abdominal aorta and inferior vena cava assures that adequate depth penetration has been attained to image the pancreas.

Sagittal scanning begins in the midline, identifying the great vessels and procedes to the right until the right kidney is seen and left to the splenic hilum (or until the pancreas is obscured by gas in the stomach or colon) to ensure visualization of as much of the organ as possible.

In both scan planes steady, firm pressure gradually applied will frequently eliminate interposed bowel gas and allow pancreatic imaging; several minutes of scanning with compression maintained may be necessary. Additionally, having the patient drink 250–500 cc of water may replace stomach gas and provide a window into the pancreas. The semi-erect position may also prove useful. If the patient is in pain, water ingestion with the semi-erect position may be most effective at the beginning of the examination to avoid excessive swallowing of air which frequently accompanies pain. Placing the patient in a steep oblique position with the right side down following water ingestion may well fill the second portion of the duodenum with fluid and provide excellent visualization of the contour of the head of the pancreas.

NORMAL ANATOMY

The pancreas lies in the retroperitoneum in the anterior pararenal fascial space anterior to the aorta and inferior vena cava. More specifically, the pancreas is generally found at a level just below the take-off of the superior mesenteric artery (SMA); the SMA is surrounded by the brightly echogenic fat at the root of the mesentery and lies posterior to the body of the pancreas. The celiac axis takes off the aorta generally at the superior border of the gland. Anterior to the SMA and seen in its transverse course is the splenic vein forming the dorsal border of the pancreas from the splenic hilum to its confluence with the superior mesenteric vein at the neck of the pancreas. At this point, the head and uncinate process of the pancreas actually wrap around the venous confluence which forms the portal vein, and pancreatic tissue is seen both anterior and posterior to the vein. The superior mesenteric vessels are considered the markers of division between the head and body of the pancreas (Figures 1–3).

The right margin of the pancreas is formed by the second portion of the duodenum (the C-loop); better visualization of the head of the pancreas is provided by having the patient drink 250–500 ml of water and positioning right side down to fill the C-loop with water,

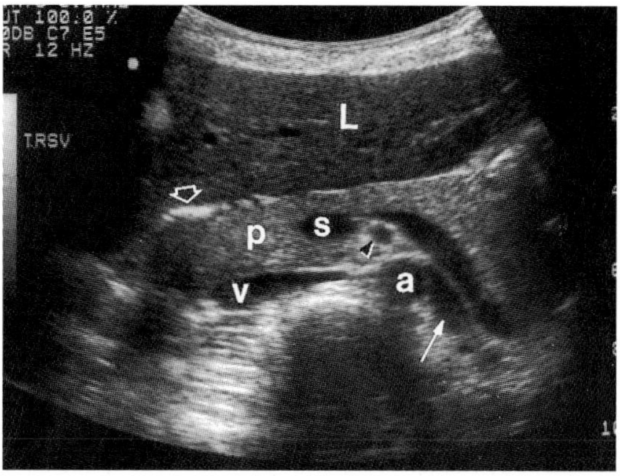

Figure 1 *Transverse view demonstrates pancreas (p) with a homogeneous texture, more echogenic than that of liver (L). The splenic vein (s) forms the dorsal border of the gland. Note that the pancreas actually wraps around the confluence of the splenic and superior mesenteric veins (on this scan coinciding with the "s") with the uncinate process lying posterior to the vein. Small arrowhead indicates the superior mesenteric artery (SMA), open arrow the gas-filled second portion of duodenum, and the white arrow the left renal vein. a = aorta; v = inferior vena cava*

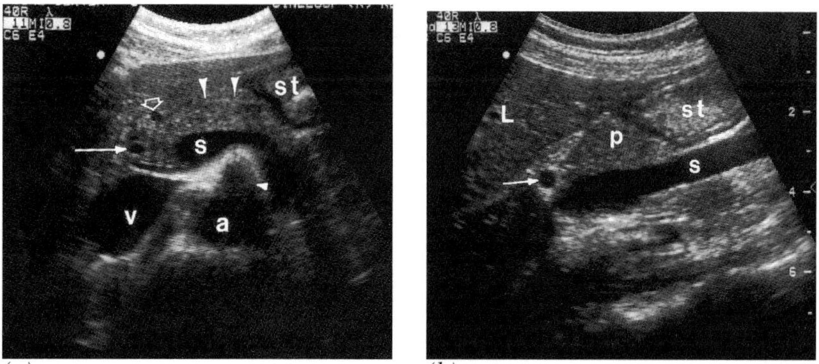

(a) *(b)*

Figure 2 a *Transverse scan in which are visible the gastroduodenal artery (open arrow) anterior to the neck of the pancreas and the common bile duct (thin white arrow) in the posterior aspect of the head of the pancreas. The duct should not exceed 10 mm in internal diameter at this level.*
Large arrowheads = body of pancreas; st = stomach; small arrowhead = take-off of superior mesenteric artery; a = aorta; v = inferior vena cava.
Figure 2 b *Sagittal scan. The pancreas (p) lies anterior to the superior mesenteric vein (s) and posterior to the stomach (st) and left lobe of liver (L). Arrow denotes the hepatic artery which has just branched off the celiac axis.*

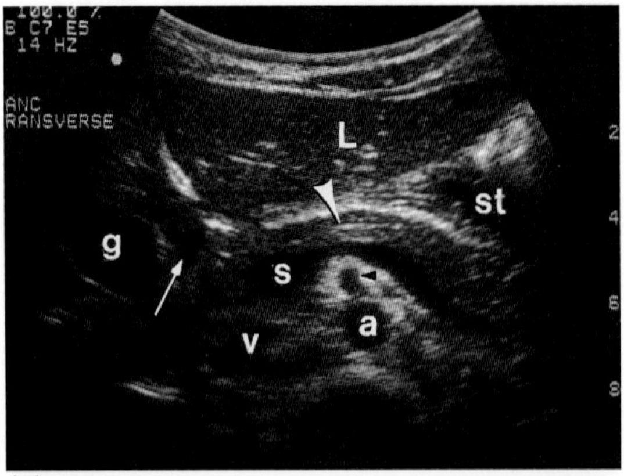

(a)

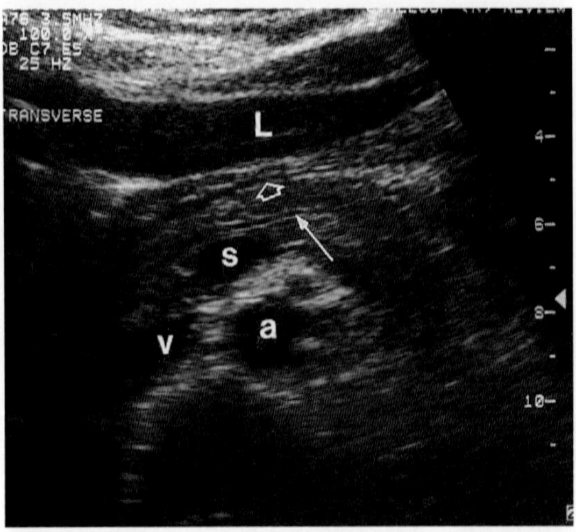

(b)

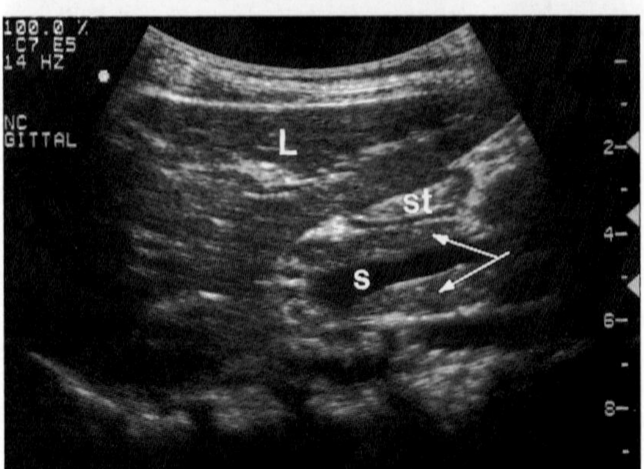

(c)

Figure 3 a *Normal pancreas seen on transverse scan with visualization of the pancreatic duct (arrowhead) as a single line. Again are seen the stomach (st), left lobe of liver (L), aorta (a) and inferior vena cava (v). The fluid-filled second portion of the duodenum (arrow) is seen adjacent to the pancreatic head; the gallbladder (g) is immediately lateral.*

Figure 3 b *In this transverse scan, the pancreatic duct (arrow) is seen as a tube rather than a single echogenic line; as long as the internal diameter does not exceed 2–2.5 mm and the walls are parallel, this is still considered normal. Note that the posterior wall of the stomach (open arrow) looks almost identical to the pancreatic duct; care must be taken not to confuse the two. a = aorta; v = inferior vena cava; L = liver.*

Figure 3 c *Sagittal scan demonstrates normal pancreatic tissue (arrows) anterior (head) and posterior (uncinate process) to the superior mesenteric vein (s). L = liver; st = stomach.*

outlining the pancreatic head with the water-filled bowel. This technique will prove particularly useful in patients in whom the collapsed duodenum may simulate a mass in the head of the pancreas.

The tail of the pancreas, which is frequently somewhat more cephalad than the head (i.e. the long axis will often be oriented more along a 2 o'clock – 8 o'clock line than simply horizontal (3 o'clock – 9 o'clock) and lies in close approximation to the hilum of the spleen. Water in the stomach may facilitate visualization of the distal body and tail; occasionally, scanning from posteriorly through the left kidney and/or spleen may provide a window into the distal body and tail.

Anterior to the pancreas lies the lesser sac which, under normal circumstances is only a potential space and thus not visible, and the stomach, identified by the alternating hyper- and hypoechoic layers of its mucosa and muscularis, respectively. The left lobe of the liver lies anterior to the stomach and is, perhaps, the single most important factor in producing a window into the pancreatic bed even in obese patients (1).

The normal size of the pancreas is a matter of some debate. Most authors who provide measurements of the gland consider normal AP measurements of the head, neck, body and tail to be in the range of 3.5 cm, 2.0 cm, 2.5 cm and 2.5 cm, respectively. In actual practice, focal enlargement or localized change in texture carries much more significance than an aberrant measurement (2).

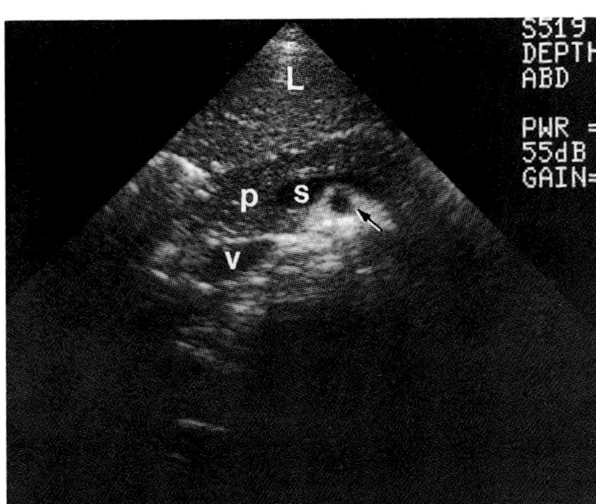

Figure 4 *Transverse scan in a young child. Note that the normal size pancreas (p) appears less echogenic than the liver (L). Predominance of glandular tissue and paucity of fat and fibrous stroma at this age make this a normal finding. s = splenic vein; v = inferior vena cava; arrow = superior mesenteric artery.*

The texture of the pancreas varies with age. In the infant and young child the gland may be hypoechoic as compared with the normal liver. This is attributed to the preponderance of glandular tissue and relative paucity of both fat and fibrous elements (Figure 4). In the adult, the echogenicity of the pancreas is taken to be normal if it is equal to or greater than that of the liver assuming, of course, that organ to be normal. Clear definition of the collagen and fat in the portal triads coupled with hepatic parenchyma which is slightly more echogenic than the adjacent renal cortex is reasonable assurance that the liver can be used as a normal internal standard (Figure 5).

At and beyond the fifth decade, replacement of glandular tissue with fat and fibrosis produces a diffuse, homogeneous increase in the echogenicity of the pancreas; it is not uncommon for the pancreas to reach a level of echogenicity at which it is indistinguishable from the contiguous retroperitoneal fat. These changes are considered a product of normal aging and are not associated with pancreatic insufficiency (3) (Figure 6).

Within the substance of the pancreas several normal structures may be visualized and evaluated most readily on the transverse scans. In the posterior aspect of the head of the pancreas is seen a circular lucency representing the termination of the common bile duct; it should measure no more than 10 mm in internal diameter. A second, usually smaller cystic structure is seen contiguous with the anterior margin of the neck of the pancreas; this is the end-on view of the gastroduodenal artery which can easily be identified as such with Doppler investigation.

A circular or ovoid lucency similar to the gastroduodenal artery may occasionally be seen in the distal body or tail of the pancreas. This represents a turn of the normally tortuous splenic artery which may mimic a cyst within the pancreatic parenchyma. Color or spectral Doppler will easily identify this structure as a portion of the normal splenic artery.

The pancreatic duct may be seen as a single echogenic line within the gland; occasionally the duct contains sufficient fluid to appear tubular with both echogenic walls imaged. This is still considered normal so long as the internal diameter of the duct does not exceed 2–2.5 mm. A caveat here is the fact that the muscular layer of the posterior wall of the stomach may mimic the pancreat-

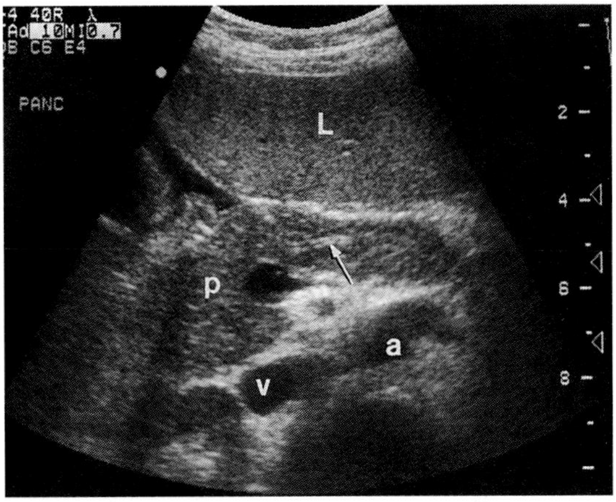

Figure 5 *The pancreas (p) appears somewhat hypoechoic as compared with the liver (L). This is due to increased echogenicity of the liver (fatty infiltration) rather than edema of the pancreas which is normal in this patient. Arrow = normal pancreatic duct; a = aorta; v = inferior vena cava.*

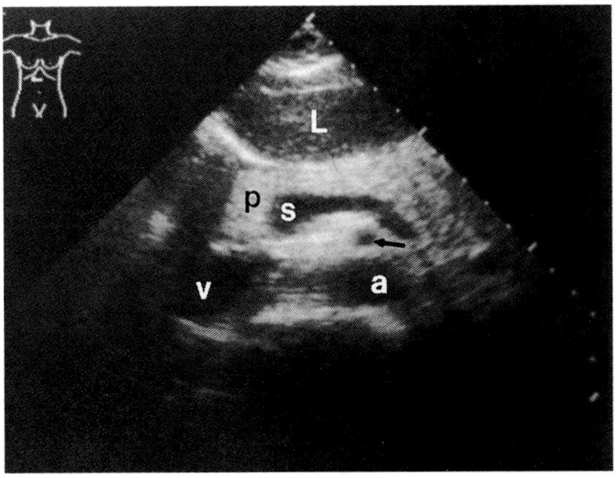

Figure 6 *The pancreas (p) in this elderly patient is markedly echogenic, becoming essentially isoechoic with the fat at the root of the mesentery which surrounds the superior mesenteric artery (arrow). This is a consequence of replacement of glandular tissue with fat and represents a normal aging change. s = splenic vein; a = aorta; v = inferior vena cava; L = liver.*

ic duct in size, configuration and echogenicity; motion may help to identify the gastric wall as such. The pancreatic duct will be bounded anteriorly and posteriorly by recognizable pancreatic tissue. Visualization of the normal duct has been reported in up to 86 % of normal subjects (4, 5) (see Figure 3 b).

PATHOLOGIC CONDITIONS

Acute pancreatitis

Acute inflammation of the pancreas may result from alcohol abuse, biliary tract disease, trauma, or familial predisposition.

Generally, the history will provide strong indications of the etiology but sonographic evaluation of the biliary tree is frequently requested to establish primary or secondary involvement (e.g. biliary tract obstruction by pseudocyst or inflammatory mass).

The classic sonographic findings in acute pancreatitis should involve diffuse enlargement of the gland with a generalized decrease in its echogenicity. Hypoechoic focal enlargement of the pancreas is also possible in acute inflammation; this is generally confined to the head, and focal enlargement confined to the tail would be unusual in pancreatitis and much more worrisome for neoplasm (6) (Figures 7, 8). It is also not uncommon to detect dilatation of the pancreatic duct to greater than 2 mm internal dia-

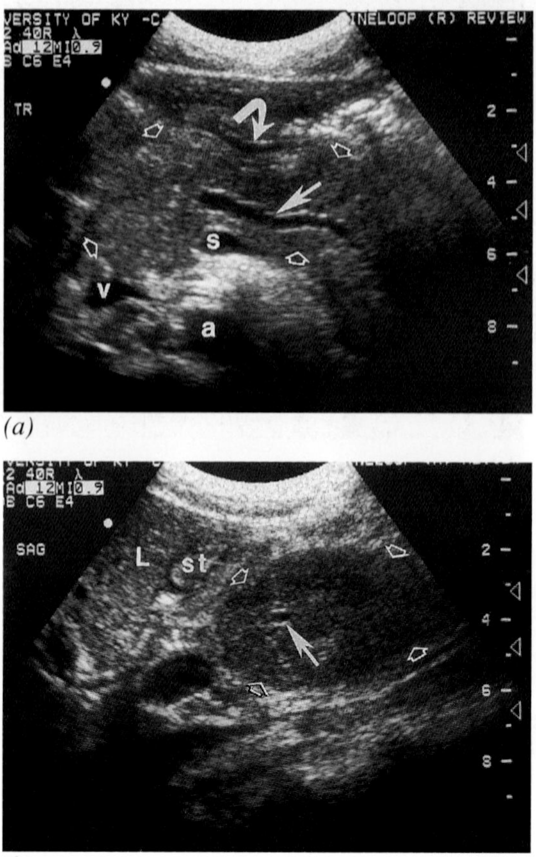

(a)

(b)

Figure 7 *Transverse (a) and sagittal (b) views of a diffusely enlarged pancreas (open arrows) whose echogenicity is considerably less than that of the liver (L). The dilated pancreatic duct (large arrow) is seen in both projections. Curved arrow = posterior wall of stomach; a = aorta; v = inferior vena cava; st = stomach; s = splenic vein.*

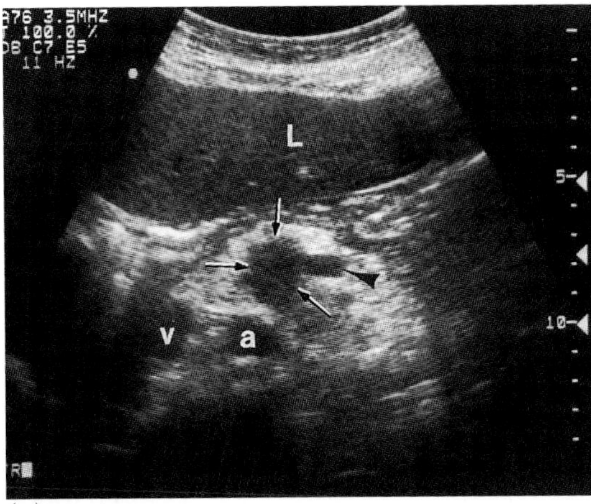

(a)

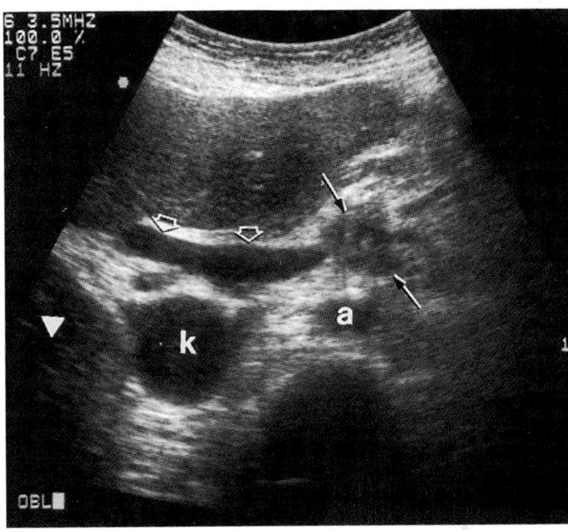

(b)

Figure 8 a *Focal hypoechoic enlargement of the head of the pancreas (arrows) may produce a sonograhpic appearance indistinguishable from carcinoma. Arrowhead = dilated pancreatic duct; L = liver; a = aorta, v = inferior vena cava.*
Figure 8 b *Oblique view again demonstrates focal enlargement of the head (arrows) with consequent dilatation of the common bile duct (open arrows). k = upper pole of right kidney; a = aorta.*

meter in patients with acute pancreatitis; the duct will most often return to normal as the inflammation regresses (7).

Comparison between the pancreas and liver will demonstrate a decrease in echogenicity of the pancreas. Whenever possible, it is preferable to compare the parenchymal textures on the sagittal scan; this provides views of hepatic and pancreatic parenchyma at equal distances from the transducer obviating differential attenuation by interposed tissues. A caution here is that the hyperechoic liver (as in fatty infiltration) will make the pancreas appear to be hypoechoic giving the false impression of acute pancreatitis.

It is important to assess hepatic echogenicity (i.e. can the normal echoes about the portal triads be seen? is the relationship of hepatic and renal cortical echogenicity maintained?) to ensure that it does represent a proper internal standard by which to judge the pancreatic texture.

A common finding with acute pancreatitis is the presence of small amounts of fluid in proximity to the pancreas, frequently in the lesser sac or elsewhere about the pancreas. These collections of pancreatic fluid, rich in enzymes, are said to occur in some 40 % of patients with acute pancreatitis; they resolve spontaneously in about 50 % of cases. Those which persist for more than four weeks are considered pseudocysts, half of which may resolve spontaneously. Morphologic characteristics do not allow separation of transient peripancreatic fluid collections from pseudocysts except by their serial behavior, i.e. the persistence of pseudocysts (8).

Pseudocysts

Persistence of fluid collections in or about the pancreas or lesser sac heralds the development of a pseudocyst which, by definition, is a collection of pancreatic fluid contained by a fibrous wall or capsule. They vary in size from only 2–3 cms to 10–15 cms in diameter. Although they are most commonly found in the peri-

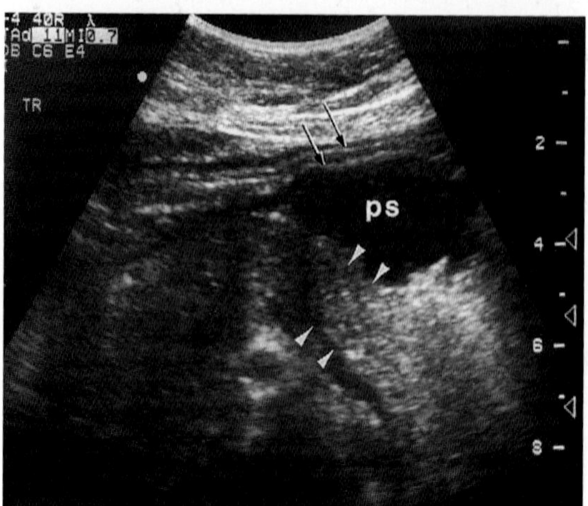

Figure 9 *A small, essentially simple pseudocyst, is seen anterior to the distal body and tail of the pancreas (arrowheads) and posterior to the stomach (arrows denote both gastric walls) lies within the lesser sac. Although pseudocysts may be found almost anywhere, this is the most common site.*

pancreatic region or lesser sac, pseudocysts have been described in a variety of locations including Gerota's fascia, the porta hepatis, and the mediastinum (Figure 9). They frequently contain gravity-dependent debris or irregular septations as a result of tissue necrosis or hemorrhage. The more extensive the internal echoes within a pseudocyst, the greater the chances of a superimposed infection (9). The distinction between a simple pancreatic pseudocyst and an infected pseudocyst (or pancreatic abscess) is not easily or confidently made at ultrasound alone; if the patient's condi-

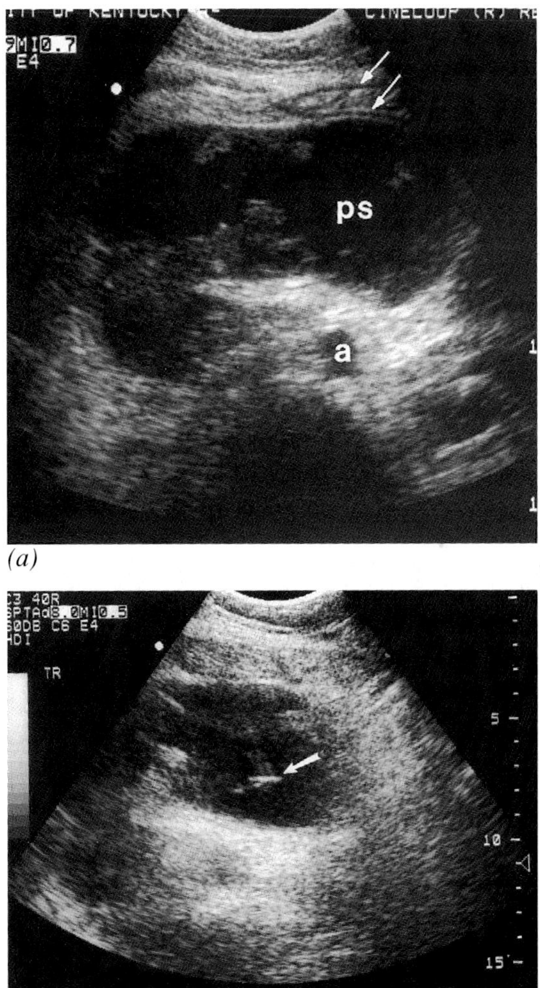

(a)

(b)

Figure 10 a *Transverse scan demonstrating a large pseudocyst (ps) containing scattered debris throughout. Both walls of the stomach (arrows) are well visualized immediately anterior to the pseudocyst indicating its location in the lesser sac; a = aorta.*
Figure 10 b *A somewhat oblique view through the same pseudocyst; a 22 gauge needle (arrow) is in place to determine the presence or absence of superiomposed infection.*

tion suggests the possibility of infected pseudocyst /abscess formation, diagnostic aspiration under sonographic guidance using a 22 gauge needle is appropriate and readily accomplished. Such an infected collection left undrained carries a mortality rate in excess of 50 % (10) (Figure 10).

Sonographic documentation of the presence of a peripancreatic fluid collection, presumably a pseudocyst, for several weeks should serve as the indicator for surgical or percutaneous intervention. Five to six weeks is considered appropriate because by that time the walls of the pseudocyst are relatively well-formed and the chances for spontaneous regression have diminished. Then, too, the possibility of superimposed complications such as bleeding, infection, and spontaneous rupture begins to rise substantially. Formation of pseudoaneurysms of vessels about the pancreas which may accompany pseudocyst formation can be detected with either color or spectral Doppler interrogation (11).

Percutaneous intervention

A multiciplity of techniques and guidance modalities have been described in the approach to percutaneous drainage of pancreatic pseudocysts and abscesses. CT is a frequently employed and effective method for placement of drainage tubes. The combined use of real-time ultrasound and fluoroscopy offers several attractive features. Ultrasound is considerably less costly and generally more widely and readily available. Then, too, ultrasound permits continuous monitoring of the puncturing needle (or trochar-catheter device) to insure its proper placement within the fluid collection. The supplemental use of fluoroscopy to follow guide wires and catheters during the introduction process serves to minimize chances for kinking of wires or tubes. We have found the combined use of sonographic and fluoroscopic monitoring of fluid drainage to provide the most cost effective, rapid, and readily available approach (8, 12–18).

Chronic pancreatitis

Recurrent bouts of acute pancreatitis will produce sonographically demonstrable signs of chronic inflammation, including irregular

Figure 11 *Transverse (a) and sagittal (b) scans of a patient with chronic calcific pancreatitis. Multiple shadowing calculi (arrows in a) are seen distributed throughout the gland. The conglomerate calcifications produce a large area of shadowing (arrowheads in b). The gland is outlined by short white arrows in b. A = aorta.*

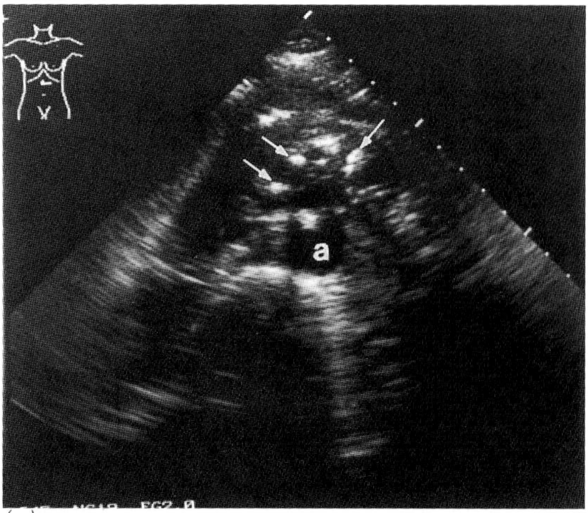

(a)

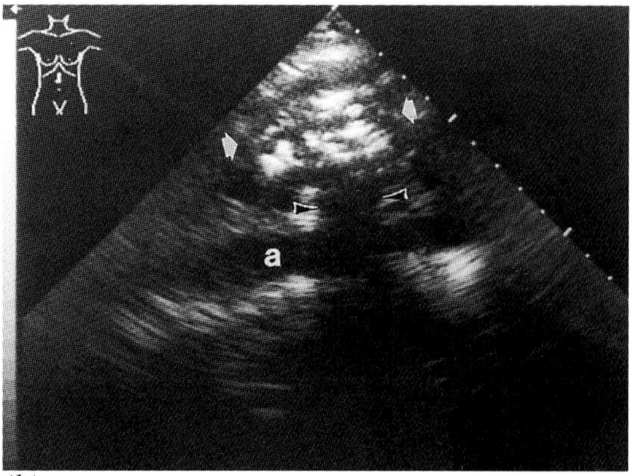

(b)

areas of increased echogenicity representing fibrosis and/or calcification. The increase in echogenicity in chronic pancreatitis is patchy and heterogeneous in contrast to the normal homogeneous increase in echotexture of the pancreas which results from fatty replacement of glandular tissue. In chronic pancreatitis the gland is usually diminished in volume and often difficult to outline. Pseudocyst formation has been reported in 25–60 % of patients with chronic pancreatitis as well (19) (Figure 11).

Dilatation of the pancreatic duct may also be a result of chronic inflammation; the dilatation is often described as irregular or "string of beads" as a consequence of alternating areas of dilatation and fibrotic stricture. This appearance is sometimes offered as

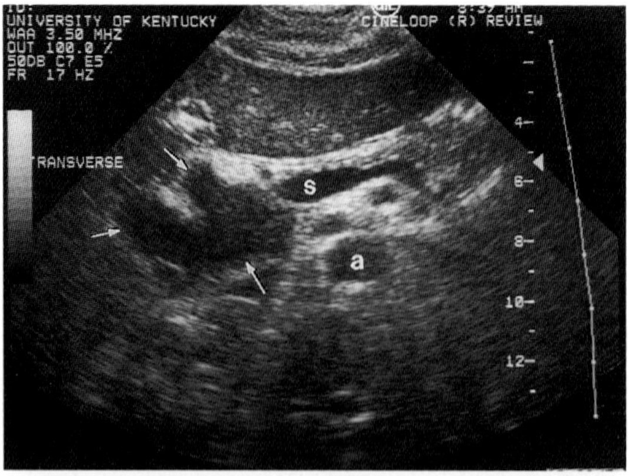

Figure 18 *Lobular enlargement and obscuration of the head of the pancreas (arrows) is produced by metastases to peripancreatic nodes from ovarian carcinoma. a = aorta; s = splenic vein.*

serve to distinguish peripancreatic adenopathy from primary neoplasm (Figure 18).

INTRAOPERATIVE ULTRASOUND

One of the most useful applications of intraoperative ultrasound in the pancreas is the location of the small, endocrinologically active tumors described above. Employing transducer frequencies of 5–10 MHz and either direct contact or water bath scanning of the exposed pancreas makes possible the identification of tumors as small as 3 mm and greatly facilitates the search for multiple tumors as in the case of gastrinoma. If frozen section provides pathological indication of a malignant tumor, intraoperative ultrasound examination should be extended to the liver to search for possible metastastic foci (33–38) (Figure 19).

Another intraoperative application for ultrasound is the identification and location of the dilated pancreatic duct. In cases in which the surgeon wishes to cannulate the duct (frequently as a preliminary step in the eventual performance of a pancreaticojejunostomy), a needle is inserted into the duct under sonographic control (a 10 MHz linear transducer is most effective) and dissection then carried out following the needle down to the duct.

The occasional small intrapancreatic pseudocyst and the much less common true cyst of the pancreas which are not readily visible or palpable at surgery can be easily located with intraoperative ultrasound.

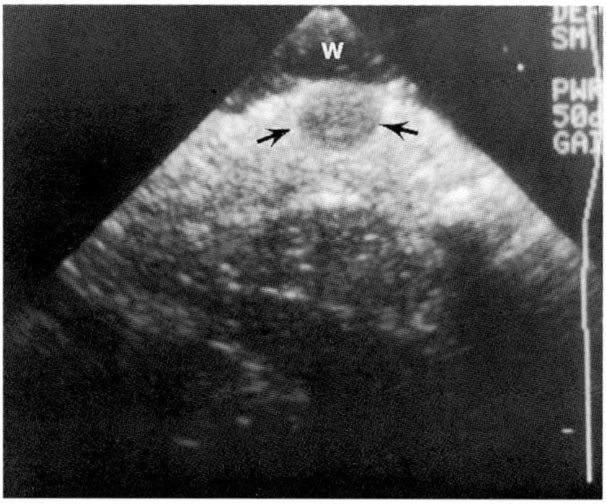

Figure 19 *Intraoperative localization of small (1.3 cm) insulinoma (arrows). The pancreas is scanned through a water bath (w) created by simply filling the abdomen with warm saline.*

ENDOSCOPIC ULTRASOUND

Still available only on a limited basis, the technique of endoscopic ultrasound (EUS) provides unique capabilities in the evaluation of the pancreas and biliary tract. Employing transducers with frequencies at and above 10 MHz integrated into an endoscope, endoscopic ultrasound produces exquisite resolution of small masses, adjacent lymph nodes and the pancreatic and biliary ducts. The drawbacks to the technique include the high cost and limited availability (and applicability) of the equipment and the expertise required of both the endoscopist and the ultrasonologist (as well as the difficulty of scheduling both in the same room simultaneously). Technical limitations include the limited depth of penetration which comes with such high frequencies and the unusual (and frequently changing) orientation of the images. These difficulties notwithstanding, EUS is a promising adaptation of well-proven technology and provides clinically useful information not otherwise available (39–41).

REFERENCES

1. Atri M, Finnegan PW. The pancreas in diagnostic ultrasound. Rumack CM, Wilson SR, Charboneau JW (eds): Mosby Yearbook, St Louis, 1991:145–154.

2. Niederau C, Sonnenberg A, Muller JE et al. Sonographic measurements of the normal liver, spleen, pancreas and portal vein. Radiology 1983;149:537–540.
3. Patel S, Bellon EM, Haaga J et al. Fat replacement of the exocrine pancreas. AJR 1980;135:843–845.
4. Bryan PJ. Appearance of normal pancreatic duct: a study using real-time ultrasound. J Clin Ultrasound 1982;10:63–66.
5. Hadidi A. Pancreatic duct diameter: sonographic measurement in normal subjects. J Clin Ultrasound 1983;11:17–22.
6. Neff CC, Simeone JF, Wittenberg J et al. Inflammatory pancreatic masses: problems in differentiating focal pancreatitis from carcinoma. Radiology 1984;150:35–40.
7. Jeffrey R B Jr. Sonography in acute pancreatitis. Radiol Clin N Am 1989;27:5–17.
8. Balthazar EJ, Freeny PC, vanSonnenberg E. Imaging and intervention in acute pancreatitis. Radiology 1994;193:297–306.
9. Lee CM, Chang-Chien CS, Lim DY et al. Real-time ultrasonography of pancreatic pseudocyst: comparison of infected and uninfected pseudocysts. J Clin Ultrasound 1988; 16:393–397.
10. Ros PR, Hamrick-Turner JE, Chiechi MV et al. Cystic masses of the pancreas. Radiographics 1992;12:673.
11. Falkoff GE, Taylor KJW, Morse SS. Hepatic artery pseudoaneurysm: diagnosis with real-time and pulsed Doppler ultrasound. Radiology 1986;58:55–56.
12. vanSonnenberg E, D'Agostino HB, Casola G et al. Percutaneous abscess drainage: current concepts. Radiology 1991;181:617.
13. Lambiase RE, Deyoe L, Cronan JJ et al. Percutaneous drainage of 335 consecutive abscesses: results of primary drainage with 1-year follow-up. Radiology 1992;184:167.
14. Feig BW, Pomerantz RA, Vogelzang R et al. Treatment of peripancreatic fluid collections in patients with complicated acute pancreatitis. Surg Gynecol Obstet 1992;175:429–436.
15. Jeffrey RB, Laing FC, Wing VW. Extrapancreatic spread of acute pancreatitis: new observations with real-time ultrasound. Radiology 1986;159:707–711.
16. vanSonnenberg E, Wittich GR, Casola G et al. Percutaneous drainage of infected and noninfected pancreatic pseudocysts: experience in 101 cases. Radiology 1989;170:757–761.
17. Bradley EL, Clements JL, Gonzalez AC. The natural history of pancreatic pseudocysts: a unified concept of management. Am J Surg 1979;137:135–141.
18. Lee MJ, Rattner DW, Legemate DA et al. Acute complicated pancreatitis: redefining the role of interventional radiology. Radiology 1992;183:171–174.

19. Bolondi L, LiBassi S, Gaiani S et al. Sonography of chronic pancreatitis. Radiol Clin N Amer 1989;27:815–833.
20. Swobodnik W, Wolf A, Wechsler JG et al. Ultrasound characteristics of the pancreas in children with cystic fibrosis. J Clin Ultrasound 1985;13:469–474.
21. Choyke PL, Filling-Katz MR, Shawker TH et al. von Hippel-Lindau disease: radiologic screening for visceral manifestataions. Radiology 1990;174:815.
22. Ekberg O, Bergenfeldt M, Aspelin P et al. Reliability of ultrasound-guided fine-needle biopsy of pancreatic masses. Acta Radiologica 1988;29:535–539.
23. Brandt KR, Charboneau JW, Stephens DH et al. CT- and US-guided biopsy of the pancreas. Radiology 1993;187:99.
24. Campbell JP, Wilson S. Pancreatic neoplasms: how useful is evaluation with ultrasound? Radiology 1988;167:341–344.
25. Buck JL, Hayes WS. From the archives of the AFIP. microcystic adenoma of the pancreas. Radiographics 1990;10:313.
26. Padovani B, Neuveut P, Chanalet S et al. Microcystic adenoma of the pancreas: report on four cases and review of the literature. Gastrointest Radiol 1991;16:62.
27. Phillips GWL, Chou ST, Mulhauser J. Papillary cystic tumour of the pancreas: findings at computed tomography and ultrasound. Br J Radiol 1991;64:367.
28. Johnson CD, Stephens DH, Charboneau JW et al. Cystic pancreatic tumors: computed tomography and sonographic assessment. AJR 1988;151:1133–1138.
29. Mathieu D, Guigui B, Valette PJ et al. Pancreatic cystic neoplasms. Radiol Clin N Am 1989: 27:163–176.
30. Fugazzola C, Procacci C, Andreis IAB et al. Contribution of ultrasonography and computed tomograhy in the diagnosis of nonfunctioning islet cell tumors of the pancreas. Gastrointest Radiol 1990;15:139.
31. London JF, Shawker TH, Doppman JL et al. Zollinger-Ellison syndrome: prospective assessment of abdominal US in the localization of gastrinomas. Radiology 1991;178:763.
32. Rossi P, Allison DJ, Bezzi M et al. Endocrine tumors of the pancreas. Radiol Clin N Am 1989;27:129–161.
33. Clyne CAC, Greene WJ, Paisey RB. Intra-operative ultrasound localization of an insulinoma undetected pre-operatively. JCU 1991;19:419.
34. Norton JA, Shawker TH, Doppman JL et al. Localization and surgical treatment of occult insulinomas. Ann Surg 1990;212:615–620.
35. Grant CS, van Heerden J, Charboneau JW et al. Insulinoma: the value of intraoperative ultrasonograhy. Arch Surg 1988;123:843–848.
36. Galiber AK, Reading CC, Charboneau JW et al. Localization of pancreatic insulinoma: comparison of pre- and intraoperative ultrasound with computed tomography and angiography. Radiology 1988;16:405–408.

37. Norton JA, Cromack DT, Shawker TH. Intraoperative ultrasonographic localization of islet cell tumors. Ann Surg 1988;207:160–168.
38. Shawker TH, Doppman JL. Intraoperative US. Radiology 1988;166:568–569.
39. Yamada M, Komoto E, Naito Y et al. Endoscopic ultrasonography in the diagnosis of pancreatic islet cell tumors. J Ultrasound Med 1991;10:271.
40. Lightdale CJ, Botet JF, Woodruff JM et al. Localization of endocrine tumors of the pancreas with endoscopic ultrasonography. Cancer 1991;68:1815–1820.
41. Yasuda K, Mukai H, Fujimoto S et al. The diagnosis of pancreatic cancer by endoscopic ultrasonography. Gastrointest Endosc 1988;34:1–8.

CHAPTER 6

The Spleen, Abdominal Vessels and Lymph Nodes

Keith Dewbury, MD, FRCR

THE SPLEEN

The spleen normally lies in the left upper quadrant of the abdomen between the 9th and 11th ribs. It is the largest lymphoid gland in the body with a mean weight of 150–180 grams. The long axis of the spleen is normally less than 13 cms, some departments use 12 cms as their maximum length.

Technique

No special preparation is required for examination of the spleen which forms an integral part of the full examination of the upper abdomen. The spleen is initially examined with the patient lying supine, the transducer being placed between the ribs in or near the mid axillary line to produce coronal and transverse images. Scanning is performed throughout quiet respiration. A deep inspiration often produces poor images by extending the pulmonary sulcus. Visualisation of the normal sized spleen may be improved by the patient lying in the right lateral decubitus position. A posterior or rarely an anterior approach can be useful.

Normal anatomy

The borders of the spleen are well defined and smooth. It is convex along its superior and lateral borders where it is covered by the diaphragm. Inferiorly it is related to the splenic flexure of the colon and the left kidney which produce concave impressions upon the spleen. Medially it is adjacent to the gastric fundus and pancreas. The hilar region is normally lobulated where the vascular pedicle attaches. Simple measurements of maximum splenic length is all that is performed in most departments. The normal adult spleen is usually less than 13 cms in its long axis (1). In children the splenic length is less than 7 cm below one year, increasing to 10 cms by 10 years (2). The normal splenic parenchyma displays a homogeneous pattern which consists in the main of low level echoes. The splenic hilum unlike the splenic substance returns higher level echoes. The normal splenic tissue is generally of slightly lower reflectivity than hepatic tissue, however, it may occasionally be more reflective in normal subjects. The internal vasculature of the spleen is not usually identified at any great distance from the hilum of the spleen.

Anomalies

Accessory spleen

The incidence of accessory spleen is approximately 10 %. They are almost always single but occasionally two or more may be present. Characteristically they are smooth rounded nodules 1–2 cms in diameter situated at or near the splenic hilum (Figure 1).

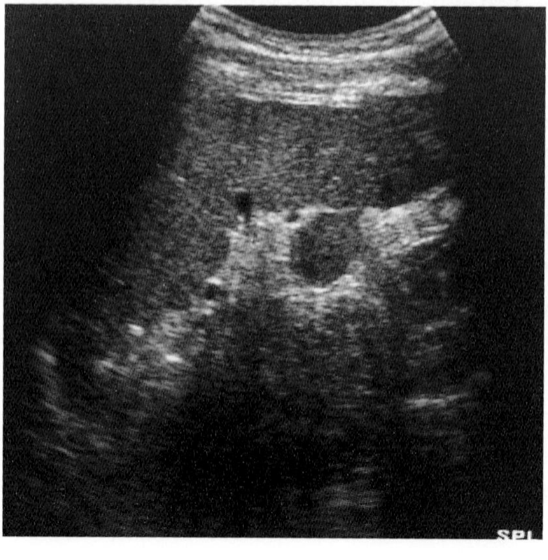

Figure 1 *Accessory spleen. Oblique intercostal scans showing the length of the spleen. The rounded accessory spleen or splenunculus lies at the hilum of the spleen and has the same echo texture as the spleen itself.*

Diagnosis is made from their position and texture. Hypertrophy of an accessory spleen in post splenectomy patients with haematological disease is a well recorded observation.

Polysplenia

Polysplenia is a rare syndrome characterised by multiple individual splenules in a retrogastric position. There is association with cardiac defects, biliary atresia and interposition of the IVC (3, 4).

Asplenia

Asplenia is a rare anomaly associated with congenital immune deficiency. Howell-Jolly bodies may be present in the peripheral blood.

Pathology

Diffuse splenic disease

Diffuse diseases may change the size or the echo pattern of the spleen or both. In practice, in the majority of cases analysis of the splenic echo texture is not particularly helpful as it is dependent on a number of factors including the vascularity of the organ or reactive changes and so is very non-specific.

Splenic enlargement occurs in a wide range of systemic or focal diseases (Figure 2): infections such as malaria and tuberculosis, blood dyscrasias, hereditary storage diseases such as Gaucher's, infiltration such as amyloid and sarcoid, chronic liver disease and portal vein thrombosis. Lymphoma is the commonest malignant tumour affecting the spleen and involvement may be diffuse or focal. Homogeneous splenic enlargement is frequently found during staging and the spleen may be echo poor or have increased reflectivity. More frequently, however, splenic reflectivity appears normal. Detection of splenomegaly is not reliable evidence of splenic involvement nor does a normal sized spleen exclude involvement with lymphoma. If splenic hilar adenopathy is present the likelihood of splenic involvement whatever the echo pattern is significantly increased.

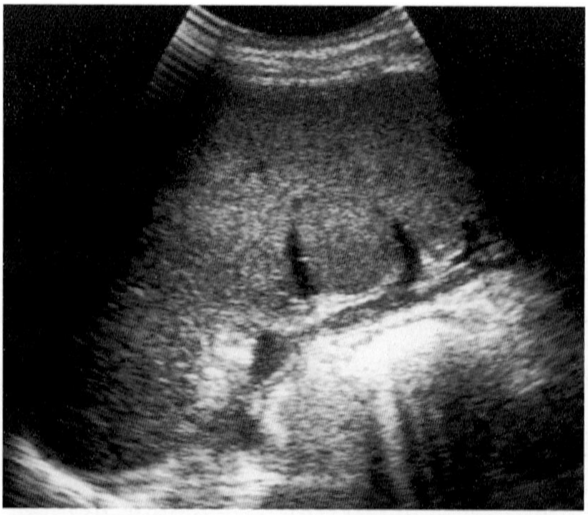

Figure 2 *Longitudinal scan of an enlarged spleen in a patient with myelofibrosis. The texture of the spleen is normal although it is considerably enlarged measuring some 20 cm in length. The vessels at the splenic hilum are correspondingly enlarged.*

Focal splenic disease

Ultrasound is sensitive in detecting focal splenic lesions, which are rarer than focal liver masses, but it lacks specificity.

Cysts

Non-parasitic cysts of the spleen are classified as primary or true cysts and false cysts or posttraumatic cysts (5, 6). True cysts have a cellular lining which may be mesothelial or epidermoid. On ultrasound, true cysts are indistinguishable from more commonly seen posttraumatic cysts. The cyst wall may occasionally calcify. Splenic cysts are often incidental asymptomatic findings but may occasionally produce discomfort or pain in the left upper quadrant of the abdomen. Most cysts are small but larger cysts are seen and may compress or distort the adjacent anatomy. Splenic cysts may be filled with cholesterol crystals which may make the lesion appear solid. Haemorrhage into the cyst may also produce debris and even septations within the cyst. Symptomatic splenic cysts may be decompressed percutaneously under ultrasound guidance. Spontaneous rupture of large cysts has been reported (7).

Hydatid cysts of the spleen are very uncommon being found in up to 2 % of all patients with echinococcus. Hydatid cysts may produce a typical appearance when multiple daughter cysts are present. However, the ultrasound findings of splenic hydatid cysts

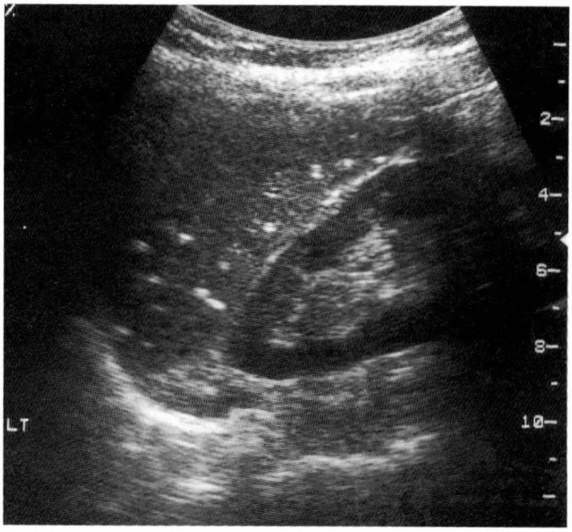

Figure 3 *Calcified splenic granulomas. Multiple small highly reflective foci are seen in this asymptomatic patient. The foci were considered to be due to healed tuberculous granulomas.*

are frequently non-specific, a simple unilocular cyst being the most usual finding.

Inflammatory and infectious diseases

Calcified granuloma are infrequent incidental findings. They are ascribed to previous granulomatous infection, such as tuberculosis or histoplasmosis. The appearances are often striking with multiple small highly reflective foci often with posterior shadowing (Figure 3). Splenic abscesses are uncommon, they are usually caused by haematogenous spread of infection that may develop after trauma or infection (8, 9). Patients that are immunocompromised and those with bacterial endocarditis are particularly at risk. The usual bacteria are streptococci, staphylococci, and salmonella. The ultrasound appearances are very variable as in liver abscess, typically they appear as a focal echo poor defect or as lesions with solid and cystic components.

In fungal abscesses of the spleen (splenic candidiasis) four patterns have been described: "wheel within wheel" lesions seen early on in the process, bullseye lesions, uniformly echo poor lesions and finally reflective foci with variable degrees of acoustic shadowing (10) (Figure 4). Many tropical parasitic diseases can produce non-specific splenomgaly. The commonest is chronic malaria.

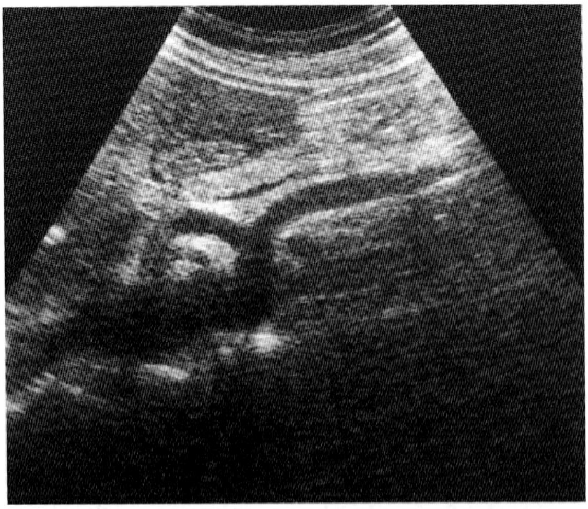

Figure 10 *A longitudinal scan through the abdominal aorta showing origin of the right hepatic artery from the superior mesenteric artery trunk.*

rior to the portal vein before entering the liver groove. The IVC tilts anteriorly before piercing the diaphragm to enter the right atrium of the heart. The major branches are the hepatic and renal veins all of which are usually well visualized.

The size of the IVC changes with respiration and cardiac cycles and with patient position. The size of the IVC is usually decreased with inspiration and Valsalva maneouvre and increased with expiration and suspended respiration after maximum inspiration.

Congenital anomalies

Congenital anomalies of the aorta are extremely rare; in situs inversus all the abdominal contents are transposed so that the aorta lies on the right side. Apart from its position the appearances are normal. Anomalies of the anterior aortic branches may be seen (Figure 10). Congenital anomalies of the IVC are not commonly identified on ultrasound but are important to define, prevent misdiagnosis and prior to abdominal surgery:

a. Interrupted IVC with azygos continuation. In this anomaly the suprarenal IVC fails to develop and venous drainage from below the diaphragm is shunted in the azygos and hemi-azygos veins which lie posteriorly to the crus. The azygos vein passes into the chest to empty into the superior vena cava in the usual way. The hepatic vein confluence drains directly into the right atrium.
b. Retro-aortic left renal vein.

c. Left-sided IVC. The upper part of the IVC is normal but the lower part does not develop from the right supracardinal vein, instead the left supracardinal vein remains patent forming a left sided IVC which crosses the midline at the level of the renal veins to continue cranially in a normal position (Figure 11 a, b).

Figure 11
Left sided IVC.
a. A right coronal section showing a left sided IVC discharging into the left renal vein and crossing the midline to continue in the normal position.
b. Transverse scans with a left image taken above the level of the left renal vein showing a normal right sided IVC. The right image shown below the level of the renal vein shows the continuation of the IVC to the left of the aorta.

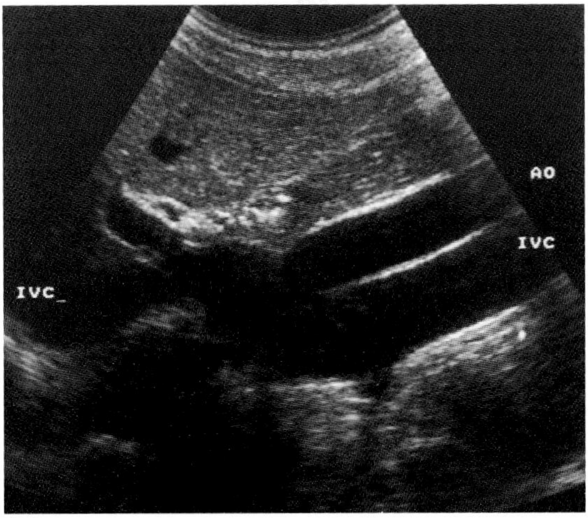

(a)

(b)
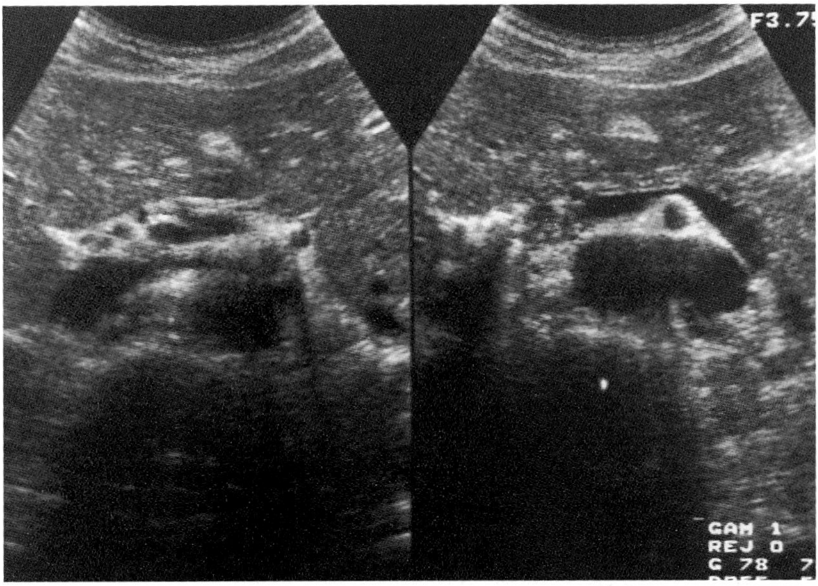

d. Duplication of the IVC which is a combination of a normal IVC and a left sided IVC as described above.

Pathology

Aorta

Atherosclerosis and ectasia

In atheroma the normally thin smooth endothelial lining of the aorta thickens and becomes irregular, often with calcification.

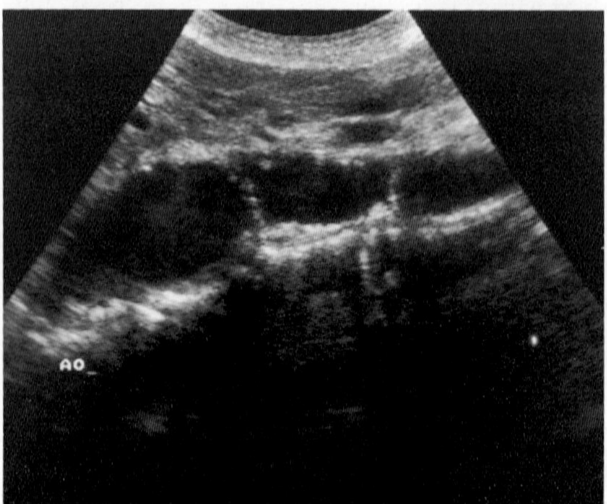

(a)

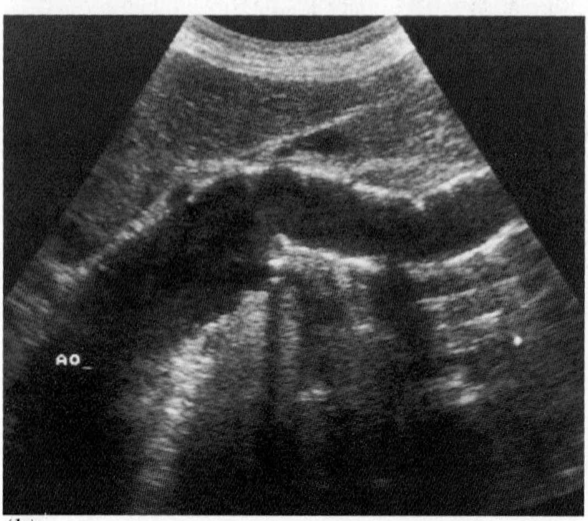

(b)

Figure 12 ***Ectatic aorta.***
a. Longitudinal section showing apparent "septations" within the aorta.
b. Coronal section showing the tortuosity of the ectatic aorta which has produced this appearance.

Larger plaques may impinge into the lumen. The aorta may also dilate slightly so that it looses its normal tapering configuration. Such ectatic aortas may produce a pulsatile epigastric "mass" that suggests an aneurysm. Ultrasound readily makes the distinction. The ectatic aorta may become very tortuous and may produce a somewhat confusing appearance occasionally (Figure 12).

Aortic aneurysm

Ultrasound has long been established as the procedure of choice for the evaluation of abdominal aortic aneurysms (19, 20). It is used initially to confirm the diagnosis and to differentiate it from other causes of a pulsatile mass such as a tortuous ectatic aorta, a hyperdynamic aorta in a thin patient or a para-aortic nodal mass. An aneurysm is diagnosed when the aortic diameter is greater than 3.0 cm (Figure 13). The majority are due to atherosclerosis although a small number are due to syphilis or trauma. Aneurysms are commoner in men and commoner in people over 55. The majority of aneurysms involve the middle and lower part of the aorta arising below the renal arteries. A distal aneurysm may extend into the iliac arteries. The diameter of the aneurysm is measured from outer wall to outer wall. Large aneurysms will usually contain a

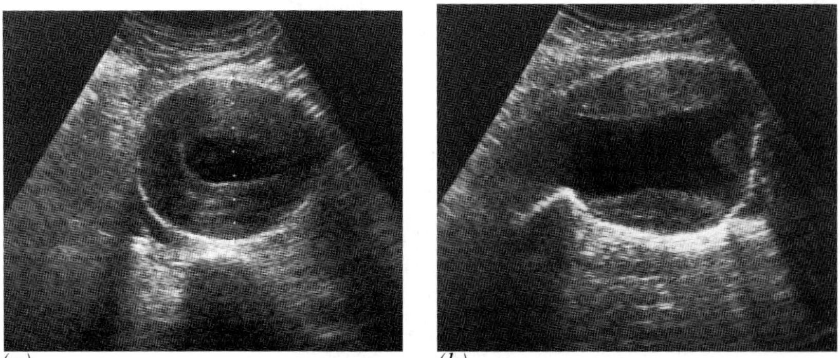

(a) (b)

Figure 13
a. Transverse section of a large aortic aneurysm measuring 7 × 9 cm in diameter. There is a large rim of concentric thrombus within the aneurysm.
b. A coronal section of the aneurysm showing its origin below the renal vessels and no extension into the iliac vessels.

crescent of thrombus within the lumen. The rupture rate for aneurysms less than 5 cm is less than 1 %. If the aneurysm is greater than 6 cm there is a 50 % one year mortality. The mortality for elective surgery is approximately 5 % and lower in specialist units. Aneuryms below 5 cms are usually scanned at yearly intervals. The average growth rate is 0.25 cms per year.

If expansion is more than 1 cm per year this is an indication for surgery. Elective surgery is usually recommended in aneurysms over 5 cms in diameter. In aortic dissection the intimal lining of the aorta separates from the rest of the wall (21). Ultrasound demonstrates a thin intra-luminal flap that moves with aortic pulsations (Figure 14).

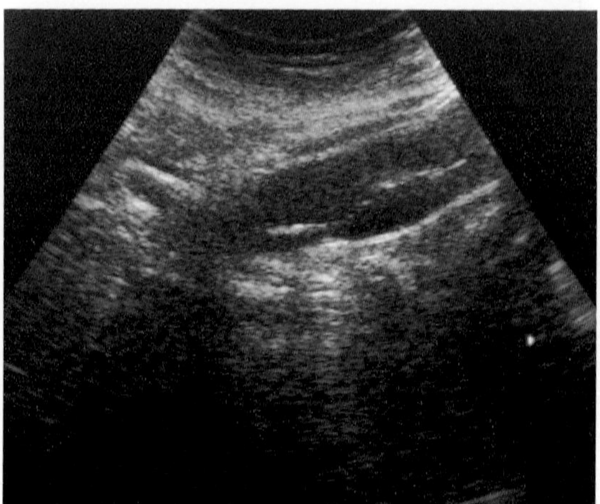

(a)

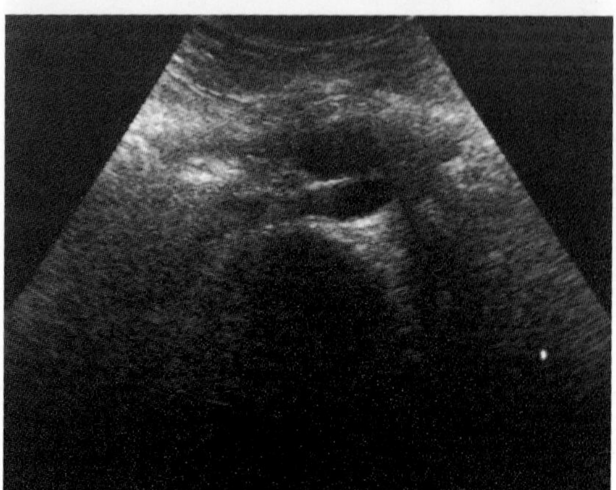

(b)

Figure 14
Aortic dissection.
a. Longitudinal scan, and b. transverse scan. The intimal flap is visualised as a fine mobile linear structure within the lumen. The differing flow patterns on either side of the flap can be demonstrated with colour Doppler.

Aortic grafts are identified by their typical sharply definied parallel reflective walls. The aneurysm sac is commonly wrapped around the aortic graft and not removed. The development of a new fluid collection around the graft may be due to haematoma, seroma or abscess. If bubbles of gas are present this suggests an abscess but needle aspiration may be necessary for differentiation. In graft occlusion, as with aortic occlusion the only ultrasound sign may be a lack of pulsatility so Doppler is required for a definitive diagnosis. One of the biggest problems for aortic ultrasound is measuring the aneurysm size in sequential scans in a consistent and accurate fashion. The width of the anerysm is less accurate than the AP diameter because the beam is parallel to the lateral aortic walls and so the lateral walls are often poorly defined. The aneurysm width however, is often the maximum diameter of the aneurysm. Inflammation around an aneurysm sac may produce a peri-aortitis which is associated with a retroperitoneal fibrosis (22).

Inferior Caval Vein (IVC)

IVC dilatation The IVC may enlarge because of proximal obstruction from many causes including right heart failure, chronic pulmonary disease, pericardial effusion with tamponade and constrictive pericarditis. With proximal obstruction the normal respiratory variation of IVC calibre will be lost and blood flow is slow.

IVC thrombus and tumour

Tumours arising around the IVC may compress or displace the IVC without invasion through the wall. This is most commonly seen with adrenal tumours and retroperitoneal lymphadenopathy. Extrinsic tumours may appear to obliterate the lumen. Direct invasion of the IVC wall is very uncommon but can be seen with retroperitoneal sarcoma and renal cell carcinoma. Even more rarely a primary leiomyosarcoma may arise in the IVC wall.

Primary renal cell carcinomas commonly have venous extension into the renal veins and IVC and this is reported in between 10 and 30 % of cases (Figure 15 a, b). Tumour extension into the

ileum by contrast is relatively featureless. The colon may appear sacculated particularly on the right side or in the transverse colon by the presence of haustra.

TECHNIQUE

With the advent of real time ultrasound the technique of examination of the solid organs in particular has become anatomically directed. Sections of the liver, for example, are produced in oblique fashion to follow the line of the portal vein and common bile duct. By contrast, evaluation of the peritoneal cavity and the bowel requires a return to the almost slavish production of sequential slices (6). Although with real time these are produced as a continuum nonetheless the entire surface of the abdomen must be covered by the passage of the probe. Typical frequencies used are between 3.5 and 5.0 MHz, although it may be possible to use higher frequencies to visualise superficially placed loops of bowel in an attempt to characterise wall layers. The advent of curved array transducers represents probably the ideal approach to scanning although both sector and linear array may be used and the linear array is of particular value in graded compression of the appendix for example. Scans are performed in longitudinal and transverse sections covering the entire abdomen if the purpose of the examination is to screen for an intraperitoneal abnormality. However, more frequently the examination is likely to be directed. For example, if there is a palpable right iliac fossa mass and pathology of the cecum is suspected then the attention of the sonologist should be directed to this area and then subsequently to the rest of the peritoneal cavity to assess complications such as ascites and to the liver to look for metastatic disease. Similarly, if the suspected diagnosis is a fluid collection such as an abscess then a number of factors will influence the way in which the examination is conducted. Abscesses are frequently post-operative and the post-operative wound and the presence of drain tubes may well limit access. The operator then has to be somewhat resourceful if he is to achieve visualisation of the whole of the peritoneal cavity. However, the nature of the surgery will also act to direct the process of scanning. Thus, if the patient has had a gastrectomy then the commonest site for the collection of fluid will be the left upper quadrant. Furthermore, features from other investigative techniques such as a raised hemidiaphragm on a chest or abdominal x-ray will also direct the sonologist to the most appropriate site for investigation. Occasionally, however, there is no such guidance. The patient presenting for example with fever, abdominal pain and a high white cell count but with no localising features will require examination of the entire peritoneal cavity. Nonetheless the examination should still be directed. In this situation, it is important to recognise the common sites for collection of peritoneal fluid. These are usually the dependant parts of the peritoneum: the Pouch of Douglas and Morrison's Pouch. These areas should be examined first, subsequently evaluating the subphrenic, subhepatic and perisplenic spaces before examining the paracolic gutters and finally the central abdomen since this will be the least common site for a fluid collection and incidentally the least reliable for diagnosis by ultrasound.

Examination of the peritoneal cavity and of the bowel requires a slight variation from normal ultrasound technique. The first is the process by which coronal scans of the abdomen are produced. Normally, when examining the flanks the patient is turned into a lateral decubitus position. When examining the peritoneum the patient should remain supine. Indeed, occasionally it is advisable to turn the patient slightly towards the transducer. There are two reasons for this. The first is that fluid will tend to collect in the more dependant part of the abdomen and therefore if the patient is turned away from the side of the examining transducer then fluid will collect on the contralateral side and possibly be missed. Similarly, a number of fluid collections may contain gas. Gas tends to rise to the top of a fluid collection and if the patient is in the decubitus position the change in position of the gas may continue to obscure a collection missed when the patient was scanned in longitudinal and transverse planes in supine position. The second technical feature concerns the use of compression. While graded compression (the gradual increase of abdominal pressure through the transducer) was described initially for the evaluation of suspected appendix pathology (7), it is applied to the evaluation of bowel throughout the abdomen. Because bowel can exist in so many different states a mixture of fluid, gas and/or faeces can occasionally produce the appearance of a pseudotumor. Compression by the transducer will displace gas allowing visualisation of deeper structures and will compress fluid and other bowel contents but not bowel pathologies.

Finally, careful attention needs to be given to the movement of bowel. Observation of peristalsis, an awareness of normal peristaltic patterns and an appreciation of increased, decreased or abnormal patterns of peristalsis are all important for the detection of not only bowel but also general peritoneal pathology.

INDICATIONS FOR ULTRASOUND EXAMINATION IN SUSPECTED BOWEL OR PERITONEAL PATHOLOGY

Ultrasound is an extremely sensitive tool for detecting free intra-abdominal fluid. As little as 100 cc of ascites may be detected, particularly if a dependant part of the abdomen is examined (6) (Figure 6). Ultrasound should therefore be the investigation of first choice in the evaluation of suspected ascites. Although characterisation of fluid versus solid has long been a feature of ultrasound examination, its role in the investigation of other abdominal fluid collections has been partly eclipsed by the advent of other imaging techniques. It must therefore be considered as complimentary to other investigative procedures. This clearly depends upon local availability and expertise but abdominal CT is likely to

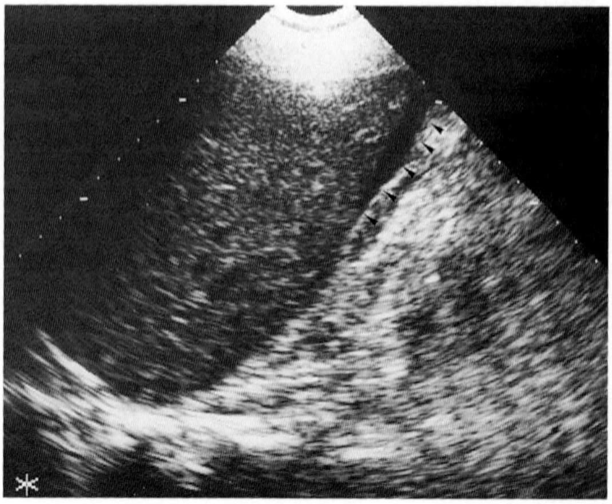

Figure 6 *Early ascites. A small thin collection is noted on the inferior margin of the liver (arrowheads).*

be more sensitive than ultrasound in the detection of abscesses and haematomas. Isotope imaging is also of particular value in the detection and location of inflammatory processes, especially when the origin is obscure (8). Similarly, ultrasound rarely will be used as the primary investigative means in the evaluation of suspected bowel pathology. For the most part the demonstration and characterisation of bowel pathology is consequent upon incidental findings – for example of bowel wall thickening. There are, however, exceptions: infantile hypertrophic pyloric stenosis, suspected appendicitis and intussusception are all clinical situations where ultrasound may be considered a first line investigation. Moreover, in the latter the use of saline per rectum may allow the ultrasound-guided hydrostatic reduction of an intussusception without the use of radiation exposure.

The use of fluid per rectum as a contrast medium is a further modification of ultrasound technique. First described in an attempt to differentiate true and pseudo masses of the rectum, others have developed the technique to allow complete evaluation of the colon, so called hydrocolonic sonography (9). In this situation it offers an alternative to barium studies and in some instances may provide greater information so that for example the depth of invasion of a tumour of the bowel can be identified.

PATHOLOGY OF THE PERITONEAL CAVITY

Abdominal collections and ascitic fluid

Ascites may occur in a number of pathological conditions. Classic ascitic fluid is categorised as exudative or transudative depending upon the etiology. Ultrasound appearances of ascitic fluid may infer whether it is a transudate or an exudate. The fluid when simple is echo-free, freely mobile in the peritoneal cavity on change in patient position, predominantly located in dependant parts of the abdomen and causing bowel loops to float freely within the centre of the abdomen (10) (Figure 7). When there are very small amounts of ascitic fluid these are rather more difficult to detect and subtle signs should be sought. Commonly, in these situations fluid collects in a thin film over the surface of the liver and around

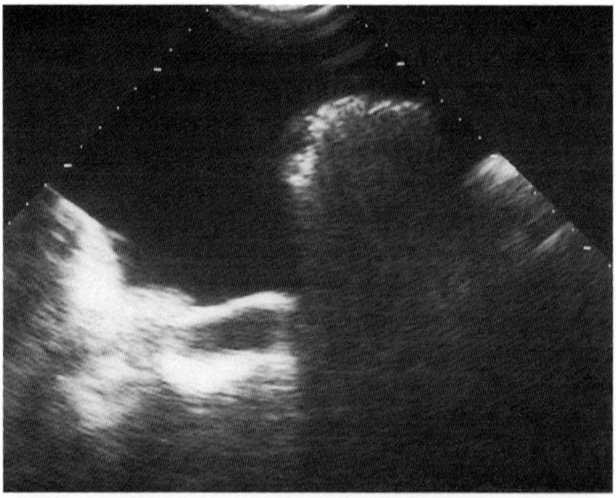

Figure 7 *Ascites. A large volume of echo free fluid is noted. There are floating bowel loops with distal acoustic shadowing.*

the gallbladder. Careful attention to these structures and to the spleen, particularly if the patient has been lying on the left hand side will allow the visualisation of very small amounts of ascitic fluid as an echo-free film on the margin of the organ. When the ascitic fluid is complicated the classical features previously described are often lost, thus the fluid may no longer be echo free but may contain multiple fine echoes which may even be seen to move upon compression with the transducer (Figure 8). The degree of echogenicity of the fluid may be used to predict transudate versus exudate, the latter only rarely being echo-free (11). Free motion of the fluid may be reduced or even absent with loculation of collections by adhesions (Figure 9). There may also be fixity of the bowel as a result of these adhesions and also because of thickening of the mesenteries fixing bowel to the posterior abdominal

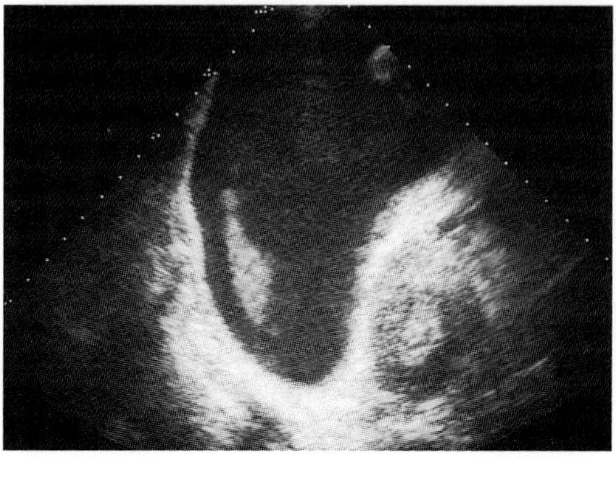

Figure 8
Complicated ascites. Transverse scan through the upper abdomen showing the inferior margin of the right lobe of the liver surrounded by echogenic fluid.

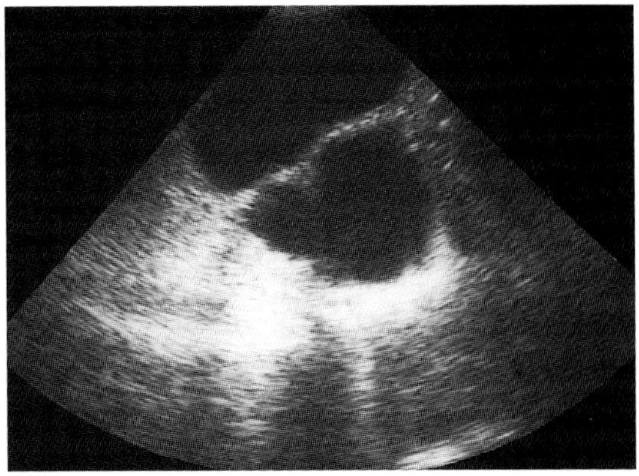

Figure 9
Complicated ascites. The fluid is loculated by a moderately thick septum.

wall so that it no longer floats freely in the ascitic fluid.

It was suggested that the presence of gallbladder wall thickening in ascites was a measure of hypoproteinaemia and therefore indicated a non-malignant exudate. However, the relationship between hypoproteinaemia and gallbladder wall thickening is inconstant and cannot therefore be used as a reliable indicator of the presence or absence of malignant pathology. Rather if the fluid appears simple then malignant pathology is unlikely while much more likely if complicated fluid has been demonstrated (6). Occasionally, when ascitic fluid is loculated it may produce a mass effect thus distorting adjacent solid organs such as the liver (12).

Haematomas, abscesses, etc

Classically, abscesses were described as oval or spherical structures containing echo poor fluid with multiple fine regular echoes. Haematomata were said to exhibit similar regular margins but contain coarser echogenic particles corresponding to aggregated clot. Fluid collections in the peritoneum rarely follow these "rules". The echo characteristics of the fluid not surprisingly depend upon the physical state of contents. Thus, haematomas may be echo free, contain fine echoes or aggregated material dependant upon the status of the blood within the cavity. Similarly abscesses may contain fine low level echoes when the pus is thin but may be grossly irregular with thickened walls and coarse aggregated echoes when the pus is thicker (Figures 10–17).

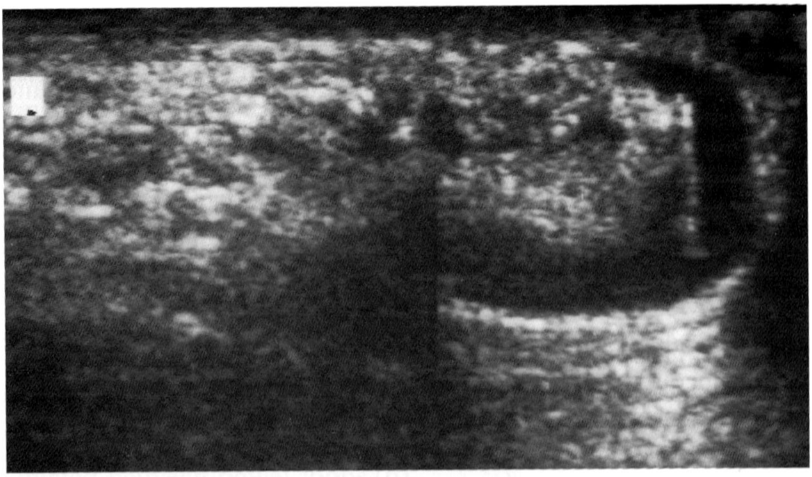

Figure 19 *Inguinal hernia. Bowel and mesentery is demonstrated along the length of the hernial sac.*

of the hernial orifices with high resolution high frequency ultrasound of the order of 7 MHz or above can demonstrate gas within the hernial sac or occasionally thickened bowel and mesentery (6) (Figure 19).

It is not suggested that ultrasound should replace the plain abdominal x-ray in situations where intestinal obstruction is suspected. Rather there are certain specific indications where ultrasound is of particular value. In infants and young children it may be of particular value in assessing the "gasless" abdomen. Similarly in closed loop obstruction the plain abdominal film may be negative for obstruction because of the absence of gas within the dilated loops.

Nonetheless, careful ultrasound examination will significantly augment the sensitivity and specificity of investigation in all cases of suspected bowel obstructions. One series suggests that diagnostic accuracy of ultrasound in this clinical situation is 89 % while that of the plain abdominal film only 71 % (13).

The atypical target or pseudo-kidney sign

Thickening of the bowel wall produces an alteration of the mucus pattern that has been described above. This has been termed the

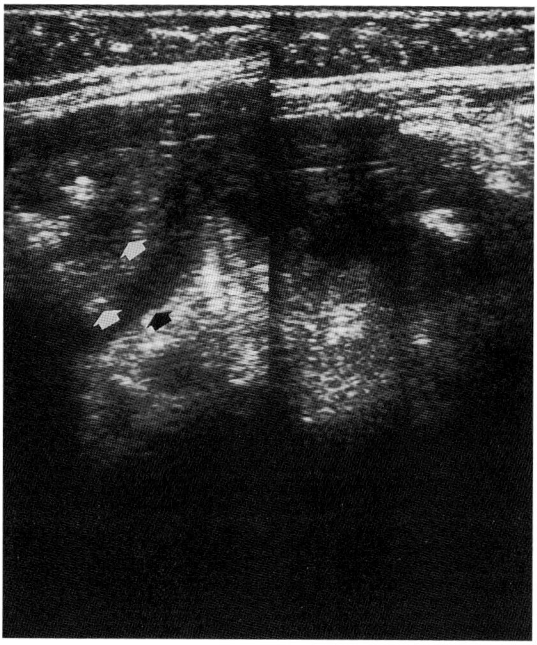

Figure 20 *Extensive bowel wall thickening in Crohn's disease. There is thickening of all the layers (arrowheads).*

atypical target sign or the pseudo-kidney sign particularly when an affected segment of bowel is viewed in longitudinal section and where the wall thickening is particularly marked. The normal thickness of the bowel wall is usually less than 4.0 mm in the collapsed state. Therefore, bowel wall thickness in excess of 5.0 mm is highly specific for bowel pathology (14) (Figure 20). However, to a very large degree the features of bowel wall thickening cannot be used to differentiate between different pathologies involving the intestinal wall. While inflammatory pathologies tend to involve long segments of bowel and neoplastic pathologies rather shorter segments, exceptions to this rule are found in intestinal lymphoma and with "kissing carcinomas". Furthermore, the inflammatory response that occurs in many intestinal neoplasms may obscure the underlying pathology. Certain authors have suggested that differentiation of inflammatory from malignant pathology can be based on the degree of bowel wall thickening implying that the thickest bowel wall is seen in malignant pathology. Our work would not confirm this with bowel wall thicknesses in Crohn's disease for example in excess of 20 mm. Other workers have suggested that the differentiation of different bowel layers, preserved in inflammatory disease but lost in malignant processes, will allow the identification of specific bowel processes (Figure 21). This suggestion is confounded by the relative infrequency in normal patients and particularly in the obese of different bowel layers, even in well defined inflammatory processes. However, early work suggests that hydrocolonic sonography may facilitate the differentiation of bowel wall layers and thus allow greater specificity in diagnosis of bowel pathology (15).

Although for the large part the demonstration of an atypical target appearance is a non-specific sign of disease of the bowel requiring further investigation perhaps by contrast studies there are certain circumstances in which ultrasound has a major role to play and where a specific diagnosis may be possible.

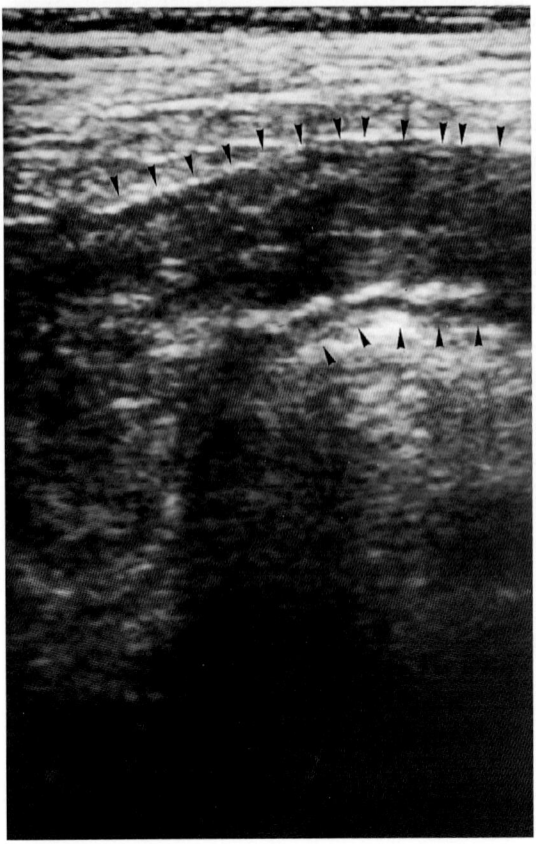

Figure 21 *Diffuse bowel wall thickening (arrowheads) without a clearly identified lumen in ulcerative colitis.*

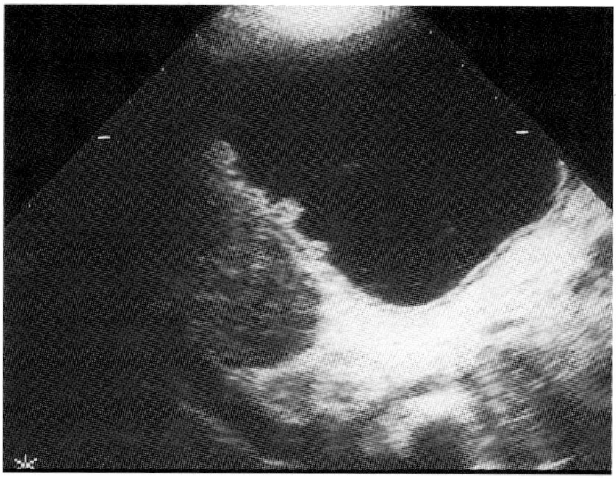

Figure 22 *Distended stomach in a patient with gastric outflow obstruction consequent upon peptic ulceration.*

Peptic ulcers

Peptic ulcers produce thickening of the gastric or duodenal wall with occasional demonstration of an ulcer crater (16). When seen in association with gastric distention the features are highly suggestive.

Gastric carcinoma

Endoscopic and endoluminal ultrasound techniques occupy pride of place in the investigation of gastric carcinoma. Nonetheless, antral carcinomas in particular can be demonstrated in excess of 70 % of cases particularly if oral contrast is used to improve gastric wall visualisation (17). In the investigation of the epigastric mass this is clearly of differential diagnostic importance. Furthermore, the demonstration of enlarged coeliac lymph nodes and/or hepatic metastases will allow prompt staging of the tumour and allow the avoidance of further more invasive procedures (Figure 23).

The use of ingested fluid to improve gastric wall visualisation has hitherto been less successful than hydrocolonic sonography. Most attempts have failed to eliminate ingested gas. However, it appears that the use of oral cellulose may have significant advantages for ultrasound imaging (18).

Hypertrophic infantile pyloric stenosis

The infant who presents with projectile vomiting and an epigastric mass can now be investigated by ultrasound evaluation alone

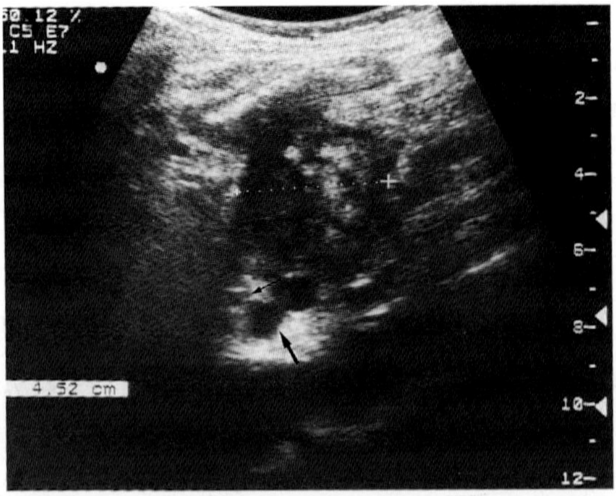

Figure 23 *Gastric tumour with lymphadenopathy. There is an irregular bowel associated mass in the epigastrium with asymmetric thickening (cursors identify measurement of the bowel mass). At least two lymph nodes situated posterior to the main body of the mass (arrows).*

without recourse to barium studies. Many surgeons are prepared to operate on infants in whom ultrasound has demonstrated a mass in the region of the pyloric canal measuring in excess of 8.0 mm in width and 12.0 mm in length (6).

However, occasionally the antropyloric muscle may not demonstrate thickening on ultrasound examination. Therefore, when the clinical suspicion is high other investigations should be performed if ultrasound is normal (19).

Intussusception

It is now considered almost invariably unnecessary to perform contrast enema for diagnosis of intussusception (2). The appearances on ultrasound are quite characteristic. While there is thickening of the bowel in the region of the intussusceptum this is demonstrated as concentric circles on a transverse scan of the bowel loop and as the "trident" or "hayfork" sign of the intussuscipiens and intussusceptum on a scan in a plane along the long axis of the affected loop of bowel (Figure 24). Certain authors have also used colour flow Doppler to assess the viability and reducibility of the bowel loop implying that the absence of a Doppler signal indicate a condition that is unlikely to be amenable to hydrostatic reduction (21). The presence of free intraperitoneal fluid is a non-specific finding and although it decreases the likelihood of hydrostatic reduction it should not be used as a reason not to attempt reduc-

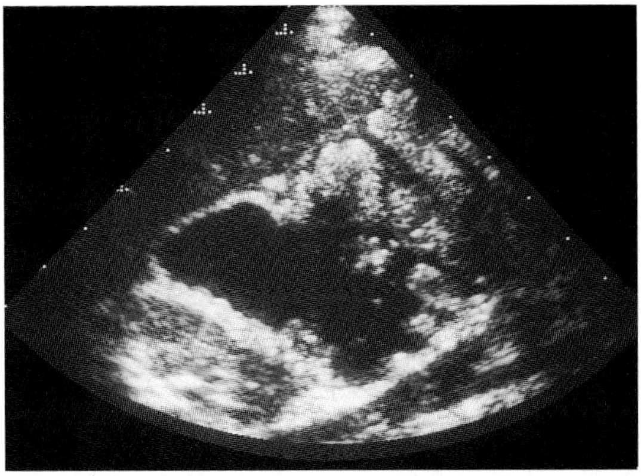

Figure 24
Intussusception. There is dilated bowel proximal to a bowel associated mass.

tion prior to surgery (22). The process of hydrostatic reduction may now be achieved simply by the use of saline under ultrasound rather than x-ray image intensification control. Isotonic saline infused into the rectum will allow the demonstration of movement of the intussusceptum and finally reflux of saline into the small bowel.

Acute appendicitis (7, 23)

Although the normal appendix is only infrequently visualized on even high frequency abdominal ultrasound examination (probably less than 30 % of cases) the abnormal appendix is clearly visible. The technique for visualisation of appendiceal pathology is a modification of compression techniques applied elsewhere in the abdomen. The ultrasound probe is applied to McBurney's point and a gradual increase in the pressure applied to the transducer. This gradual increase in pressure allows the displacement of gas while minimising patient discomfort. It is important to remember not to release the pressure rapidly since the technique is not applied to demonstrate peritonism which has already presumably been painfully elicited by the physician or surgeon. Appendiceal pathology is characterised by thickening of the appendix to > 6.0 mm (Figure 25), the presence of thickened echogenic omentum and frequently also the presence of a focal fluid collection either in the right iliac fossa or in the Pouch of Douglas or rectovesical pouch. Clearly in appendiceal perforation free intraperitoneal fluid

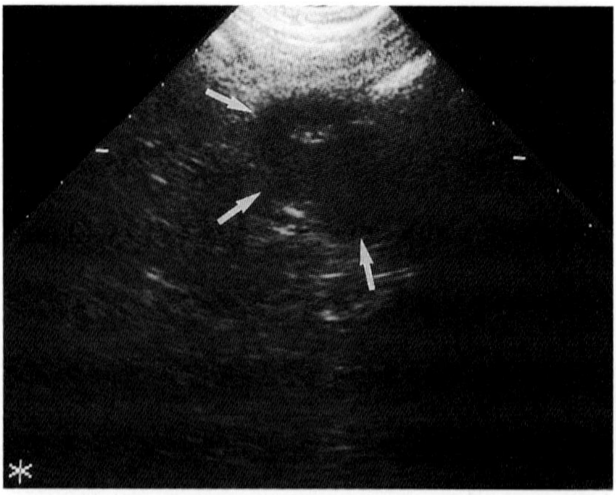

Figure 25
Acute appendicitis. There is a bowel associated mass in the right iliac fossa (arrows). In this situation it is not possible to distinguish this from other causes of bowel wall thickening.

may be demonstrated. An appendicolith may occasionally be demonstrated in the neck of the appendix.

Although frequently appendiceal thickening per se is demonstrated occasionally simply a bowel associated mass is identified in the right iliac fossa with or without a focal fluid collection. In this situation it is not possible to differentiate between an acute appendicitis and other diseases of the cecum and appendix including cecal tumour, cecal tuberculosis, etc.

Inflammatory bowel disease (24)

The inflammatory bowel diseaseases: Crohn's disease and ulcerative colitis, may produce bowel wall thickening which is diffuse and extensive. The thickening is normally greater in Crohn's disease than in ulcerative colitis reflecting the transmural nature of the pathology. Also in Crohn's disease it may be possible to demonstrate the involvement of intestine by skip lesions, i.e. non contiguous loops of affected bowel. Complications such as pericolic abscesses and mucocutaneous fistulae can also be demonstrated. Differentiation of different inflammatory diseases of the bowel by demonstration of loss or preservation of bowel wall layers is unreliable with transabdominal ultrasound (Figure 26). However, Limberg and Osswald claim that using hydrocolonic sonography such distinction is possible with the layered structure being lost in Crohn's but preserved in U.C. (15).

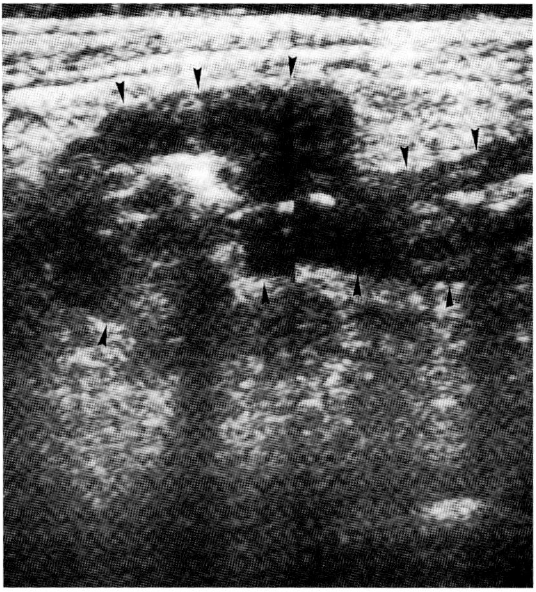

Figure 26
Crohn's disease. Diffuse irregular thickening of bowel (arrowheads).

Diverticular disease will produce similar features of segmental bowel wall thickening. The circular muscle hypertrophy that occurs in diverticular disease will occasionally produce a pattern which has been described as a "concertina". Other causes of diffuse bowel inflammation include antibiotic related enteropathy. The features are often indistinguishable from the other diffuse inflammatory processes of the bowel and may also mimic diffuse bowel ischaemia.

MISCELLANEOUS

The demonstration of bowel wall thickening is the mainstay of diagnosis of bowel pathology. While the finding is non-specific in terms of the nature of intestinal pathology, seen for example in carcinoma and lymphoma, inflammatory processes such as Crohn's disease, appendicitis, chronic granulomatous disease of childhood, tuberculosis, ischaemic colitis, etc., it may also be seen in other conditions. These include portal hypertension, intestinal haemorrhage such as in Henoch Schönlein Purpura. In all of these conditions appropriate ultrasound may be used to monitor the progress of treatment. This is particularly important in childhood where the repeated use of ionising radiation is to be discouraged.

The importance of the demonstration of bowel wall thickening is that the positive predictive value of finding a pseudo-kidney sign is as high as 86 % (25).

Ultrasound is finding application in other pathologies within the abdomen. Although of clear value in the assessement of infants with persistent vomiting to demonstrate or exclude the diagnosis of IHPS (26), it also appears to be of value in the diagnosis of gastro-oesophageal reflux in the same group of infants. It appears that the length of the abdominal oesophagus is fundamental for the production of gastro-oesophageal reflux and ultrasound is a sensitive technique for the measurement and evaluation of this portion of the oesophagus (27).

Although intraluminal air has been considered to be an impediment to the diagnosis both of bowel and other intra-abdominal pathology, the greater understanding of the distribution of bowel and contents within the abdomen and its demonstration by ultrasound has allowed the detection and characterisation of gas elsewhere. Thus free gas in association with fluid within the peritoneum either on the surface of the liver or close to one of the hemidiaphragms appears to refine the sensitivity for the diagnosis of perforation of a hollow viscus (24), but also it is possible to demonstrate a "bright ring" appearance of affected bowel in the presence of intramural gas indicating bowel necrosis. Since ultrasound forms the primary diagnostic technique in many situations the recognition of such findings is critical for proper management of the patient (28).

The combination of ultrasound with other investigative techniques such as contrast studies may enhance the demonstration of small bowel tumours and improve the demonstration of extent and invasion.

DOPPLER TECHNIQUE IN BOWEL DISEASE

At present, neither pulsed nor colour flow Doppler have an established role in the investigation of intestinal disease. While hyperaemia may be demonstrated in superficial bowel loops in the presence of inflammatory processes and occasionally also in neoplasia visualisation of these features is inconstant and therefore not reliable for specific diagnosis. Similarly, hyperaemic patterns in the superior mesenteric and inferior mesenteric artery in Crohn's and other inflammatory processes are only infrequently demonstrated. Moreover, the demonstration of acute bowel ischaemia, critical for this life threatening condition is not reliably achieved by transabdominal Doppler techniques.

However, the activity of certain pathologies such as Crohn's disease may be inferred from colour flow Doppler patterns of mucosal perfusion and the loss of perfusion may be used as a predictor of the need for surgical intervention in for example intussusception (21) (Figure 27).

Furthermore, in chronic mesenteric ischaemia – intestinal angina duplex evaluation of compromise of flow in the coeliac axis and superior mesenteric artery appear highly sensitive in predicting the results of angiography. It is possible therefore to use these techniques to screen for mesenteric angina (24).

Figure 27 *Colour Doppler energy (Doppler angio) of a patient with acute active Crohn's disease demonstrating the hyperaemia.*

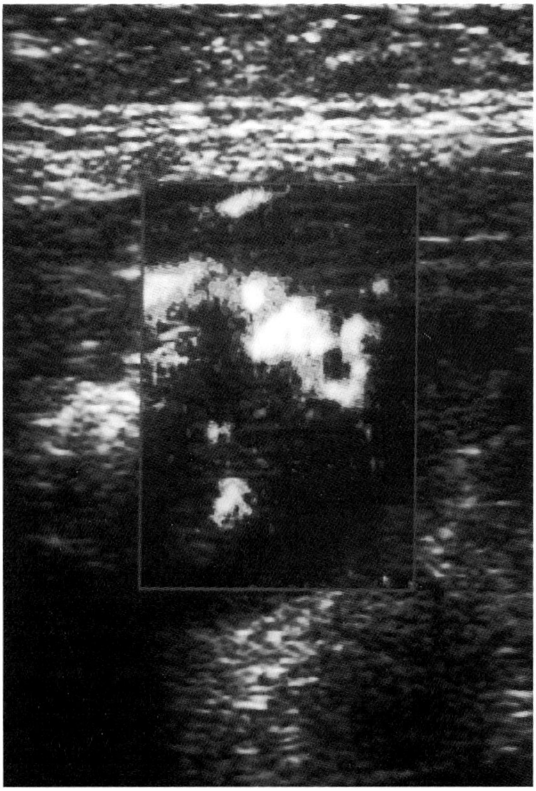

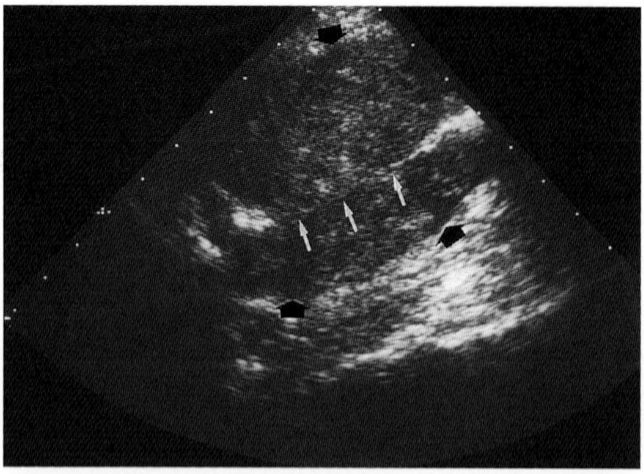

Figure 28 *Carcinoma of the left colon demonstrating complete obliteration of the bowel lumen (arrows) by a large mass anterior to the ilio-psoas muscles (arrowheads).*

SUMMARY

Ultrasound occupies a central role as the first procedure in a variety of different pathological conditions. Because of this intestinal pathology will frequently be discovered during the course of an examination of the abdomen (Figure 28). There are certain pathological conditions of the gastrointestinal tract in which ultrasound is indicated as the first and sometimes only investigation necessary for diagnosis and management. In other situations ultrasound will form part of the diagnostic pathway guiding subsequent investigations. It is, however, clear that it is no longer the case that gut simply provides an impediment to ultrasound imaging of the abdomen rather that ultrasound imaging of the gut has come of age.

REFERENCES

1. Wyburn GM. The peritoneum. In: Romanes GJ (ed). Cunningham's Textbook of Anatomy, 10th ed. Oxford University Press, 1964:403–405.
2. Weill F, Watrin J, Rohmer P et al. Ultrasound and CT of peritoneal recesses and ligaments. A pictorial essay. Ultrasound Med Biol 1986;12:977–989.
3. Meyer MA. The spread and localization of acute peritoneal effusions. Radiology 1970;95:547–554.
4. Fleischer AC, Muhletaler CA, Everett-James A. Sonographic patterns arising from normal and abnormal bowel. Radiol Clin N Am 1980;18:145–159.
5. Meiser G, Meissner K, Satlegger P. Perkutane Schichdifferenzierung der Kolonwand durch Ultraschall. Ultraschall 1988;9:41–44.
6. Dubbins PA. Gastrointestinal tract and peritoneum. In: Goldberg

BB (ed). Textbook of Abdominal Ultrasound. Williams & Wilkins, 1993:221–260 (ch 10).

7. Puylaert JBC. Acute appendicitis: US evaluation using graded compression. Radiology 1986;158:355.
8. Joseph AE. Imaging of abdominal abscesses. Br Med J 1985;291:1446–1447.
9. Limberg B. (Diagnosis of tumours of the large intestine by colonic ultrasound). In German. Ultraschall Med 1990;11:127–131.
10. Edell SL, Gefter WB. Ultrasonic differentiation of type of ascitic fluid. AJR 1979;133:111–114.
11. Mallde HM, Gandhi RD. Exudative vs. transudative ascites: differentiation based on fluid echogenicity on high resolution sonography. J Postgrad Med 1993;39:132–133.
12. Baer JW. Extraperitoneal mass effect by ascites under tension. Gastrointest Radiol 1990;15:3–8.
13. Ko YT, Lim JH, Lee DH et al. Small bowel obstruction: sonographic evaluation. Radiology 1993; 188:649–653.
14. Bozkurt T, Richter F, Lux G. Ultrasonography as a primary diagnostic tool in patients with inflammatory disease and tumors of the small intestine and large bowel. J Clin Ultrasound 1994;22:85–91.
15. Limberg B, Osswald B. Diagnosis and differential diagnosis of ulcerative colitis and Crohn's disease by hydrocolonic sonography. Am J Gastroenterol 1994;89:1051–1057.
16. Lim JH, Lee DH, Ko YT. Sonographic detection of duodenal ulcer. J Ultrasound Med 1992;11:91.
17. Miyamoto Y, Nakatani M, Ida M et al. Ultrasonographic findings in gastric cancer: in vitro and in vivo studies. J Clin Ultrasound. 1989;17:309.
18. Lund PJ, Fritz TA, Unger CA et al. Cellulose as a gastrointestinal contrast agent. Radiology 1992;185:783.
19. O'Keeffe FN, Stansberry SD, Swischuk LE, Hayden CK Jr. Antropyloric muscle thickness at US in infants: what is normal? Radiology 1991;178:827–830.
20. Shanbhogue RL, Hussain SM, Meradji M et al. Ultrasonography is accurate enough for the diagnosis of intussusception. J Ped Surg 1994; 29:324–327.
21. Avni EF, Rypens FR. Pediatric gastrointestinal tract. In: Dubbins PA, Joseph AE (eds). Ultrasound in Gastroenterology. Churchill Livingstone, 1994:27–54 (ch 2)
22. Feinstein KA, Myers M, Fernbach SK, Bhisitkul DM. Peritoneal fluid in children with intussusception: its sonographic detection and relationship to successful reduction. Abdominal Imaging 1993;18:277–279.
23. Ooms HW, Koumans RK, Ho Kang You PJ, Puylaert JB. Ultrasonography in the diagnosis of acute appendicitis. Br J Surg 1991;78:315–318.
24. Dubbins PA. Gastrointestinal ultrasound. In: Dubbins PA, Joseph AE

(eds). Ultrasound in Gastroenterology. Churchill Livingstone, 1994:55–73 (ch 3)
25. Lorentzen N, Nolsoe CP, Khattar SC et al. Gastric and duodenal wall thickening on abdominal ultrasonography: positive predictive value. J Ultrasound Med 1993;12:633–637.
26. Rollins MD, Shields MD, Quinn RJ, Wooldridge MA. Value of ultrasound in differentiating causes of persistent vomiting in infants. Gut 1991;32:612–614.
27. Gomes H, Lallemand A, Lallemand P. Ultrasound of the gastroesophageal junction. Pediatr Radiol 1993;23:94–99.
28. Bloom RA, Craciun E, Lebensart PD et al. The ultrasound appearances of intramural bowel gas: the bright ring appearance and the effervescent bowel. A report of three cases. Br J Radiol 1992;65:585–588.

CHAPTER 8

The Kidney and Adrenal Glands

Maria Chiara Bossi, MD

NORMAL ANATOMY

The kidneys, surrounded by fat, lie in the retroperitoneal space, next to the vertebral column. The left kidney is usually slightly higher than the right, as the spleen is smaller than the right lobe of the liver. Their shape is oval, or "bean shaped" in longitudinal and rounded in transverse section; their long axis diverges from the midline, therefore the lower poles are more lateral than the upper; the hilum lies more anteriorly than the lateral edge. The length of an adult kidney is 10 to 12 cm, but the range, for normal functioning kidneys, can vary from 8 to 14 cm (1). Volume measurement can be obtained through a modified three-dimensional ellipsoid formula (the length, the transverse and antero-posterior diameters are multiplied by a constant value of 0.5 (2). The kidney is surrounded by a fibrous capsule. Its parenchyma, in the outer part, is formed by the cortex which surrounds the medulla made up of pyramids, arranged around the central renal sinus which contains fat, major vessels, branches and part of the collecting system. The renal vessels can usually be visualized with color Doppler and their spectral trace obtained. Normal renal artery branches show a high diastolic flow as the renal vascular bed has low resistance; the diastolic component decreases in pathologic conditions which increase the vascular resistance (Figure 1).

Anatomical correlations

The psoas muscles are related to the medial aspect of both kidneys. The right kidney is "covered" antero-laterally by the right

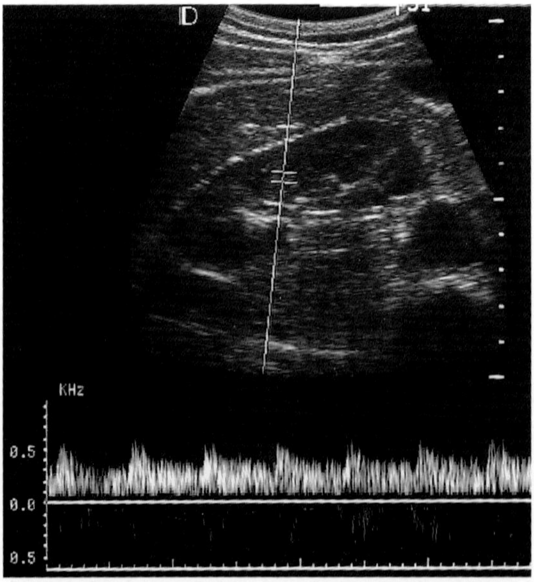

Figure 1
Normal kidney. Doppler signal from an interlobar artery, showing the normal high diastolic flow.

hepatic lobe, and relates to the right colonic flexure and the duodenum; medially, at the level of the upper pole, lies the right adrenal, while at the level of the hilum lies the inferior vena cava. The left kidney relates laterally to the spleen and inferiorly to the splenic colonic flexure, supero-medially to the left adrenal, at the level of the hilum to the pancreatic tail, depending on its shape and to the aorta, caudally to the small bowel. Both kidneys are surrounded by the renal fascia which are not seen on ultrasound (US), but determine the shape and extension of the retroperitoneal collections. Reflections of the parietal peritoneum give origin on the right to the hepato-renal space or Morrison's pouch while, on the left, the lesser sac sits in front of the kidney.

SCANNING TECHNIQUE

To image an adult kidney a curved or sector 3.5 MHz transducer is needed; in very thin patients better details of the parenchyma can be obtained with a 5 MHz probe. A linear transducer may be useful to study grossly enlarged kidneys.

To adequately image the normal kidney it is necessary to use different approaches. First, the right kidney is examined with the patient supine as the liver acts as an acoustic window: the transducer is moved subcostally, or intercostally while the patient is asked to hold a deep breath; then with the patient turned on the left side a coronal view is obtained. The posterior approach, with the patient prone, is used during interventional procedures. The left kidney is more difficult to study because the spleen is too small an acoustic window and the small bowel/left colonic flexure content can create reverberations: so it is better to start with the patient turned on his right side with the left arm raised above the head; sometimes it is also necessary to put a pillow under the right flank. The patient is then asked to take a small breath and to hold it (a very deep breath may cause the base of the lung to descend, obscuring the view). During the examination it is also important to check the normal downward movement of the kidney with inspiration, as its loss could be due to intra- or extrarenal pathological fixation. Scanning the patient while standing can help in better defining an upper pole mass, or better localizing a perirenal fluid collection and in the assessment of nephroptosis. The examination can be technically difficult in obese patients or due to overlying bowel gas.

Sonographic anatomy

The normal kidney is easily recognized, in the retroperitoneum, surrounded by the reflective fat. The normal renal cortex echogenicity is commonly less than that of the liver and spleen, assuming that they are normal: if the renal cortex reflectivity is increased, renal parenchymal disease must be excluded. The cortex can extend into the central renal sinus, between the less reflective pyramids. The column of Bertin can be prominent and simulate a tumour. The medullary pyramids are echo-poor triangular structures, regularly distributed at the inner margin of the cortex, in contact with the renal sinus. With high resolution equipment between the periphery of the pyramids and the adjacent cortex small bright foci, produced by the arcuate artery, can be seen, while deeper, towards the sinus, the interlobar and segmental arteries can be recognized, especially when using color Doppler.

Normal limits for cortical thickness are not available due to significant variation in normal kidneys but, with experience, an overall impression of renal length and cortical thickness can be assessed and related to the clinical condition. The parenchymal thickness can be focally reduced due to scarring secondary to chronic pyelonephritis, hydronephrosis, or infarcts; the scar is usually at the periphery and triangular in shape. The renal sinus, or "central echo complex" is highly reflective due to the fat that extends towards the apex of the papillae: in elderly and obese patients it can increase in size (sinus lipomatosis), however, the overall size of the kidney does not decrease as is the case with cortical atrophy. In clinically normal patients the absence of renal sinus echoes can be due to the presence of a duplex collecting system, or tumour infiltration (especially transitional cell tumour). Within the renal sinus under diuresis, or in patients with a full bladder the central component of the collecting system can become hypoechoic due to the presence of urine in the renal pelvis (3): a repeat scan, following emptying of the bladder, will usually result in emptying of the intrarenal collecting system. Dilatation of the renal pelvis can be physiologic during pregnancy and will usually disappear 48 hours after delivery. The renal pelvis, which usually lies entirely within the renal sinus, can extend outside and, when dilated, mimick a parapelvic cyst, or an extrarenal fluid collection. In a transverse section a differential diagnosis is possible as a distended extrarenal pelvis will connect with the calyces.

CONGENITAL VARIANTS

Fetal lobulations present as bulges along the cortical surface, with normal echotexture. On the left side the spleen can produce distortion (hump) of the upper lateral aspect; however, the thickness between the outer border of the hump and the renal sinus is homogeneous with the remaining kidney, therefore excluding a mass. With a *duplex collecting system* a bridge of parenchymal tissue crosses the kidney creating two separate moieties, clearly seen when dilated (Figure 2). A *column of Bertin* has already been mentioned as downwards projection of the cortex into the renal sinus (4). *Ectopic kidneys* are found along the fetal urogenital ridge, next to the psoas muscle, down to the pelvis and inferior iliac fossa, on the left side in 80 % of cases. Their size and shape is usual-

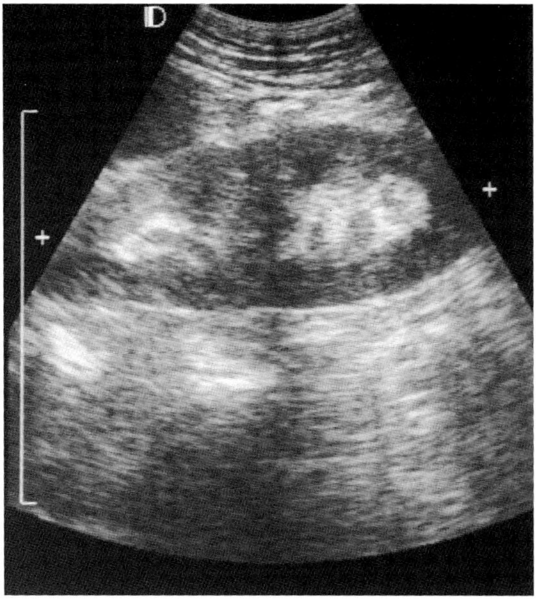

Figure 2 *Duplex collecting system – longitudinal scan. A column of cortex separates the renal sinus echoes into two parts.*

ly similar to any normal kidney but the degree of tilting in the pelvis may be confusing and can be misinterpreted as a mass, especially when the empty renal fossa is occupied by the colon which may give the false impression of an in situ normal kidney ("pseudo-kidney"). An ectopic kidney can lie on the opposite side (crossed renal ectopia) and may be fused to the other kidney (crossed fused renal ectopia). In the latter case, a reniform mass with two separated renal sinus complexes may be seen. Fused ectopic kidneys lying across the midline are known as *pancake kidneys*. Kidneys fused at the level of their lower poles by a bridge of parenchymal or connective tissue are known as *horseshoe kidneys*. In this case, the renal axis is medially placed and the lower pole lies in the midline with the collecting system rotated anteriorly (5). The tissue isthmus sits in front of the aorta and inferior vena cava, posing problems of differential diagnosis with a nodal mass, pancreatic tumour, retroperitoneal fibrosis and less commonly, with an aortic aneurysm (Figure 3). *Agenesis* is a common condition, especially on the left side. The differential diagnosis with renal ectopia is made by finding a contralateral enlarged kidney. In some cases, an atrophic kidney, when not well outlined, can mimick agenesis. *Hypoplastic kidneys* are small, but other-

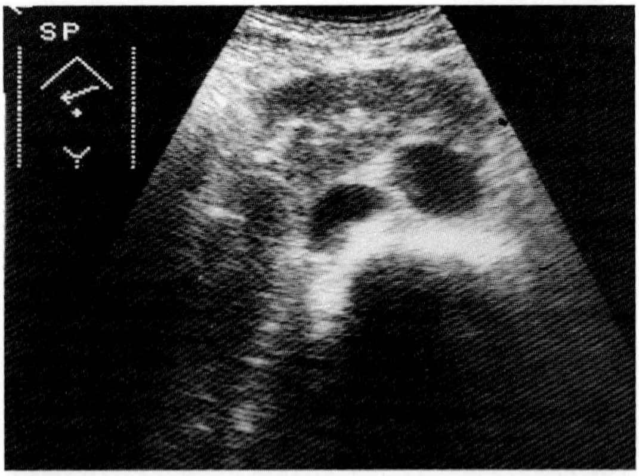

Figure 3
Horseshoe kidney. The central portion of the linked lower poles lies in front of the aorta and inferior vena cava. Within the mass bright echoes from the sinus complex are seen.

wise normal in appearance. *Atrophic kidneys*: there are often signs of cortical scarring and they are usually of increased echogenicity with loss of definition between the cortex and medullary region, as the result of chronic disease.

PATHOLOGIC CONDITIONS

Renal calculi

The US appearance is that of a highly reflective focus, with distal acoustic shadowing at the level of the sinus, but also in the dilated collecting system and in the parenchyma. The acoustic shadow may be absent, when the stone lies outside the focal zone of the transducer, or is not perpendicular to the US beam. The composition of the stones – calcium, or urate – is indistinguishable on US, but the reflectivity and distal shadowing are identical. Calculi as small as 2–3 mm in diameter can be detected, especially when using at least a 5 MHz probe, whether or not associated with regional caliceal dilatation. Differential diagnosis between papillary, or vascular calcification can be difficult, as well as between stents or clusters of stone fragments following lithotripsy, although in the latter conditions the patient's history is diagnostic. Calculi at the level of the ureter are detected only in the dilated upper or lower portion near the bladder. The mid-portion of the ureter is usually obscured by bowel gas. It is often useful to scan the patient with a full bladder to improve the chances of detecting a stone in the dis-

Figure 4
Staghorn calculi. Bright echoes with distal acoustic shadow fill the collecting system.

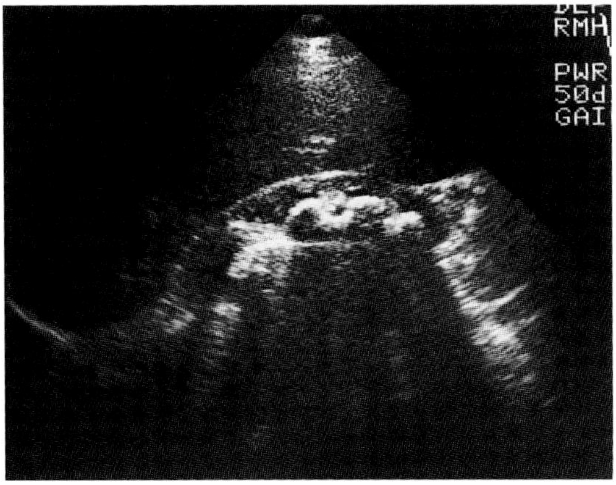

tal ureter. US plays an important role in the preliminary localization of stones for extracorporeal shock wave lithotriopsy and in the follow up of residual stone fragments, ureteric dilatation and other complications, such as adjacent hemorrhage.

Hydronephrosis

Dilatation of the collecting system can be generalised or localised. Depending on its extent *generalised dilatation* presents as a centrally placed collection of fluid which communicates with dilated calyces. The reflective renal sinus fat is displaced, around the dilated renal pelvis in the mild (grade 1°) and moderate (grade 2°) dilatation, while it disappears with marked dilatation (grade 3°). In grade 1° there is miminal calyceal dilatation, in grade 2° moderate and in grade 3° severe with associated cortical thinning. Dilated calyces can be differentiated from parapelvic cysts, which do not communicate with the pelvicalyceal system. There are multiple causes for hydronephrosis including stones, ureteral tumors, reflux, crossing vessels, retroperitoneal fibrosis and extrinsic compression by a variety of masses. In pelvi-ureteric junction obstruction the pelvis is dilated, but the upper ureter can not be visualized. The sensitivity of US can be very low in acute obstruction or with dehydration. Dilatation can be obscured by "staghorn" calculus which completely fills the collecting system (Figure 4) (8). A distended urinary bladder can "dilate" a normal pelvicalyceal system and thus the patient should be rescanned with an empty bladder. Various causes such as a prominent extrarenal pelvis, a parapelvic cyst, renal artery aneurysm, reflux, congenital megacalyces, or papillary necrosis may mimick an obstruction of the collecting system. When infection develops within the hydronephrotic fluid (pyonephrosis), debris is seen within the fluid of various degrees of reflectivity which often layers in the dependant portion of the collecting system. When no echoes are seen, it can not be differentiated from simple hydronephrosis (9). Blood clots within a dilated renal pelvis may have a similar appearance to pyonephrosis.

Localised calyceal dilatation presents as a focal fluid-filled space which can be related to obstruction due to a stone, stricture, transitional cell carcinoma, tuberculosis, or to such non-obstructive conditions as megacalyces, calyceal diverticulum or papillary necrosis (Figure 5).

US is considered the method of choice in guiding a needle for the puncture of the dilated collecting system (Figure 6). After local anaesthetic injection, a 20 or 22 gauge needle is inserted while the patient holds his/her breath in deep inspiration (10). Depending on the degree of dilatation just a puncture for urine analysis can be performed, or a drainage catheter left in situ in which case fluoroscopy is used.

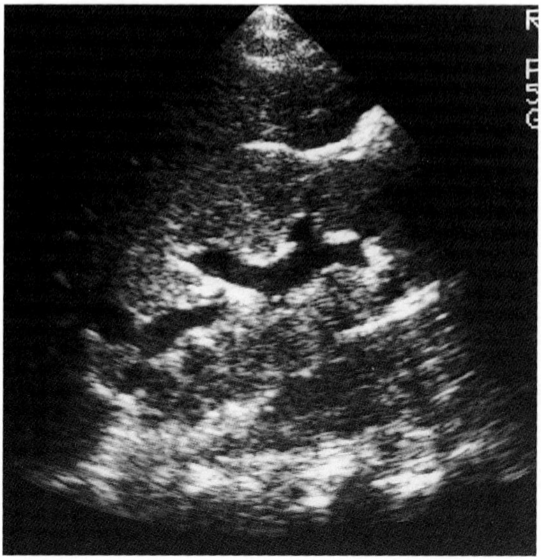

Figure 5 *Mild collecting system dilatation. The upper pole shows thinning and scarring in a patient with reflux nephropathy.*

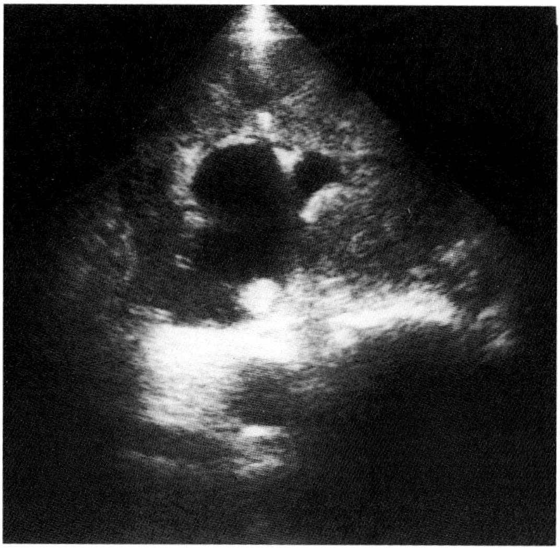

Figure 6 *Moderate collecting system dilatation. A stent is placed in the renal pelvis (seen as a bright, round echo).*

Renal cystic masses

Simple renal cysts

Simple renal cysts are a common, incidental finding during US examination, in approximately 25 % of asymptomatic adults over 50 years and they tend to increase in size and number with age (11). The US features are those of a simple cyst elsewhere in the body: smooth outline, echofree content, distal acoustic enhancement, round or oval shape. The finding of accessory features such as internal echoes, septations, irregular walls, solid projections, and calcification, requires further investigation. Cysts arise in the renal cortex, due to obstruction of tubules, and can be single, multiple and bilateral. In the differential diagnosis various fluid-filled space occupying lesions have to be included: a) calyceal diverticula, b) hydrocalyx; c) aneurysm, or d) pseudoaneurysm. Doppler can be used to identify flow within aneurysms or posttraumatic pseudoaneurysm.

Complex cysts

Internal septae are suspicious only when thick and irregular (13). Haemorrhagic cysts may contain dependant debris, septae or wall nodules which can mimick a necrotic tumour: follow-up or other investigation including aspiration are necessary to exclude malignancy.

Cysts with calcified walls, especially when the rim is thick, can obscure a portion of the cyst itself and in 20 % of cases can be associated with a malignant tumour, therefore further investigation is necessary. Infected cysts, usually clinically symptomatic, present with debris, often dependant. If thick walled, their appearance is indistinguishable from abscess. If the infection is due to gas forming organisms, highly reflective echoes can be seen.

Multiple simple cysts

Such cysts can be differentiated from polycystic kidneys, since the kidney is usually of normal size with intact parenchyma.

Renal sinus cysts

These arise in the central portion of the kidney and stretch the pelvicalyceal system. Parapelvic cysts lie in the deeper cortex, extend into the sinus and are single, while peripelvic cysts are usually multiple and originate from hilar lymphatic ectasia (12).

Diffuse renal cystic disease

This presentation deals with adult diseases only.

Adult polycystic disease is a bilateral, autosomal dominant inherited condition, with 100 % penetrance. The kidneys are enlarged, distorted, sometimes completely replaced by cysts which can bleed and sometimes calcify (Figure 7). It usually presents clinically in the fourth decade with hypertension, haematuria, renal impairment, abdominal pain, or mass. The liver is involved in 30 % and the pancreas in 10 % of the cases. A screening program on the patient's relatives should be performed using US (14).

Medullary cystic disease is recessive and rare. It affects adolescents. Both kidneys are small with increased reflectivity with small cysts seen at the cortico-medullary junction. The clinical presentation is with severe uraemia (15).

Tuberose sclerosis: the kidneys contain multiple cysts and associated angiomyolipoma which result in a highly reflective renal pattern (16).

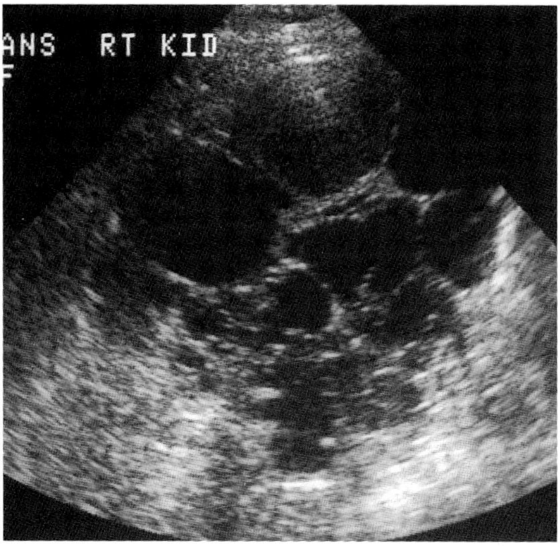

Figure 7
Adult polycystic kidney disease. Typical appearance with multiple cysts which replace the sinus echoes, medulla and cortex.

von Hippel-Lindau disease is an autosomal dominant condition, with variable penetrance. The cysts are an early sign of the disease which in 1/3 of cases is associated with adenomas or adenocarcinomas (17).

Medullary sponge kidney and *acquired cystic disease* of the kidney will be discussed under medical diseases.

Solid renal masses

This includes both benign and malignant adult tumours.

Benign tumours

Adenoma: usually very small, often detected at autopsy, with non-specific US features of a solid lesion.

Angiomyolipoma is more often seen in women over 40. It is usually asymptomatic, unless bleeding occurs. The most typical US pattern is that of a highly reflective, round lesion. However, it may have a mixed reflectivity or even a central fluid space, the result of haemorrhage. US follow-up or CT confirmation is suggested, even in the pathognomonic homogeneous predominantly fatty lesions since a small percentage of adenocarcinomas may look identical.

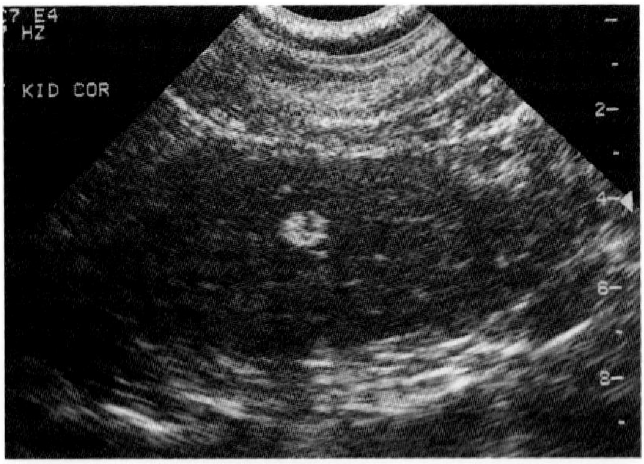

Figure 8
Angiomyolipoma. Typical round, hyperechogenic mass.

US is able to detect even very small angiomyolipoma (a few mm in diameter), because the highly echogenic lesions stand out against the relatively low reflective renal cortex (Figure 8) (18).

Oncocytoma most often affects males in their 50s to 60s. It is usually asymptomatic, but may be painful when haemorrhage occurs. The classic US appearance is that of a solid, low reflective mass with a central highly reflective scar. The sonographic diagnosis is best confirmed using CT (19).

Multilocular cystic nephroma mainly occurs in females and consists of multiple cysts contained within a thick capsule with internal septae and calcifications. US features resembles a bunch of cysts enclosed in a dense capsule, not unlike hydatid disease with daughter cysts, or a multilocular cystic adenocarcinoma (20).

Malignant tumours

Renal adenocarcinoma is the most common primary malignant tumour in adults, accounting for 85 % of the cases. The clinical presentation is usually with heamaturia, flank pain, or mass, sometimes with systemic symptoms and metastases. US is on occasion able to detect asymptomatic masses as small as 1 cm in diameter. The characteristic US finding is that of a solid, well encapsulated mass, with a reflectivity slightly less than, greater than, or similar to normal renal parenchyma. The texture can be heterogeneous, especially when necrosis or bleeding occurs. In 20 % of the cases the mass is highly reflective thus posing a differential diagnostic problem relative to angiomyolipomas. In 10 % of the cases, calcium may be present. When assessing a renal cyst with atypical US features the possibility of a cystic renal adenocarcinoma must be kept in mind. The sensitivity of US in detecting a solid mass, ranging in diameter between 1 and 2 cm is approximately 65 %. This increases to 85 % in 2 to 3 diameter masses. A prominent column of Bertin, focal infection, or focal hypertrophy in a scarred kidney can have an appearance similar to an adenocarcinoma. Of course, when ancillary malignant features, such as renal vein-inferior vena cava invasion, liver metastases or retroperitoneal lymph node involvement are detected, the diagnosis is confirmed. Renal vein involvement occurs in 30 % of the cases, while inferior vena cava extension, especially from a right-sided carcinona is seen in 10 %. A neoplastic thrombus looks like a solid, homogeneous projection which fills the lumen and tends to enlarge it (Figure 9) (22). In some cases, a helpful sign of malignancy, using Doppler, is the change in flow signal obtained from within the mass, from its edge and from the ipsilateral renal artery, showing high peak systolic velocity, broadening of the spectrum and turbulence (23).

Transitional cell carcinoma: small lesions are more readily detected by urography. With US larger lesions are seen as solid low reflective masses within the collecting system, surrounded by sinus echoes. Blood clots, fungus balls and pus may simulate a tumour mass.

Wilm's tumour is very rare in adults. It appears as a solid mass which may undergo necrosis and calcifications.

Sarcoma is rare and appears as a solid, heterogeneous mass, with focal calcification.

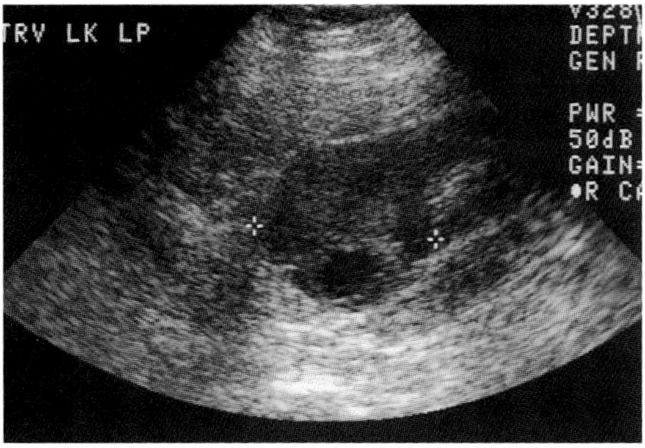

Figure 9
Renal adenocarcinoma. Typical heterogeneous solid upper pole mass with a reflectivity similar to the normal parenchyma.

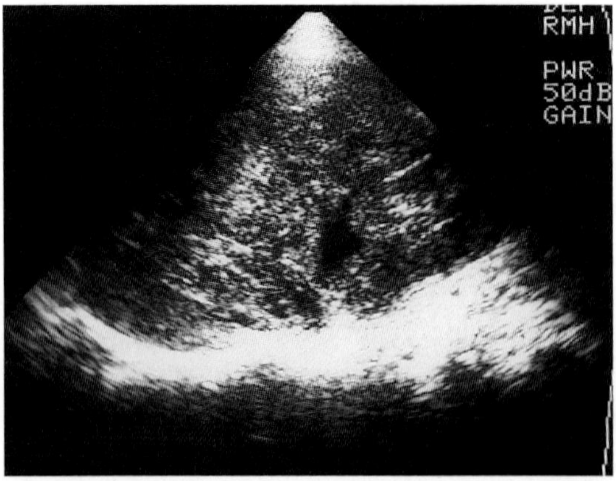

Figure 10
Non-Hodgkin lymphoma.
The kidney is enlarged with loss of the normal architecture due to diffuse involvement.

Lymphoma: renal lymphoma mainly occurs with non-Hodgkin lymphoma. It can present as hypoechogenic, solitary or multiple discrete masses. However, diffuse spread causing renal enlargement with generalized replacement and loss of the cortico-medullary distinction can occur (Figure 10). The detection of retroperitoneal nodal masses is helpful in making a diagnosis (24).

Metastases: they are usually multiple and hypoechogenic. The most common primary sites are breast, lung, kidney and colon. When a metastasis is solitary, the differentiation from a primary renal tumour is impossible.

Medical diseases

US is the method of choice in the assessment of patients with acute or chronic failure from any cause. Even if the findings are non-specific, US readily detects any sign of obstruction and can also determine the renal size, as well as echogenicity of the cortex and pyramids. Doppler US is also able to assess the vascular flow including renal vessel patency. Unfortunately, US does not differentiate the various causes of acute or chronic renal impairment. However, as a general statement in acute disorders the renal overall size is usually increased, due to inflamed or oedematous parenchyma with resulting reduction in the cortical reflectivity. With chronic disease the kidney tends to contract as fibrotic changes occur (26).

Glomerulonephritis: the US appearance do not relate to the degree of renal failure. In the acute stage the renal size is usually

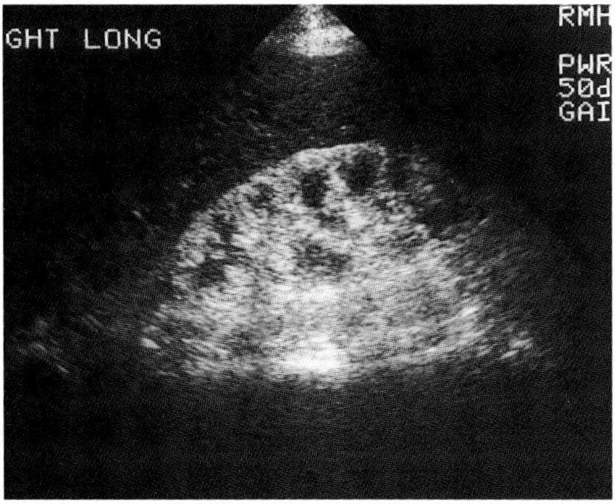

Figure 11
Glomerulonephritis. The parenchyma is highly reflective in contrast with the echo-poor renal pyramids.

normal, but it may be increased. With progression of the disease the kidney shrinks and the cortico-medullary differentiation is lost (Figure 11). A more specific appearance may be seen in post-streptococcal glomerulonephritis with multiple hypoechoic lesions separated by thin, echogenic bands of tissue (27).

Acute tubular necrosis (ATN) is the most common cause of acute renal failure and its aetiology includes sepsis, drugs, hypotension, dehydration. US shows an increase in renal size, particularly in the antero-posterior diameter, as well as prominent pyramids due to an increase in cortical reflectivity (28, 29).

Renal papillary necrosis: the medullary pyramids become necrotic due to analgesic intake, diabetes, sickle cell anemia, or vesico-ureteric reflux. US delineates the region of total papillary necrosis as small cystic areas with calcified spots at the apex of the pyramids. When chronic, the renal outline becomes irregular with some loss of volume (30).

Medullary sponge kidney: it is probably due to a developmental anomaly with ectatic tubules in the papillary tips. The disease is asymptomatic until stone formation, which can be focal or diffuse, unilateral or bilateral (31). US show focal areas of increased echogenicity having a medullary distribution.

Nephrocalcinosis: the aetiology of this condition includes renal tubular acidosis, primary hyperoxaluria, hyperparathyroidism, hypercalaemia, sarcoid, or it can be idiopathic. The deposition of calcification is usually medullary and rarely cortical. US shows

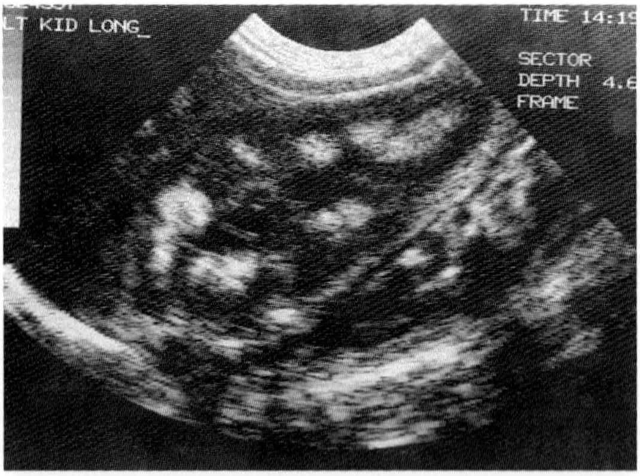

Figure 12
Nephrocalcinosis. Dense calcium deposition is seen within the region of the pyramids which are hyperechogenic.

focal areas of high reflectivity in the region of the pyramids. Acoustic shadowing can be absent, depending on the size of the stones (Figure 12) (32).

Amyloidosis: there is cortical deposition of insoluble fibrillar protein material. The kidneys are involved in 90 % of cases of systemic amyloidosis and the patients present with proteinuria and azotaemia with a 30 % of them having nephrotic syndrome. US, in the acute phase, shows a swollen kidney with a diffuse or patchy incrase in cortical reflectivity. The pyramids remain normal and therefore cortico-medullary differentiation is preserved. In the chronic phase the kidney decreases in size and become contracted (33).

Diabetes mellitus: the kidney is affected through vascular changes. The US findings are non-specific, but in the early stage there can be a minimal increase in renal volume. In the chronic phase the size is mildly reduced and the reflectivity slightly increased (34).

Connective tissue disorders: in systemic lupus erythematosus, systemic sclerosis and rheumatoid arthritis the kidney is affected with vasculitis and glomerulonephritis. The US appearance is non-specific with a decrease in renal volume and an increase in reflectivity in some cases (35).

Acquired immunodeficiency syndrome (AIDS): the symptoms are proteinuria and uraemia. The US features are non-specific with an increase in cortical reflectivity. Some patients present with large kidneys and pathognomonic focal nephrocalcinosis, associated with a mycobacterium infection (36).

Vascular disorders

Renal artery occlusion: it is usually a unilateral event due to an atheroma, aortic dissection or embolus. While the ultrasound image is usually unhelpful, Doppler can demonstrate the loss of flow. In its early stage there may be minimal increase in size of the affected kidney. In the long term the kidney slowly shrinks. Segmental occlusion will produce a focal scar.

Renal artery stenosis is due to an atheroma, vessel wall dysplasia, arteritis, emboli, or trauma. In unilateral stenosis the kidney may be slightly smaller with normal reflectivity. Dopper usually demonstrates an increased peak velocity at the level of the main artery. Measurement of the true velocity is difficult as an angle correction is not always possible (37).

Renal vein thrombosis is often associated with underlying renal disorders, such as the nephrotic syndrome, the intake of steroids, trauma and dehydration in hot climates. Renal adenocarcinoma can invade and occlude the vein and extend into the vena cava. The US features are related to the degree of occlusion and collateral formation. In acute complete occlusion, during the first 24 hours, the kidney enlarges and become hypoechogenic. Focal infarcted hypoechogenic areas can also develop. Over time the kidney starts to shrink and the cortico-medullary differentiation is lost. Eventually, the kidney becomes small and hyperechogenic (38). Doppler is useful in confirming the absence of venous flow at the level of the renal vein and within the parenchyma.

Dialysis and acquired cystic disease of the kidney

The severity of acquired cystic changes is related to the period on dialysis and, following a successful transplant, the cysts may even disappear. The usefulness of US in patients who require dialysis is both in haemodialysis, using Doppler to estimate the flow at the level of the arteriovenous shunt and in the artery above, or to detect stenoses and thrombus (39). Also complications occuring during continuous ambulatory peritoneal dialysis can be followed up by US including collections at the site of the catheter insertion, in the anterior abdominal wall and intraperitoneal pockets of fluid. Thickening of the mesentery (sclerosing peritonitis) can also occur (40).

Renal biopsy

In patients who need a biopsy for proper assessment and therapeutic planning, US plays a major role by being able to guide the tip of the cutting needle to the biopsy site, usually the lower pole of the kidney (41). Post biopsy complications, mainly subcapsular or perirenal haematomas can also be detected and monitored until resolved. Pseudoaneurysms and arteriovenous fistulas can be detected using Doppler ultrasound.

Renal infections

Patients present with flank pain, fever, frequency, and haematuria. Infections more commonly reach the kidneys by an ascending route to colonise the renal pelvis and interstitium, less frequently by haematogenous or lymphatic spread. Factors predisposing to renal infections are: obstruction of the collecting system, renal stones, vesico-ureteric reflux, neurogenic bladder, diabetes, anomalies of the urinary tract, catheter insertion and altered immunity. The classification of renal infections can be simplified and based on the renal portion primarily involved:

– pathological conditions involving the renal interstitium and collecting system (acute pyelonephritis, acute bacterial and focal bacterial nephritis, pyonephrosis, emphysematous pyelonephritis, renal abscess, xanthogranulomatous pyelonephritis, tuberculosis, fungal and hydatid infection);

– conditions involving the perinephric tissue (perinephric abscess) (42, 43).

Acute pyelonephritis: the infection (in 90 % of cases the organism is E. coli) ascends from the lower urinary tract. It is particularly common in women, elderly males with prostatic disease, or following catheter insertion. In adults who promptly respond to antibiotic treatment US is usually not required and can be normal. However, abnormal findings include renal enlargement, diffuse decreased reflectivity with multiple, scattered low reflective foci, due to severe inflammation and loss of cortico-medullary definition (44).

Acute bacterial nephritis: this is the progression of a non-responding acute pyelonephritis. The purpose of US is to detect the underlying cause such as stones, or sloughed papilla in diabetics. The infection involves the renal parenchyma which can appear less reflective, sometimes posing a differential diagnostic problem with renal lymphoma. The wall of the renal pelvis and calyceal system in severe cases may be thickened up to 8 mm and differentiation from transitional cell carcinoma must be kept in mind (45).

Focal bacterial nephritis (lobar nephronia): the causative agent is mainly E. coli, but can also occur with Klebsiella and Proteus. The infection is more common in children who have vesico-ureteric reflux. US may demonstrate a localised oedematous renal segment which appears as a low reflective mass with ill defined boundaries. There may be disruption of the cortico-medullary junction (Figure 13). The mass

Figure 13
Lobar nephronia.
In the medial aspect of the left kidney there is an echo-poor lesion with a regional loss of the normal cortico-medullary differentiation.

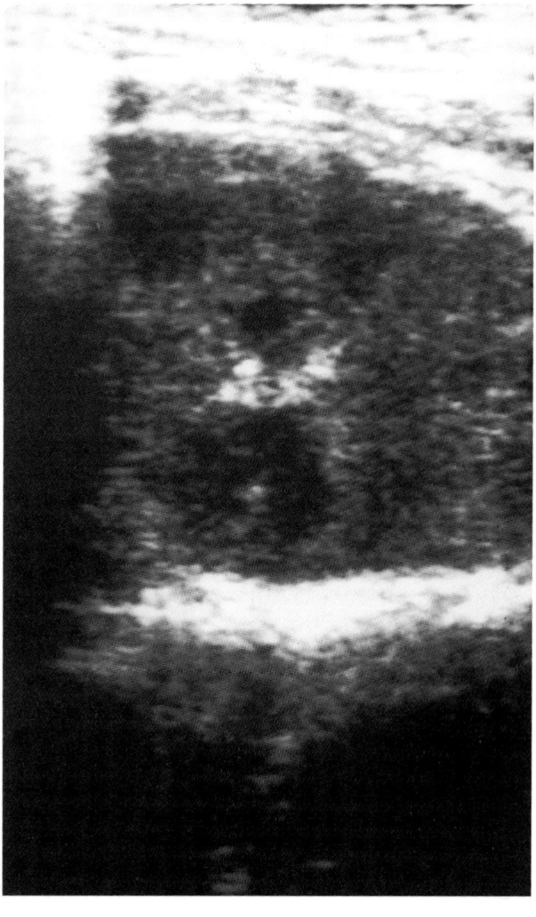

may resolve without scarring or may result in the formation of an abscess (46). In adults the differential diagnosis includes infected or haemorrhagic cysts, lymphoma and necrotic carcinoma.

Pyonephrosis: obstruction of the renal collecting system, whether due to congenital anomalies, stones, or neoplasms is a predisposing factor. US is accurate only when the infected material contains debris, which can be imaged, otherwise it cannot be distinguished from an uncomplicated hydronephrosis. The US appearance is variable including the detection of weak dependent echoes within a dilated collecting system; a fluid debris level which shifts with patient re-positioning; strong echoes with distal acoustic shadow due to gas formation or complete filling of the collecting system with low reflective, homogeneous echoes (47).

Emphysematous pyelonephritis is a rare, but severe complication of acute pyelonephritis which predominantly occurs in diabetics with gas production in the renal parenchyma and collecting system. US demonstrates highly reflective foci, due to the gas spread in the parenchyma, often with distal "dirty" shadowing and "comet-tail" artifacts (48).

Renal abscess: the infection may be introduced in a retrograde fashion from the lower urinary tract, due to E. coli and Klebsiella. Less commonly it is from haematogenous spread or from focal bacterial nephritis. There is a strong association with diabetes, stones and drug abuse. In the acute phase there are signs of generalised sepsis with flank pain, tenderness, and dysuria. US shows the typical findings of an abscess anywhere in the abdomen, i.e. a complete mass with thick, irregular walls and weak internal echoes with good sound transmission. The degree of reflectivity increases when gas bubbles develop. Septations and fluid-fluid levels may also be seen. The differential diagnosis is with infected or haemorrhagic cysts or necrotic tumours (49).

Xanthogranulomatous pyelonephritis: this is an unusual chronic renal infection which occurs in an obstructed kidney. Female and diabetics are predominantly affected. Proteus mirabilis is the most common pathogen. The mass lesion tends to diffuse and to extend into the perirenal space. The calyces are filled with debris. US demonstrates a unilateral enlarged kidney with loss of the normal architecture. There is often acoustic shadowing from stones. Dif-

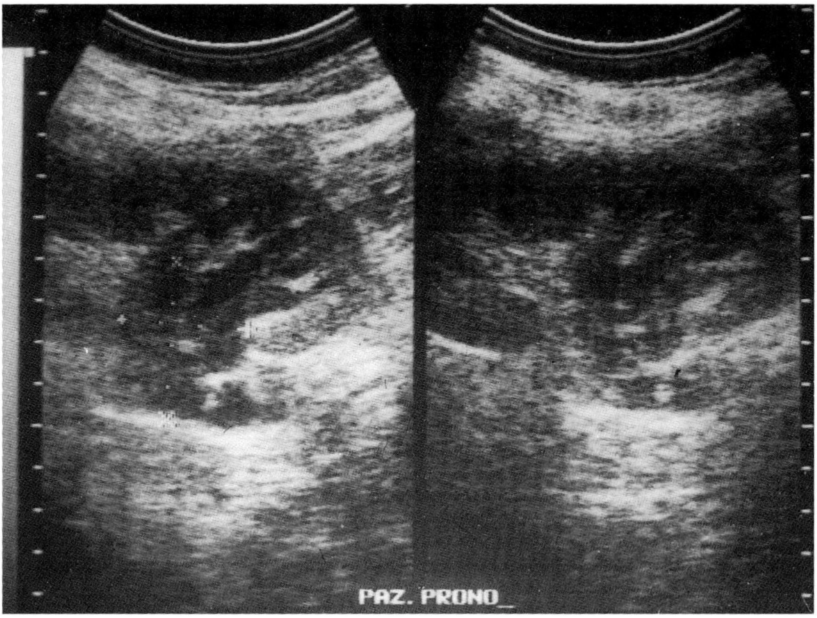

Figure 14 *Xanthogranulomatous pyelonephritis. Mild dilatation of the calyces which are filled with reflective debris, as well as two small bright foci due to stones.*

ferential diagnosis includes malignancy, pyonephrosis and tuberculosis (Figure 14) (50).

Tuberculosis: the infection usually follows haematogenous spread. Clinically it presents with dysuria and haematuria. Forty percent of patients have evidence of previous pulmonary tuberculosis. US may show localised calyceal dilatation or generalised hydronephrosis with calcification and debris in the collecting system. In severe cases there can be parenchymal destruction. Differential diagnosis includes infected cysts, malignancy, and abscess (51).

Fungal infection: the most common pathogens are Aspergillus, Candida, and Actinomyces, with Candida most commonly seen in immunosuppressed patients. In generalised infection, US may show a highly reflective renal parenchyma. "Fungus ball" of mycelia may be delineated within the calyces (Figure 15).

Hydatid disease: Echinococcus larvae may infect the kidney and produce typical masses either simple or thick walled cysts with daughter cysts attached to the inferior wall. With chronic dis-

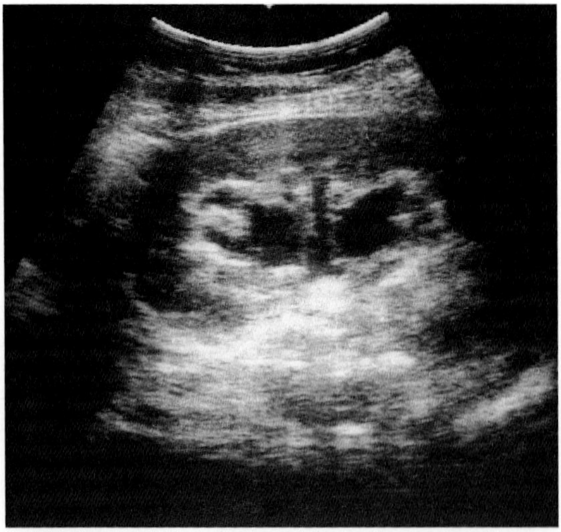

Figure 15
Candida infection. A fungus ball is seen as a reflective lesion projecting into the upper portion of mildly dilated upper calyces.

ease the wall may calcify. A diagnostic clue is the detection of hydatid cysts in the liver.

Perinephric abscess: they are produced by either haematogenous spread (88 %), direct extension of renal inflammation, or from trauma. The abscesss is usually confined between the renal capsule and Gerota's fascia, but the infection may extend posterolaterally and extend down to the iliac fossa or ascend into the subphrenic space. A subcapsular abscess tends to compress the renal parenchyma, while an extracapsular abscess often forms an elongated mass. US shows a low reflective mass with good sound transmission which may contain bright foci due to gas formation.

Percutaneous abscess drainage is considerd a safe procedure under US guidance for any kind of renal, perirenal or pararenal collection. The advantage of US is that it can be performed at the patient's bedside. US can be used to guide the needle for diagnostic purposes in order to withdraw some pus and for guiding the catheter placement. US is also used to monitor the drainage procedure and to follow response to treatment (52).

Renal trauma

The damage to the kidney may arise from a blunt or a penetrating injury. The patient can present with haematuria, pain, shock or flank ecchymosis. US can detect lacerations and fracture of a portion of the parenchyma, damage to the vascular pedicle and to the pelvi-ureteric junction. Although US cannot provide functional information relative to parenchymal damage, perinephric bleeding or urine collection (urinoma) can be obtained. Lacerations may be seen as reflective bands throughout the parenchyma. Acute subcapsular haematomas compress the renal outline and present as a complex cystic mass (Figure 16). Clot within the renal pelvis can be seen as reflective echoes. Doppler may be able to detect vascular pedicle injuries. US follow-up examinations may show healing of small parenchymal tears, scarring, calcification, arteriovenous fistula and pseudocyst formation (53).

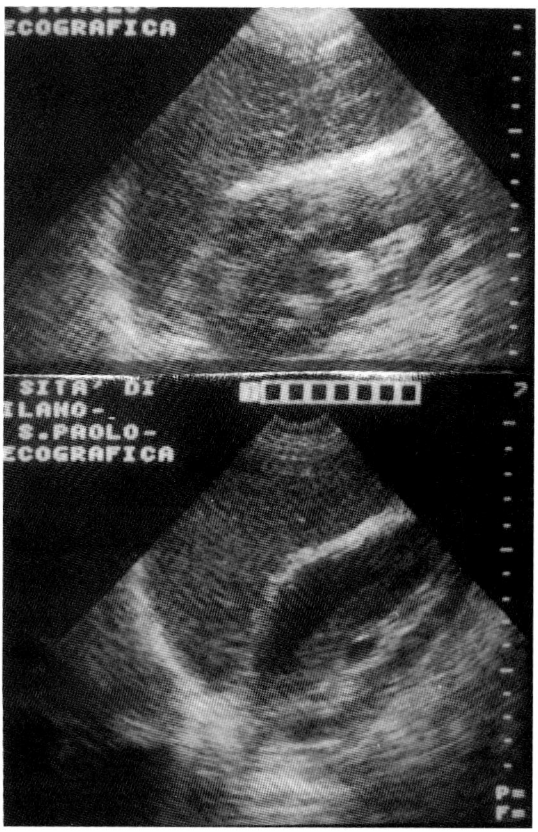

Figure 16 *Renal trauma: post motorbike accident.*
Top: acute subcapsular haemorrhage
Bottom: follow-up at day 10 shows liquefaction of the haematoma, presenting as an echo-free region.

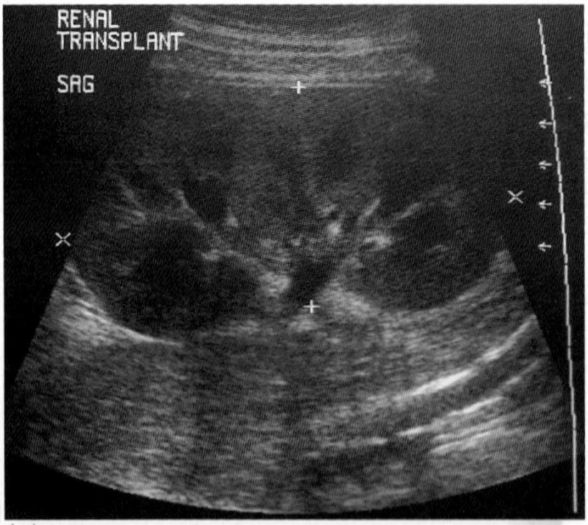

(a)

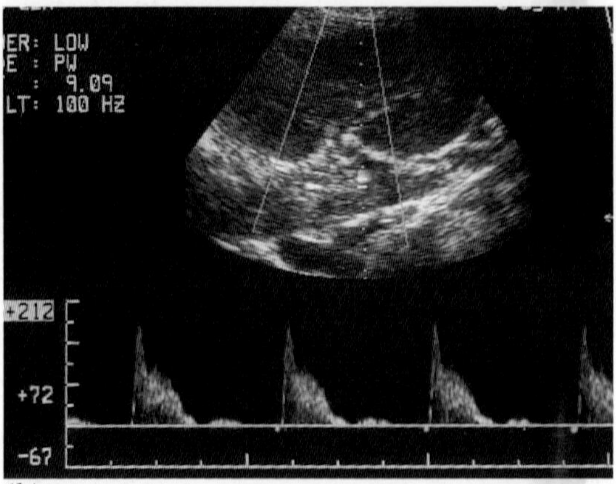

(b)

Figure 17
A. Renal transplant (exam peformed with a 5 MHz longitudinal probe) shows changes of acute rejection: the kidney is swollen with partial loss of the cortico-medullary junction.
B. Typical Doppler patterns of rejection with absence of diastolic flow.

Renal transplants

Transplant rejection may be due to medical or to surgical complications many of which are detectable by US including Doppler (54). Since US is cost effective and easy to perform at the patient's bedside, it is accepted as imaging modality of choice when graft rejection is suspected. Furthermore, it can be used to diagnose perirenal collections, to guide nephrostomy tubes and catheter insertions and to perform biopsies. Since renal grafts lie superficially in the iliac fossa, a 5 or 7.5 MHz transducer should be used. The US appearance of a normal functioning transplant kidney is similar to a normal native kidney.

Medical complications

These consist of acute tubular necrosis (ATN), acute and chronic rejection, as well as drug toxicity (cyclosporin A). Transplant size is an indicator of acute rejection with a cross-sectional increase of at least 10 % in area at the level of the hilum, considered to be significant. Morphological signs of rejection such as thickening of the renal cortex with increased prominence of the medullary pyramids and reduced echogenicity of the renal sinus are seen late in rejection and tend to persist when biochemical recovery is already on the way (Figure 17) (55). Chronic rejection features include increased echogenicity of the cortex with increased definition of the cortico-medullary junction. With end disease the kidney shrinks and becomes highly reflective without differentiation between the cortex renal pyramids and sinus. The use of spectral Doppler in acute rejection can be helpful. Increased resistance to perfusion results in a decrease in the diastolic flow which, in severe cases, may be absent or even reverse (56).

Surgical complications

Obstructive renal disease: The ureter, which has been reimplanted into the bladder, may be dilated, usually due to a stricture.

Vascular compromise includes stenosis or occlusion at the site of the anastomosis.

a) With stenosis there is a typical Doppler spectrum with dampered systolic flow near the stenosis, increased velocity across the stenosis and reduction of systolic flow downstream. Color Doppler is useful in detecting segmental infarcts.

b) In renal artery occlusion, Doppler flow within the main artery and its branches is absent.

c) In renal vein thrombosis the flow in the main vein is absent. With renal vein occlusion the renal artery Doppler spectrum shows no forward flow during diastole.

d) Arteriovenous fistulae and psdueoaneurysms are post biopsy complications that can be detected with color and spectral Doppler. They usually have no haemodynamic significance and usually resolve.

Peritransplant fluid collections present as an echofree or complex fluid area adjacent to the graft. Large collections may compress the kidney, ureter or adjacent vessels. Lymphoceles are often loculated, while haematomas commonly contain echogenic clots. Urinomas are usually completely fluid. These collections may become infected. Abscesses present with diffuse low reflective echoes within the collection. US can guide needles or catheters to collections (57).

ADRENAL ULTRASOUND

Normal anatomy

Each adrenal gland lies in the perinephric space and is firmly attached to the Gerota's fascia by fibrous bands; it seats on the renal upper pole. The shape of the gland is triangular with a medial and a lateral wing. The right gland is posterior to the inferior vena cava, lateral to the crus of the diaphragm and medial to the posterior margin of the right lobe of the liver. The left adrenal is posterior to the pancreas and to the aorta, lateral to the left crus of the diaphragm. Its shape is more crescentic than the opposite adrenal.

Scanning technique

A 3.5 or 5 MHz convex or sector probe is preferable to detect such a small structure as the approach of choice is intercostal with the patient lying supine, or on his side. The left gland is more difficult to scan, because the spleen is a small acoustic window. The renal upper pole is a most reliable landmark.

Sonographic anatomy

The gland's cortex is echopoor with a thin, central, more reflective medullary region. Overall, the adrenal appears as an hypoechoic structure compared to the surrounding fat (Figure 18). The right crus of the diaphragm can be mistaken for the medial wing of the gland. The normal dimensions of the gland are 3 to 5 cm in length, 1 to 3 cm in width and 2 to 6 cm in thickness. Using high

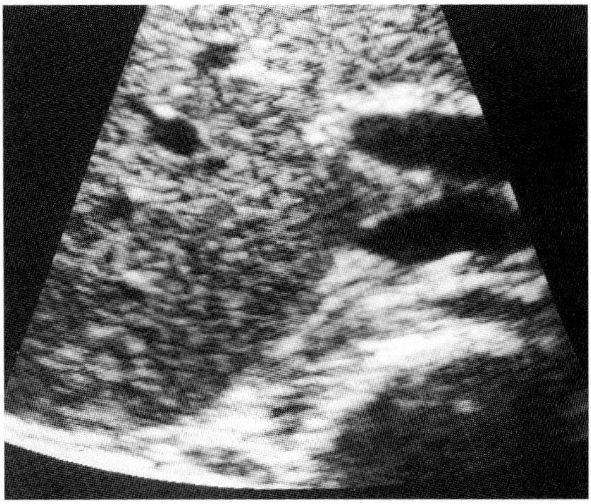

Figure 18 *Right adrenal gland – transverse section. The two gland's wings are clearly seen posterior to the inferior vena cava and lateral to the crus of the diaphragm.*

resolution real time scanning the right adrenal gland can be demonstrated in 92 % of patients and the left in 71 % (58). The contour of the normal gland is straight and any convexity should be looked at with suspicion.

Pathologic conditions

Cystic lesions

These are asymptomatic and usually found as an incidental finding. The most common are endothelial in origin, the other being the result of haemorrhage sequelae. The US appearance is typical: well defined walls, anechoic content, and acoustic distal enhancement (Figure 19). The wall may calcify. The differential diagnosis of simple cysts does not pose any problem. However, cystic wall irregularities may mimick a necrotic tumour.

Adrenal haemorrhage

This condition is commonly encountered in neonates. In adults haematomas can occur in hypertrophy or under anticoagulant therapy. With US, haemorrhage is echofree in its early stage, then can become echogenic and even calcify. It can also resolve over time.

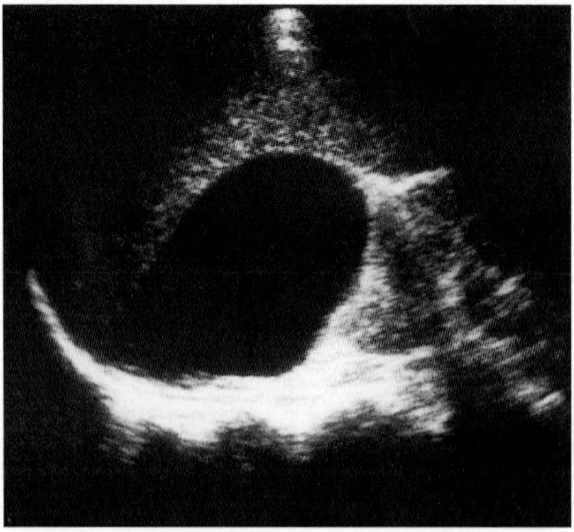

Figure 19 *Large right adrenal simple cyst posterior to the liver and cranial to the upper pole of the right kidney.*

Adrenal hyperplasia

Adrenal hyperplasia is usually bilateral and can be difficult to detect on US unless there is significant enlargement. The appearance is of a central reflective medullary region, which is well delineated, surrounded by the prominent enlarged peripheral cortex. This criteria helps in differentiate it from diffuse infiltrative diseases, such as lymphoma (59).

Adrenal cortical tumours

The gland is usually diffusely enlarged and of irregular echotexture. The overall accuracy of US in the detection of adrenal masses is 95 %. In order to differentiate an adrenal from a kidney mass, a separating interface must be detected (60). A large adrenal mass can displace the kidney infero-laterally and can even indent the liver (see Figure 20).

Adenoma: The patient may present with Cushing's or adrenogenital syndrome. It is almost always unilateral, while adrenal hyperplasia is bilateral. On US it usually appears as a low reflective small, well defined mass. The differential diagnosis is with hyperplasia and metastases.

Myelolipoma: is a rare non-functioning, non-malignant tumour, composed of fat and bone marrow elements. On US it is highly re-

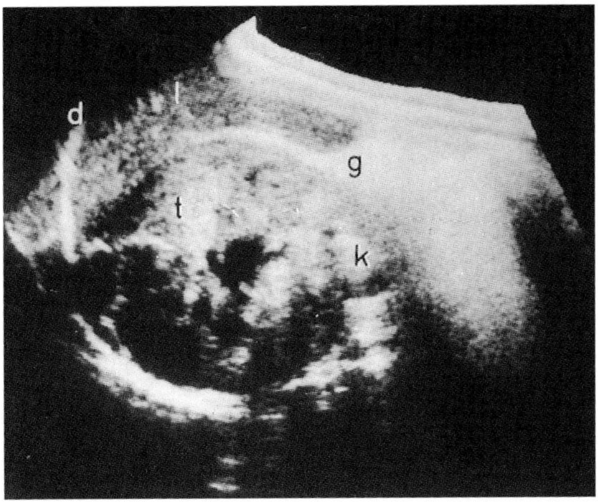

Figure 20 *Large right adrenal carcinoma with heterogeneous echotexture.*
t = tumour; k = right kidney; l = liver; d = diaphragm; g = bowel gas.

flective and homogeneous due to the fatty component. When large, it may bleed and become heterogeneous (61). Differentiation from lipoma and liposarcoma may be difficult.

Carcinoma is usually asymptomatic and therefore tends to grow very large. Metastases can reach the liver and upper para-aortic nodes through the adrenal vein. Depending on the size, it may appear homogeneous or necrotic, rarely with calcification (Figure 20). When fixed to adjacent organs, during respiration, no mass movement can be detected (62, 63).

Adrenal medullary tumours

Phaeochromocytoma: The patient often presents with paroxysmal hypertension, concurrent headaches, nose bleeds, palpitations, tremors and weight loss. In 5 % of the cases, the lesion can be malignant and bilateral. The diagnosis is confirmed by detecting catecholamines in the urine. With US small lesions are homogeneous and of low reflectivity. When large they undergo necrosis, haemorrhage and may even calcify (64). The differential diagnosis includes all solid adrenal mases.

N*euroblastoma* is one of the commonest tumours of childhood (as described in chapter 16).

A*drenal metastases*: The most common primaries include bronchial, breast or stomach carcinomas, as well as melanoma and

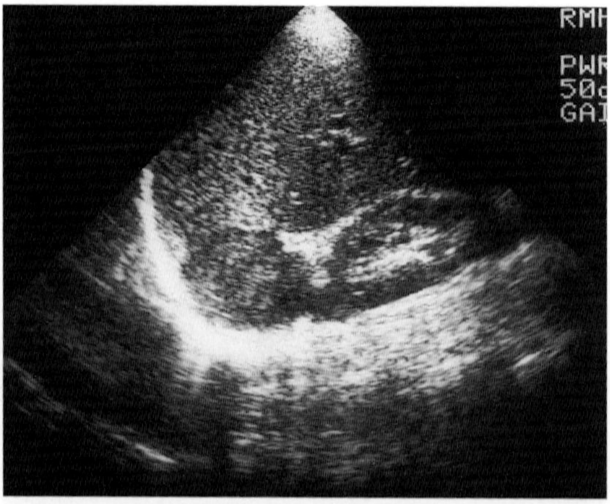

Figure 21 *Right adrenal metastases. Homogeneous mass is seen located between the liver and the upper pole of the kidney.*

non-Hodgkin lymphoma. With US they appear to be of low reflectivity and homogeneous in echotexture. When large they may bleed, calcify, or undergo necrosis (Figure 21). The differential diagnosis is with hyperplasia and adenoma.

REFERENCES

1. Brandt TD, Neimann HL, Dragowski MJ et al. Ultrasound determination of normal renal dimensions. J Ultrasound Med 1982;1:49–52.
2. Hricak H, Lieto RP. Sonographic determination of renal volume. Radiology 1983;148:311–312.
3. Morin ME, Baker DA, The influence of hydration and bladder distension on the sonographic diagnosis of hydronephrosis. J Clin Ultrasound 1979;7:192–194.
4. Mahoney BS, Brooke-Jeffrey R, Laing FC. Septa of Bertin: a sonographic pseudotumour. J Clin Ultrasound 1983;11:317–319.
5. Mindell HJ, Kupic EA. Horseshoe kidney: ultrasonic demonstration. AJR 1977;129:526–527.
6. King W, Kimme-Smith C, Winter J. Renal stone shadowing: an investigation of contributing factors. Radiology 1985;154:191–196.
7. Middleton WD, Dodds WJ, Lawson TL, Foley WD. Renal calculi: sensitivity for detection with ultrasound. Radiology 1988;167:239–244.
8. Amis ES, Cronan JJ, Pfister RC, Yoder IC. Ultrasonic inaccuracies in diagnosing renal obstruction. Urology 1982;19:101–105.
9. Jeffrey RB, Laing FC, Wing VW, Hoddick W. Sensitivity of sonography in pyonephrosis: a re-evaluation. AJR 1985;144:71–73.
10. Rickards D, Jones SN. Percutaneous interventional uroradiology. Br J Radiol 1989;62:573–581.

11. Laucks SP, McLachlan MSF. Aging and simple cysts of the kidney. Br J Radiol 1981;54:12–14.
12. Amis ES, Cronan JJ. The renal sinus: an imaging review and proposed nomenclature for sinus cysts. J Urol 1988;139:1151–1159.
13. Rosenberg ER, Korobkin M, Foster W et al. The significance of septations in a renal cyst. AJR 1985;144:593–595.
14. Bear JC, McManamon P, Morgan J. et al. Age at clinical onset and at ultrasonographic detection of adult polycystic kidney disease: data for genetic counselling. Am J Med Gen 1984;18:45–53.
15. Rego JD, Laing FC, Jeffrey RB. Ultrasonic diagnosis of medullary cystic disease. J Ultrasound Med 1983;2:433–436.
16. Mitnick JS, Bosniak MA, Hilton S et al. Cystic renal disease in tuberous sclerosis. Radiology 1983;147:85–87.
17. Jennings CM, Gaines PA. The abdominal manifestations of von Hippel-Lindau disease and a radiological screening protocol for an affected family. Clin Radiol 1988;39:363–367
18. Hartman DS, Goldman SM, Friedman AC et al. Angiomyolipoma: ultrasonic-pathologic correlation. Radiology 1981;139:451–458.
19. Quinn MJ, Hartman DS, Friedman AC et al. Renal oncocytoma: new observations. Radiology 1984;153:49–53.
20. Beck With JB. Multilocular renal cysts and cystic renal tumours. AJR 1981;136:435–436.
21. Charboneau JW, Hattery RR, ERnst EC et al. Spectrum of sonographic findings in 125 renal masses other than benign simple cyst. AJR 1983;140:87–94.
22. Webb JAW, Murray A, Bary PR, Hendry WF. The accuracy and limitations of ultrasound in the assessment of venous extension in renal carcinoma. Br J Urol 1987;60:14–17.
23. Ramos IM, Taylor KJW, Kier R et al. Tumour vascular signals in renal masses: detection with Doppler US. Radiology 1988;168:633–637.
24. Hartman DS, Davidson AJ, Davis CJ, Goldman SM. Infiltrative renal and perirenal lymphoma: a further look. Clin Radiol 1990;42:233–238.
25. Choyke PL, White EM, Zeman RK et al. Renal metastases: clinicopathologic and radiologic correlation. Radiology 1987;162:359–363.
26. Platt JF, Rubin JM, Bowerman RA, Marn CS. The inability to detect kidney disease on the basis of echogenicity. AJR 1988;151:317–319.
27. Rochester D, Aronsen AJ, Bowie JD, Kunzman A. Ultrasonic appearance of acute poststreptococcal glomerulonephritis. J Clin Ultrasound 1978;6:49–50.
28. Rosenfield A. Experimental acute tubular necrosis: ultrasound appearance. Radiology 1985;157:771–774.
29. Nomura G, Kinoshita E, Yamagata Y, Koga N. Usefulness of renal ultrasonography for assessment of severity and course of acute tubular necrosis. J Clin Ultrasound 1984;12:135–139.

CHAPTER 9

The Lower Genitourinary Tract

Dennis L. Cochlin, MB, BCh, FRCR

THE URETERS

The upper ureters are demonstrated on oblique longitudinal scans as fine structures continuous with the renal pelves. The lower ureters may be demonstrated through the full bladder, while the mid ureters are normally only seen if very dilated. The only information usually obtained from an ultrasound examination about the ureters themselves is the presence and level of dilatation. Periureteral pathology causing obstruction such as retroperitoneal fibrosis or invasive prostatic cancer may also be demonstrated.

Ureteric obstruction

Pelvi-ureteric junction obstruction may be inferred from a dilated calyceal system and pelvis, and a normal upper ureter. Dilatation of the ureter at the upper end and at the vesico-ureteric junction indicates obstruction at this level or bladder outlet obstruction. A dilated upper ureter and non dilated lower ureter infers obstruction at mid ureter level.

In retroperitoneal fibrosis the involved ureters are not usually demonstrated, but a soft tissue mass of medium echo density may be seen surrounding but not distorting the great vessels (1). Computed tomography and magnetic resonance imaging are, however, superior to ultrasound in making the diagnosis and demonstrating the extent of retroperitoneal fibrosis (2). Invasive cancer of the prostate often obstructs the lower end of the ureters and may be demonstrated transabdominally or transrectally as a mass continuous

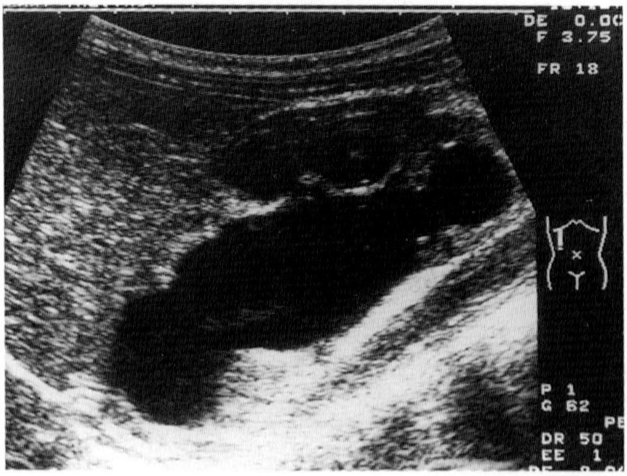

Figure 1 ***Megaureter*** *A portion of the very dilated and tortuous ureter is shown. The tortuousity often leads to the appearance of multiple apparently separate fluid filled spaces as the ureter curves into and out of the scan plane.*

with the prostate associated with a dilated ureter. Tumours involving the bladder trigone are readily demonstrated in a full bladder. Rarer causes of ureteric obstruction such as acute appendicits or endometriosis may also cause ultrasonic changes (3, 4, 5).

Intrinsic lesions of the ureters (tumours or calculi) are, however, only rarely demonstrated ultrasonically, their visualisation requires intravenous urography, antegrade or retrograde pyelography.

Megaureter

Megaureters occur in children though they may remain undetected until adulthood. They are primary or secondary to reflux and/or obstruction. These ureters are often extremely dilated and tortuous so the ultrasound appearance is often that of apparently multiple fluid filled spaces rather than a continuous tubular structure (6) (Figure 1).

Ureterocele

Ureteroceles are balloon-like dilatations of the lower end of the ureters extending into the bladder (Figure 2). They may be orthoptic (normally positioned) or ectopic, entering the lower bladder, urethra, vagina or perineum. Orthoptic ureteroceles are readily identified by their balloon-like structure and position. Ectopic ureteroceles usually drain the dilated dysplastic upper moiety of a duplex kidney though they may occur in single ureters. When they

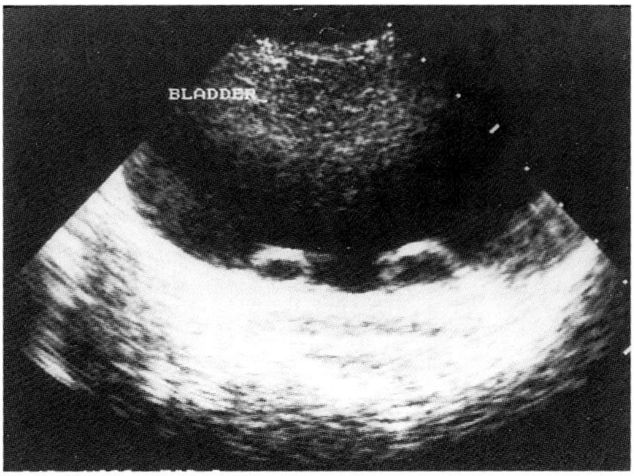

Figure 2 ***Bilateral ureteroceles***
These orthoptic (normally positioned) ureteroceles are seen as ballon-like dilatation of the ureters extending into the bladder.

are situated in the bladder they have appearances similar to orthoptic ureteroceles. Those emptying outside the bladder are not readily demonstrated ultrasonically (7, 8).

Ureteroceles may present difficulties in diagnosis if they are very large in which case they may fill the bladder, or if they invert with a full bladder. In these cases they look like diverticulae but rescanning with a half emptied bladder will provide the diagnosis.

THE BLADDER

Indications for scanning

The most common use for bladder ultrasound is the assessment of residual bladder volume in patients with outflow obstruction. Ultrasound may also be used to look for bladder tumours in cases of haematuria or high risk patients, but is inferior to cystoscopy for the detection of tumours and inferior to CT or MRI for staging. Other abnormalities such as bladder diverticulae are usually incidental findings. Ultrasonic examination of the bladder is an integral part of a renal ultrasound study.

Residual bladder volume

The bladder is scanned in transverse and midline sagittal planes, and the maximal antero-posterior, transverse and longitudinal diameters are measured (Figure 3). Various formulae have been de-

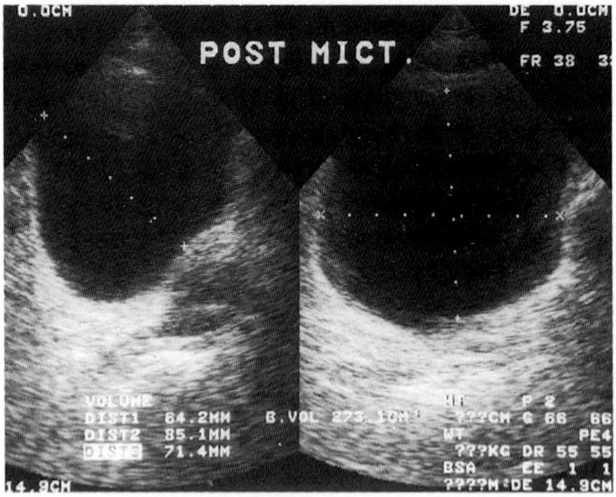

Figure 3
Measurement of post micturition residue
The bladder has been measured in three planes at right angles to each other (the right hand image is the sagittal plane, the left the axial plane). The volume is calculated from the three measurements using an appropriate formula.

vised to assess volume. None is accurate because of variation in bladder shape but in practice great accuracy is not required and any of the accepted formulae is adequate. We use the formula: AP × TS × L × pie/6 (pie/6 = 0.52). A post micturition residue of less than 20 cc in an adult is regarded as normal (9, 10).

Haematuria

Examination of the kidneys and bladder is often the first line of investigation for haematuria. A full bladder is necessary. The bladder is scanned via a suprapubic approach in transverse and longitudinal planes. Care is taken to angle caudally to visualise the bladder base and to angle cranially to show the apex. Oblique sagittal views are taken from both sides to examine the lateral bladder walls. Even with careful technique and a full bladder, the bladder base may be poorly shown, the apex may be partially obscured by overlying bowel and the lateral walls poorly seen as they lie tangential to the scan plane. Thus, the absence of demonstrable tumour on ultrasound does not totally exclude the diagnosis, the sensitivity of transabdominal ultrasound being about 90 %. Sensitivity may be improved by combining transabdominal and transrectal ultrasound though this makes the procedure invasive so that most centres prefer cystoscopy (7).

Despite its deficiencies ultrasound is used in screening for bladder tumours in high risk populations such as those with previously resected bladder or other uroepithelial tumours and patients with schistosomiasis. If used for this purpose, however, the limitations of ultrasound must be appreciated (11, 12).

Bladder tumours

Transitional cell tumours, the most common bladder tumours, are usually of medium echodensity and extend often with fronds into the bladder lumen (Figure 4). Encrustations on the surface may cause areas of shadowing and this in some cases may simulate a bladder calculus. Appearances similar to those of bladder tumour may be produced by adherent blood clot and by invasive prostatic cancer. Benign tumours are often hypoechoic compared with malignant tumours but in practice similar appearances may be produced by all these pathologies and the true diagnosis may only be reached by cystoscopic biopsy. Invasion of the bladder wall gives a hypoechoic area of discontinuity in the normal wall pattern, which may extend into the perivesical fat. Staging of bladder tumours is, however, more accurately achieved with computed tomography or magnetic resonance imaging (13).

In schistosomiasis thickening of the bladder wall occurs as part of the disease. Malignant change produces a focal area of in-

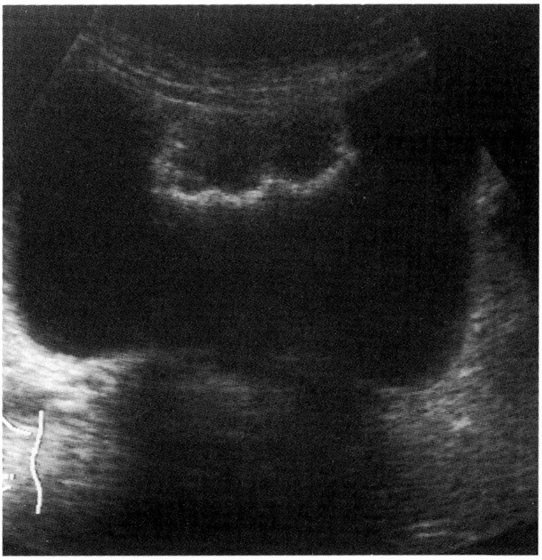

Figure 4
Bladder tumour
This is a typically lobulated tumour on the anterior wall of the bladder. There is encrustation of urine salts on its surface giving the hyperechoic line. It does not appear to extend through the bladder wall though staging is more accurately achieved by CT or MRI.

creased thickening. Non malignant change can, however, be irregular so that the diagnosis of malignancy may not be easy. All areas of focal thickening should therefore be biopsied (14).

Other bladder pathologies

Diverticulae are usually found incidentally as cystic outpouchings of the bladder (Figure 5). The neck should be carefully sought to distinguish diverticulae from cysts. If a neck is not found and there is doubt, an intravenous urogram will provide the diagnosis. Rarely, calculi or tumours may occur within diverticulae as filling defects (12).

A patent urachus may cause sinuses, fistulae or cysts. The majority are not visible ultrasonically but, when seen, an urachal cyst may appear as a cystic or solid lesion above and often bulging into the bladder fundus (15, 16).

Ureteroceles are considered in the section of the ureters.

Bladder calculi appear as an echogenic crescent with distal shadowing and move with patient position.

Cystitis may cause a diffuse thickening of the bladder wall or focal thickening which may simulate tumour. The appearances are similar whether the cause is infection, radiation or cyclophosphamide (17). The rare entity of emphysematous cystitis causes total reflection of the ultrasound beam by the gas, the diagnosis being confirmed by plain x-ray film (18).

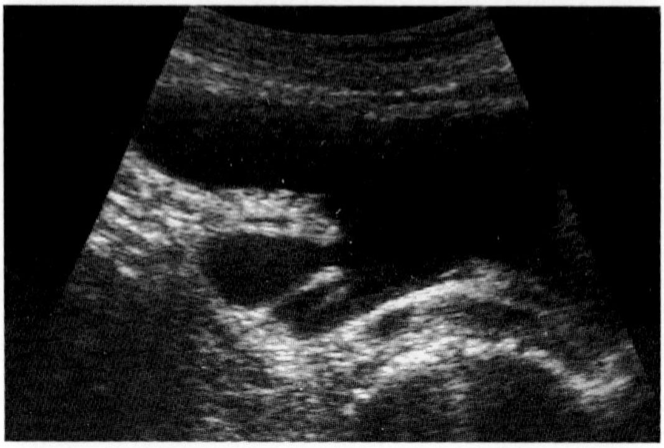

Figure 5
Bladder diverticulae
Two diverticulae are seen at the apex of the bladder. The anterior one has a wide neck, the posterior a narrower neck. Demonstration of the neck is important to distinguish diverticulae from cysts.

THE URETHA

Urethral studies for micturition disorders and urethral pathology are usually achieved by contrast urethrography. Recently, ultrasound studies have been shown to be an effective alternative that avoid the use of ionising radiation and catheterisation (19, 20). The transperineal approach may be used, but transrectal (in either sex) or transvaginal planes are preferable. The whole of the female urethra and the prostatic and membraneous male urethra are well visualised. Pathological appearances are very similar to those seen in contrast studies and interpretation is similar. The penile urethra is discussed below, in the section on the penis.

THE PENIS

Indications for ultrasound scanning

There are three indications for ultrasound studies of the penis: as part of the investigation of erectile dysfunction, where Doppler studies play a part; sonourethrography where ultrasound may be used instead of contrast urethrography to study the penile urethra; and to study penile lesions such as Peyronie's disease and tumours. The techniques differ in each case and will be discussed in their individual sections.

Erectile dysfunction

Erectile dysfunction may be due to psychogenic causes, neurological causes, arterial insufficiency or venous leakage, and sometimes a combination of more than one of these. A few cases may be due to endocrinological conditions. The vascular (arterial and venous) causes may be investigated by dynamic infusion cavernosography, which remains the "gold standard" (21).

Doppler studies are, however, less time consuming and expensive and many centres now use Doppler in the first instance reserving cavernosography for problem cases (22, 23, 24).

Doppler studies are easist to perform with a high frequency near focused linear array with duplex and preferably colour Doppler, but if these are not available, a simple continuous wave Doppler device held at a fixed angle of about 60° to the penile shaft is adequate.

First, Papaverine 45 mg (Phentolamine, or Prostaglandin, E1) is injected percutaneously into one of the corpora cavernosae. Papaverine is a smooth muscle relaxant and initiates the process of penile erection independently of psychogenic or neurologic factors. It has its maximal effect at about ten minutes. If this produces a good erection, then the arterial and venous response must be normal and the examination is complete. If there is no erection at ten minutes then Doppler measurements of the arterial response are performed. Some workers have advocated measuring the diameter of the penile arteries. An increase of more than 70 % in diameter is a normal response, less than 25 % indicates significant disease. The penile arteries are, however, small and accurate measurements are difficult. Doppler studies are therefore preferable. The systolic peak is a measure of arterial input and lowering of the diastolic curve measures the veno-occlusive mechanism. A systolic peak velocity of more than 30 cm per second is normal, while less than 25 cm per second indicates definite arterial insufficiency. Measurements are taken in both cavernosal arteries. The end-diastolic velocity normally decreases as the veins are compressed during erection. An end diastolic velocity of more than 6 cm per second or a resistance index of less than 0.7 indicates failure of the veno-occlusive mechanism. These diastolic

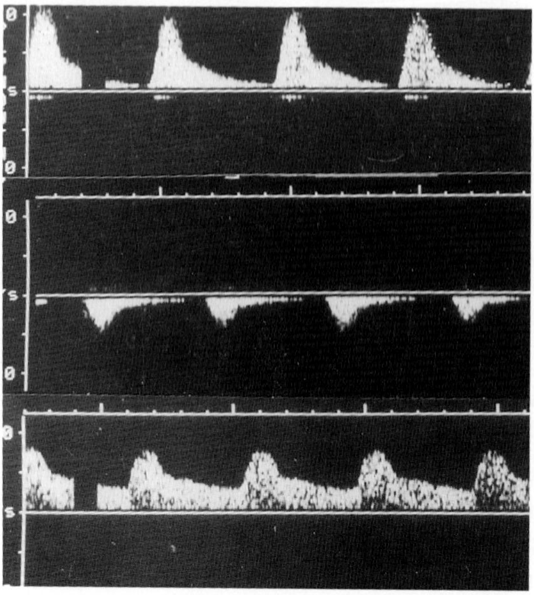

Figure 6 ***Penile Doppler studies for erectile dysfunction***
(a) Shows a normal cavernosal artery response to papaverine
(b) Shows the typical response of a patient with vasculogenic impotence
(c) Shows failure of the veno-occlusive mechanism (Reproduced with permission from: Cochlin DA, Dubbins PA: Urogenital Ultrasound – A Text Atlas. London: Martin Dunitz, 1994.)

measurements are, however, only valid if the arterial velocity is normal, as arterial insufficiency will cause insufficient pressure for venous occlusion to occur (Figure 6).

Sonourethrography

This technique may be used instead of contrast urethrography in the penile urethra, demonstrating urethral filling defects, as well as, or better than contrast studies, though it is less good at showing diverticulae, false passages or leaks.

Technique

The urethra is distended with saline using a similar technique to a contrast study or, alternatively, the patient micturates against a clamped or compressed glans. The penis is scanned using a high frequency, high definition transducer from a ventral approach, in longitudinal and transverse planes. The ultrasonic appearances are analogous to those obtained with a contrast urethrogram (25, 26) (Figure 7).

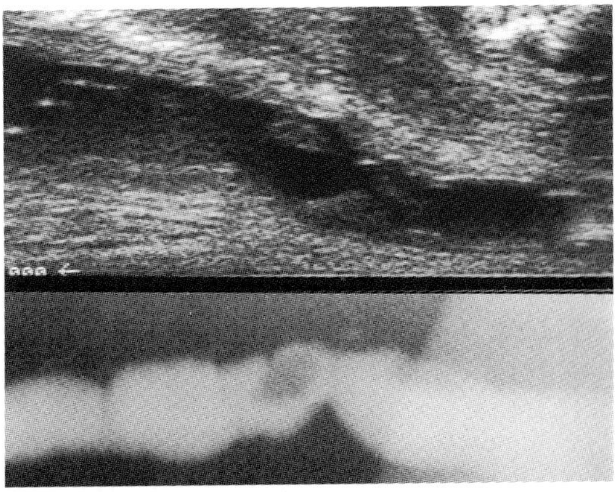

Figure 7 ***Sonourethrogram***
The study shows a long irregular urethral stricture. The ultrasound images (top) are comparable to the contrast study (bottom). The ultrasound study has the advantage of clearly distinguishing between soft tissue lesions and bubbles. (Reproduced with permission from: Cochlin DA, Dubbins PA: Urogenital Ultrasound – A Text Atlas. London: Martin Dunitz, 1994; and with thanks to Dr P Bearcroft and Dr L Berman, Addenbrooks Hospital.)

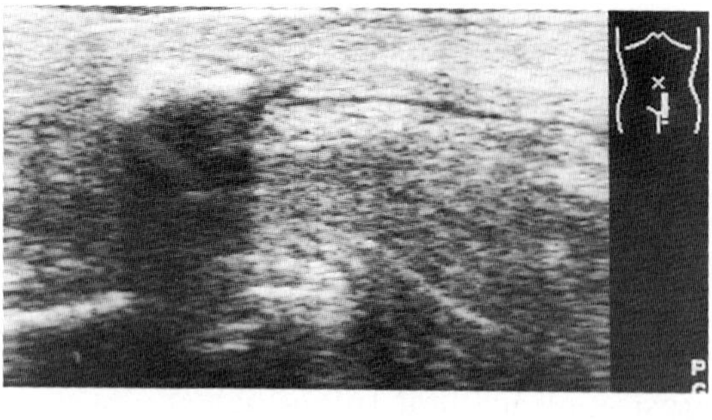

Figure 8
Peyronie's disease
A heavily calcified plaque is shown on the anterior surface of the corpus cavernosum. (Reproduced with permission from: Cochlin DL, Dubbins PA: Urogenital Ultrasound – A Text Atlas. London: Martin Dunitz, 1994.)

Other penile pathology

Peyronie's disease is particularly well suited to ultrasound studies. The plaques are well demonstrated and calcified and non-calcified plaques may be distinguished. This is important as non calcified plaques may resolve spontaneously while calcified plaques do not and may require surgical excision (27, 28) (Figure 8). In cases of penile trauma, ultrasound may be used as an alternative to contrast cavernosography to demonstrate rupture of the corpora (29).

Palpable masses within the penis may be studied by ultrasound, which will differentiate between solid tumours and cysts of Cowper's or Littre's glands (30).

Finally, ultrasound has a place to play in demonstrating the position of malplaced urethral catheters and urethral stents.

THE SCROTUM

Scrotal anatomy

The testes are almost homogeneous ovoid structures measuring about 4 × 3 × 3 cm, but varying from (3–5) × (2–3) × (2–3) cm. Blood vessels may be seen as small hypoechoic structures on high resolution scans, particularly the transmediastinal vessels that cross the testes in about 30 % of men. The mediastinum testis is only visible in about 20 % of patients in whom the rete testis appears as a group of hypoechoic tubular structures which may be barely visible or very prominent (31) (Figure 9). At the mediasti-

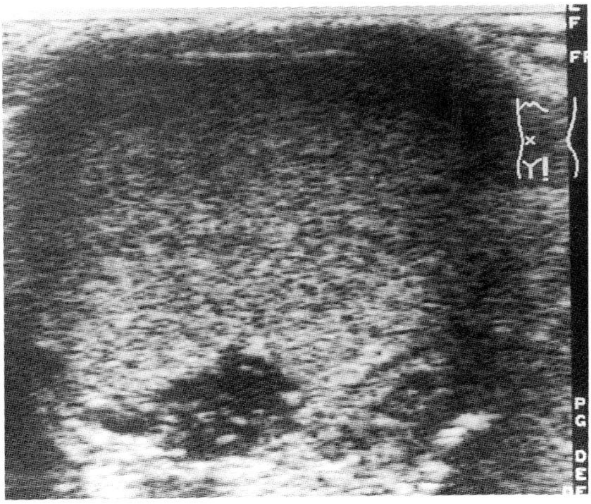

Figure 9
The rete testis
A prominent rete testis is shown (arrows). The rete testis varies from a structure barely or not visible on ultrasound images to a very prominent structure that extends well into the testis. It is important not to misinterpret a prominent rete testis as a pathological process.

num a triangular invagination of the tunica vaginalis may be seen as an echogenic linear or triangular structure, the shape depending on the angle of the scan. The testis is divided into lobules by fibrous septae. These are not normally seen though they are occasionally just visible on high resolution scans.

The testis is covered by a membrane, the tunica albuginea which surrounds most of the testis but is reflected at the bare area and continues to cover the inner wall of the scrotum. The testicular tunica is visible as an echogenic line where the ultrasound beam is at or nearly perpendicular to it. Between the two tunical layers there is fluid which varies in volume from an amount which is not visible to an appreciable crescent of fluid. If fluid is seen around more than 75 % of the testis, however, this constitutes a hydrocele.

The epididymis is a loose inhomogeneous structure. The head is always visible adjacent to the rete testis, the tail is usually visible as a more or less discrete structure but the body is often not discernable as a discrete structure unless enlarged.

The spermatic cord is often visible in transverse section as a triple tubular structure at the level of the testis, but above the testis and in the inguinal canal the cord is usually indistinguishable from surrounding fat except on colour Doppler or if enlarged. The scrotal wall is visible as a multi-layered structure, its normal thickness being less than 5 mm though often somewhat thicker in Afro-Caribbeans.

Indications for ultrasound scanning

Indications for scanning the scrotum include scrotal masses, pain, undescended testes, infertility, trauma and tumour screening in at risk patients. It is not clear, however, whether all or how many patients in each group should be scanned. Testicular masses should be scanned but masses that are clearly extratesticular on clinical examination are almost certainly (though not definitely) benign, and arguably do not need scanning. Clinically clear cut cases of epididymo-orchitis may also not need scanning, though tumours sometimes present with symptoms which masquerade as epididymo-orchitis. The trend at present is to scan all patients with scrotal masses and most of those with scrotal pain. This is undoubtedly the safest procedure, but this policy is costly and the decision as to which patients should be scanned must depend on local opinions and resources. The role of ultrasound in infertility, trauma, tumour screening and undescended testes is discussed in the relevant section.

Ultrasonic technique

For the best results a high frequency high resolution linear transducer system is necessary. Scanning with general purpose transducers is possible but fine detail will be lost. General purpose transducers require the use of a standoff gel pad to move the area of interest into the zone of maximal focus. The scrotum is supported by a folded sheet placed over and between the patients legs. Both hemiscrota are scanned in multiple longitudinal (sagittal) and transverse (axial) planes. In the axial plane images of both testes should be obtained to compare their echotexture. In cases of a very enlarged scrotum, a general purpose transducer, preferably curved linear, will give a greater depth of field allowing the whole scrotum to be examined though even in these cases it is usually worth rescanning areas of interest with a high resolution transducer. With small palpable masses, difficulty may be encountered in finding the mass on ultrasound. In these cases the sonologist should locate the mass with one hand whilst scanning with the other. The palpating finger will be seen on real time and this will enable location of the mass.

Visualisation of the epididymis often requires the use of an oblique longitudinal plane. Moving the transucer to the median raphe and angling outwards usually produces the best results, though sometimes the opposite oblique plane or scanning through the opposite testis is necessary. The head of the epididymis may also be seen by scanning cephalad from the lower pole of the testis using the testis as a sonic window. It must be appreciated that the scrotal contents are very mobile and positioning of the scrotum for scanning may distort the classical anatomical relationships. This happens particularly in a lax scrotum which may be inverted over the pubis. Also, the relationship of the epididymis to the testis is variable. The epididymis may be inverted head to tail or in the antero-posterior plane. In practice therefore, multiple scanning angles may have to be used to visualise the epididymis. Even so, while the head may always be seen, the tail is sometimes not identified and the body is most often not seen as a discrete structure.

Scrotal masses

The most important single piece of information that ultrasound can give about scrotal masses is whether they are intratesticular or extratesticular. This is not always clinically obvious. Intratesticular masses with a few exceptions must be assumed malignant until proven otherwise. Extratesticular masses, on the other hand, are nearly all benign cysts and may be treated conservatively. Solid lesions may, however, very occasionally be malignant and so should be followed or excised.

The next important ultrasonic distinction is into cystic or solid lesions. Cystic lesions of the epididymis are common. They are mostly spermatoceles or epididymal cysts. It is difficult to distinguish between these, but such distinction is academic as both are treated conservatively. Cysts are occasionally seen in the testis. Simple testicular cysts are small and have the characteristics of cysts anywhere (Figure 10). Cysts of the tunica albuginea may bulge into or out from the testis. They are usually small but may occasionally become quite large. The important point when scanning such cysts is to ensure that there are no solid elements or ir-

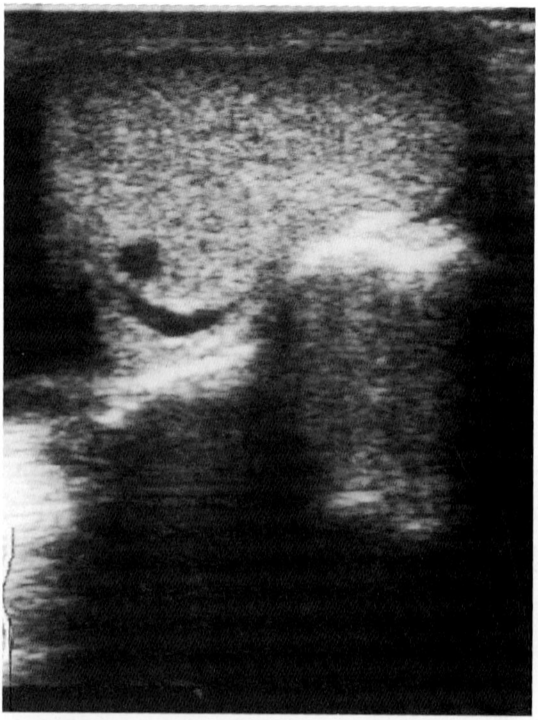

Figure 10
Testicular cyst
A typical testicular cyst is shown. It has the characteristics of any simple cyst: anechoic contents, a thin wall, no associated solid elements and posterior enhancement.

regularities in the wall. If these features are present, the lesion is probably a cystic teratoma (epidermoid cyst) (32) (Figure 11).

Solid or mixed lesions within the testis all raise the strong suspicion of malignancy. Exceptions are areas of focal orchitis and haematomas. In such cases there is a history of acute pain or trauma but such histories may be misleading and do not exclude tumour. In cases of focal orchitis, the rest of the testis is usually enlarged and inhomogeneous (31) and there are often other features of epididymitis such as an inflammatory hydrocele and an oedematous scrotal wall. In cases of tumour (with the exception of leukaemia) there is usually at least some normal remaining testicular tissue and little or no hydrocele. Testicular haematomas normally occur after severe trauma and there is often an accompanying haematocele and scrotal wall bruising. Despite these features, however, there often remains doubt as to the diagnosis. In such cases, magnetic resonance imaging may help though even this is not always definitive. The choice then is either to follow the patient carefully, measure serum tumour markers and await outcome or to proceed to radical orchidectomy. On follow-up, haematomas will become smaller and liquefy, and focal orchitis may improve with treatment, while tumours will remain unchanged or enlarge.

Testicular tumours

Although typical appearances are described for different testicular tumours, in practice there is great overlap in their appearance and the usual management, having made a diagnosis of malignant tumour, is radical orchidectomy. Subsequent treatment (radiotherapy or chemotherapy) depends on the tumour type but this may await the pathology report. For this reason the descriptions given here are brief and all the variations in appearance are not described.

Virtually all malignant testicular tumours are basically hypoechoic compared with the normal testis, though they often contain hyperechoic and cystic areas (33, 34).

Primary tumours are usually solitary though seminomas are sometimes multifocal. Typically, seminomas are of even echodensity lower than that of the normal testicular tissue, but in larger tumours haemorrhage and necrosis may cause areas of high and low echodensity. Teratomas are typically of very mixed echodensity

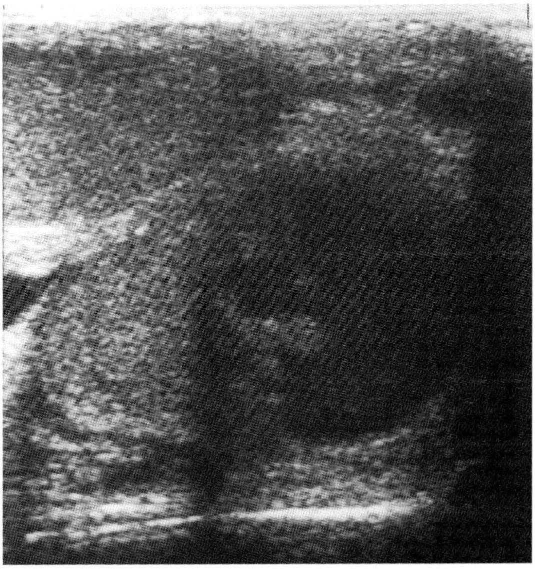

Figure 11 ***Testicular epidermoid cyst***
This cystic structure has clearly defined irregular solid elements in its wall indicating that it is an epidermoid cyst. This is part of the spectrum of teratoma tumours.

reflecting the different tissue elements within them, and often contain cystic areas. A fibrous capsule may be visible at the periphery of the tumour. Small teratomas, however, may be of fairly even low echodensity. An epidermoid cyst is really a type of teratoma in which the cystic elements predominate alongside a small solid element (32) (Figure 12).

Stromal tumours are rare and large series describing their ultrasound appearances are lacking. From available descriptions, however, it seems that they have rather variable appearances (35, 36). Lymphoma usually produces multiple hypoechoic areas in the testis (37) (Figure 13). Leukaemia may produce similar appearances but may involve the whole of the testis (Figure 14). It is the only tumour that may not leave any normal remaining testicular tissue (38). Secondary deposits are hypoechoic and may be solitary or multiple. The most common primary tumour is the prostate followed by the colon (39).

With such varied appearances, any solid lesion within the testis must be assumed to be a malignant tumour unless or until proven

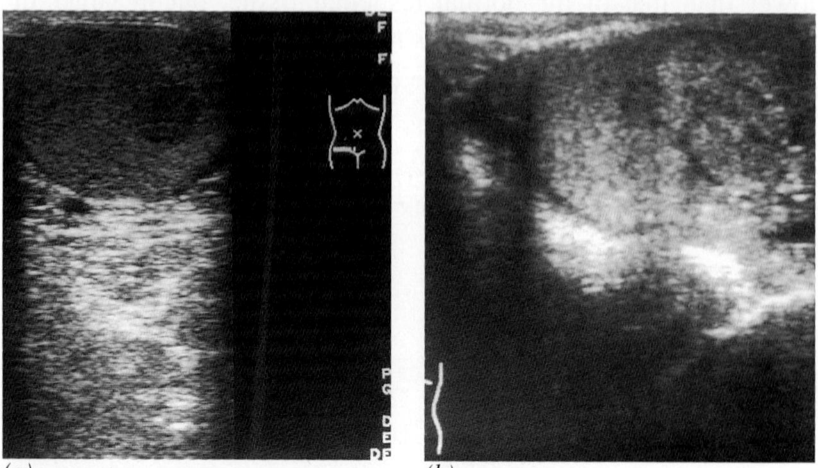

(a) *(b)*

Figure 12 ***Testicular tumours***

(a) Shows a "typical" seminoma: a uniformally hypoechoic tumour

(b) Shows a "typical" teratoma with mixed low and high echodensity areas reflecting the mixed tissues within the tumour.

In practice, there is often overlap between the appearance of these tumour types, and prediction of tissue type by ultrasound is imprecise.

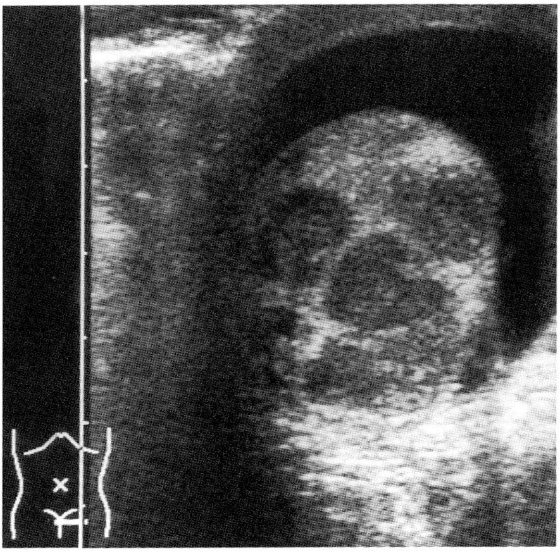

Figure 13
Lymphoma
Multiple hypoechoic areas within the testis are typical of lymphoma though similar appearances may be seen in multifocal seminoma, leukaemia and more rarely secondary deposits.

otherwise. Testicular masses in children are rare, and are usually yolk sac carcinomas, which occur in children under the age of 5 y. Their appearance is variable. They can be homogeneous or heterogeneous with or without anechoic areas. The diagnosis is inferred from the patient's age (40).

Tumour staging

Local staging is not necessary at the time of diagnosis, as this will be determined at orchidectomy. Ultrasound has no place in the assess-

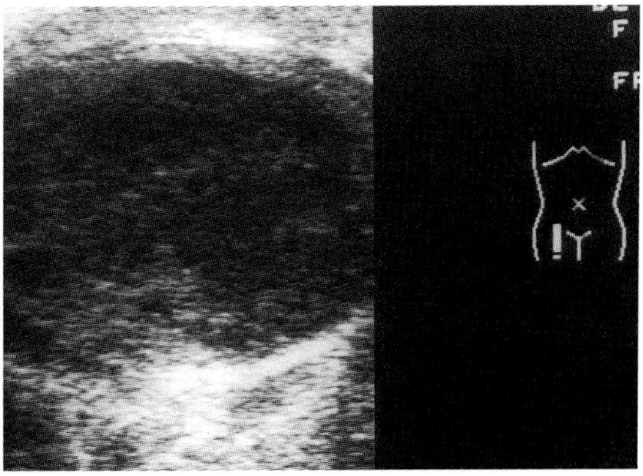

Figure 14 ***Leukaemia***
Leukaemic deposits may be multifocal or, as in this case, infiltrative. It is the only testicular tumour that may completely replace the normal testicular tissue. In this case, virtually the whole testis is involved with hypoechoic tumour but with a small portion of testicular tissue remaining inferiorly.

ment of nodal spread. For this, computed tomography or magnetic resonance imaging is necessary. Pulmonary metastases are detected by a chest x-ray plus or minus thoracic computed tomography.

Tumour screening

Certain groups of patients are at high risk of testicular malignancy. These include patients who have had an orchidectomy for tumour in whom there is increased risk of malignancy in the contralateral testis, and patients with undescended testes who even after orchidopexy, especially if this is carried out after puberty, are at increased risk of malignancy in this and the contralateral testis. Screening regimes vary. Most rely on clinical examination only, but ultrasound will detect tumours before they are clinically palpable and some centres therefore use this method.

Patients with lymphoma and leukaemia may be regularly scanned for testicular involvement, though magnetic resonance imaging has been shown to be more sensitive in these cases.

Solid epididymal lesions

The majority of solid epididymal lesions are benign, though a few are malignant (sarcomas) (41). The most common lesions are granulomas occurring after surgery or occasionally epididymitis, and so called adenomatoid tumours that usually occur in the tail of the epididymis in middle aged men (41) (Figure 15). Both lesions are small (less than 1 cm) and nearly isoechoic with the normal epididymis. Malignant tumours may reach a larger size and any lesion larger than 1.5 cm or that is shown to increase in size should be regarded as malignant. Solid tumours are far less common than cysts and some surgeons advocate excision of all solid lesions though most surgeons argue that malignancy of the epididymis is so rare that a conservative approach should be adopted initially with close follow up in lesions smaller than 1.5 cm (42).

In epididymitis the epididymis may be generally enlarged but more often the enlargement is focal, most often in the tail. Pain and tenderness suggest the diagnosis. The ultrasonic appearances are discussed more fully below.

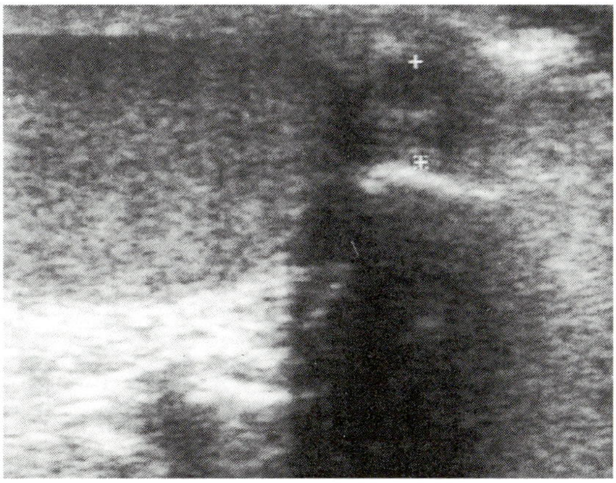

Figure 15
Adenomatoid tumour of the epididymis
A solid, only slight hypoechoic lesion is seen in the tail of the epididymis, less than 1 cm in diameter. These features are not specific but a solid lesion at this site in a middle aged man is usually assumed to be an adenomatoid tumour or a granuloma. On follow-up the lesion did not increase in size.

Painful scrotum

Acute scrotal pain may be due to orchitis or torsion. Tumours give less severe pain, though they may be initially misdiagnosed as orchitis, and are often found following a misleading history of trauma. Finally, there is the largely unexplained entity of mild chronic pain in which no cause is found. In cases of severe pain the diagnosis of torsion or epididymo-orchitis is often clinically clear. These cases may not need ultrasound scanning.

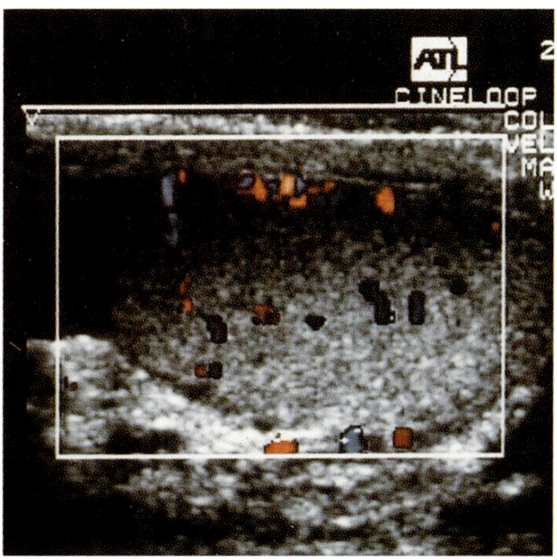

Figure 16
Normal testicular Doppler study
The normal intratesticular vessels are seen as small structures less than 1 mm in diameter. They are seen in short segments because of their spiral shape.

Suspected torsion

If a clear clinical diagnosis of torsion is made then surgery should not be delayed by imaging investigations. If there is doubt, however, an isotope scan or a Doppler study should be performed. Gray scale ultrasound appearances are non-specific (43) and Doppler, preferably with colour, is necessary. The examination requires high resolution, high frequency equipment to reliably show the small intratesticular vessels (Figure 16). Even with such equipment, some (10 to 50 %) of pre-pubertal boys will have intratesticular vessels that are too small to detect. In this group the diagnosis may be excluded by Doppler studies but not confirmed. Diagnosis depends on the exclusion of normal blood flow in the intratesticular vessels. In adults, with careful studies and appropriate equipment, specificity is near 100 %. Overall sensitivity is about 90 % (44). False negatives may be found in incomplete (less than 180°) torsion and in spontaneous detorsion (44). In cases of incomplete torsion, flow may be retained as far as the testicular hilum and sometimes slightly beyond. Spectral analysis will, however, reveals absent or reversed diastolic flow. Spontaneous detorsion may give rebound hyperaemia and this cannot be distinguished from orchitis. Such cases also give false negative results on isotope studies.

Suspected epididymo-orchitis

Epididymitis is, in the majority of cases, not associated with orchitis. Only in the most severe cases is the testis involved. Isolated orchitis (without epididymitis) occurs in mumps. The diagnosis is usually clear and not all cases require ultrasound scans. If there is clinical doubt, however, or in cases that do not resolve with treatment, ultrasound is required as testicular tumours may give similar symptoms. Severe cases need ultrasound imaging to assess the complications of abscess, pyocele, or testicular ischaemia due to a swollen cord (45).

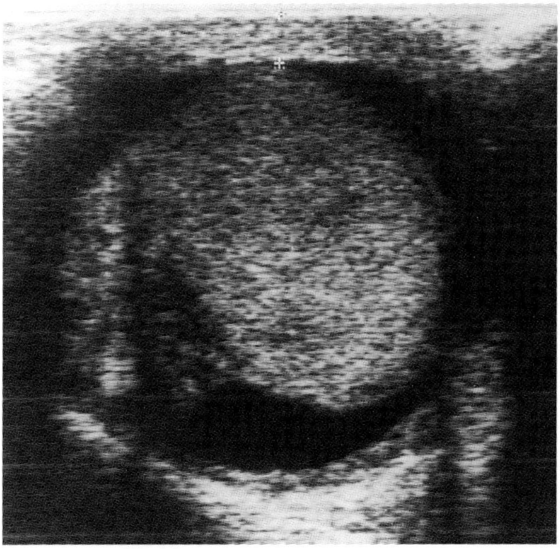

Figure 17
Epididymitis
The head and part of the body of the epididymis is enlarged with hypoechoic areas due to oedema and hyperechoic areas due to haemorrhage. There is a reactive hydrocele and slight thickening of the scrotal wall.

Ultasound appearances in epididymo-orchitis

In mild cases no abnormality may be detected. In more severe cases, the epididymis may be swollen. This may involve the whole or only part of the epididymis, most frequently the tail. The epididymis may develop mixed echodensity with hypoechoic areas due to oedema and, in severe cases hyperechoic areas due to haemorrhage (Figure 17). A very hyperechoic epididymis, however, suggests more severe haemorrhage found in torsion (46). There is of-

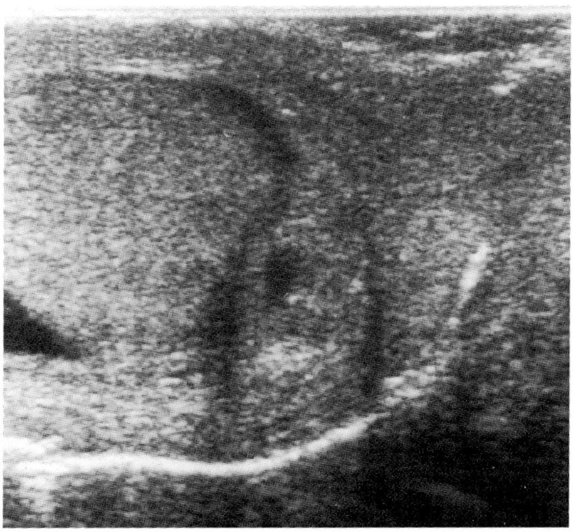

Figure 18
Epididymal abscess
A small hypoechoic area is seen in an obviously enlarged epididymal tail indicating abscess formation. Note also the very thickened scrotal wall and the reactive hydrocele.

ten an associated hydrocele which usually contains particulate material seen to swirl around on real time. In severe cases abscesses are seen as hypoechoic areas with liquefied centres (47) (Figure 18). These may rupture to give a pyocele with a fluid – fluid level. Colour Doppler studies of severe cases will show enlarged vessels in the epididymis, though mild and partially treated cases give normal Doppler appearances (Figure 19).

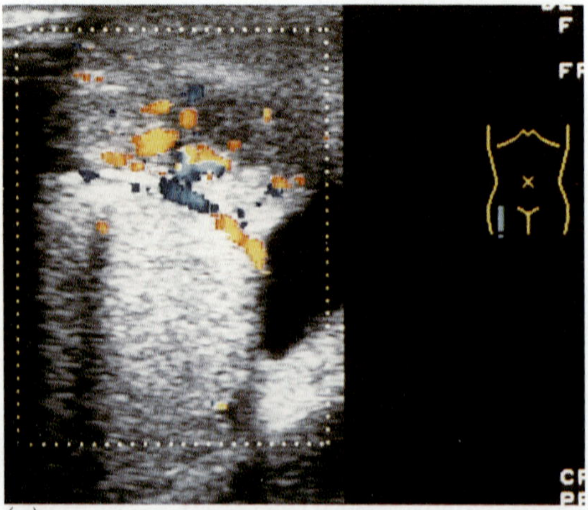

(a)

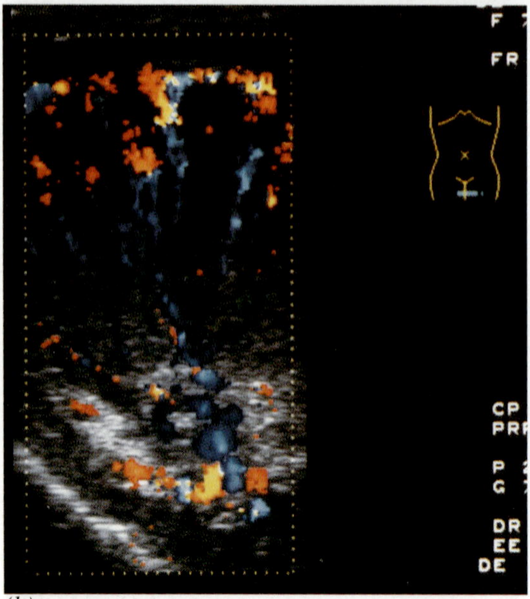

(b)

Figure 19
Doppler studies of epididymo-orchitis
(a) Shows an enlarged epididymis which is hyperaemic while the testis is normal. This indicates epididymitis without orchitis.
(b) Shows an enlarged hyperaemic testis indicating orchitis.
Hyperaemia is usually assessed by subjective comparison with the operator's experience of the normal appearances. Objective features are vessels measuring more than 1 mm in diameter and, in the testis, straightening of the normally spiral arteries so that they are shown in greater length.

Chronic scrotal pain

Chronic mild scrotal pain or discomfort is a common problem. In virtually all cases ultrasound appearances are normal or only incidental lesions such as epididymal cysts are found. It may be argued, however, that these patients need imaging because tumours may present with low grade pain. The contrary argument is that if the pain has been present for months or years, any tumour would be clinically obvious. It is therefore a local decision whether these patients should be scanned.

Hydrocele

A hydrocele is an excessive volume of fluid lying between the two layers of the tunica vaginalis. The most common type in the west is idiopathic, perhaps related to poor lymphatic drainage. Worldwide, the most common cause is parasitic; filariasis and bilharzia. Hydroceles may also occur secondary to epididymo-orchitis or secondary to testicular tumour. Ultrasonically, simple hydroceles (idiopathic or secondary to malignancy) are almost anechoic though on high resolution scans, fine echoes due to crystals may be seen. Larger echoes are seen in inflammatory and in chronic idiopathic hydroceles due to cellular debris, while filarial hydroceles may have strong multiple echoes due to masses of parasitic eggs. Septae are seen in chronic and inflammatory hydroceles but also in old liquefied haematomas (Figure 20).

Infertility, hypospermia

The role of ultrasound in infertility is to detect subclinical varicoceles (48). These are diagnosed when the veins of the pampiniform plexus measure more than 2 mm with the patient supine or 3 mm standing. Colour Doppler may be used and will show little passive flow but marked reflux flow following a cough or Valsalva manouvre.

Severe scrotal trauma

In cases of severe scrotal trauma, it is important to establish the integrity of the tunica vaginalis testis, as a ruptured tunica, if un-

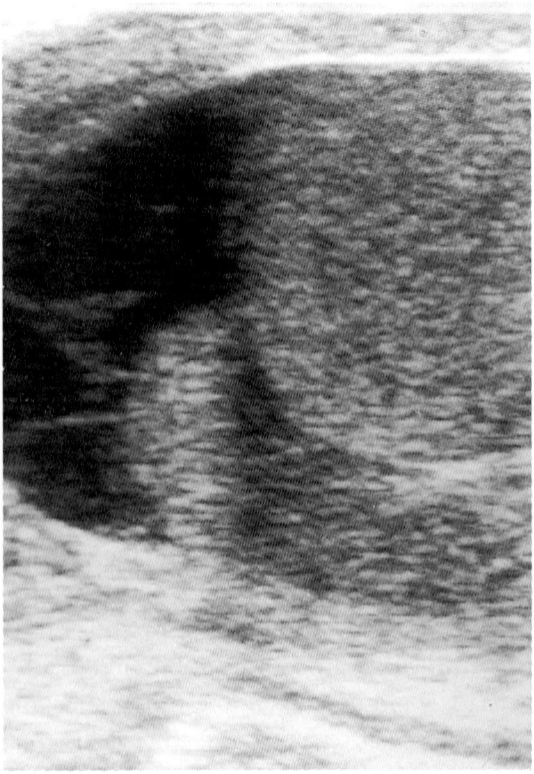

Figure 20
Chronic inflammatory hydrocele
Fine septae of fibrin bands are seen across the hydrocele. These occur in chronic hydroceles, but also form early in inflammatory hydroceles.

treated, will result in testicular atrophy, while if repaired the testicular remnant will retain its viability. Also large intratesticular haematomas may compress the testis against an intact tunica impairing the vascular supply. Extratesticular tumours if large may also cause testicular ischaemia. The size of the haematoma is readily assessed on ultrasound and ischaemia may be assessed by a Doppler study of the intratesticular vessels (49). There may be no flow, a diminished number of vessels visible, decreased or absent diastolic flow on spectral Doppler. In such cases, evacuation of the haematoma is indicated.

The undescended testis

If a testis is absent from the scrotum, it may be undescended, ectopic or congenitally absent. A large proportion (8 %) of testes are undescended in babies up to one year of age but, after this, a search should be made for the testis. The first imaging modality should be ultrasound and this will show testes in or just proximal to the inguinal ring as well as ectopic testes in the perineal region (50). These testes are small but otherwise have the characteristics of a normal testis. Abdominal ectopic testes are most often not detected by ultrasound. If a testis is not found ultrasonically then a T2 weighted MRI scan should be performed. This will show some but not all abdominal testes. Computed tomography may be used but is less sensitive. If the testis is still not demonstrated then laparoscopy is indicated. As laparoscopy is the most sensitive method for detecting abdominal testes, some centres advocate going directly to laparoscopy after a negative ultrasound scan, bypassing the MRI or CT study.

REFERENCES

1. Saunders RC, Duffy T, McLoughlin MG, Walsh PC. Sonography in the diagnosis of retroperitoneal fibrosis. J Urol 1977;118:944.
2. Fagin CJ, Larrieu AJ, Amparo EG. Retroperitoneal fibrosis: ultrasound and CT features. AJR 1979;133:239.
3. Abu-Yousef MM, Frankin EA. An overview of graded compression sonography in the diagnosis of appendicitis. Semin Ultrasound CT MR 1989;10:352.
4. Laing FC, Jacobs RP. Value of ultrasonography in the detection of retroperitoneal inflammatory masses. Radiology 1977;123:169.
5. Lucero SP, Wise HA, Kirsh G et al. Ureteric obstruction secondary to endometriosis. Report of three cases and review of the literature. Br J Urol 1988;61:201.
6. Wood BP, Ben-Ami T, Teele RF, Rabinowitz R. Ureterovesical obstruction and megaureter: diagnosis by realtime US. Radiology 1985;156:79.
7. Nussbaum AR, Dorst JP, Jeffs R et al. Ectopic ureter and ureterocele: the varied sonographic manifestations. Radiology 1986;159:227.
8. Rose JS, McCarthy J, Yeh HC. Ultrasound of ectopic ureterocele. Pediatr Radiol 1979;8:17.
9. Kiely EA, Hartnell GG, Gibson RN et al. Measurement of bladder volume by realtime ultrasound. Br J Urol 1987;60:33–35.
10. McLean GK, Edell SL. Determination of bladder volumes by grey scale ultrasonography. Radiology 1978;128:181–182.
11. Abu-Yousef MM, Narayana AS, Franken EA, Jr. et al. Urinary bladder tumours studied by cystosonography; part I: Detection. Radiology 1984;153:223–226.
12. Vallancien G, Veillon B, Charton M et al. Can transabdominal ultraso-

nography of the bladder replace cystoscopy in the follow-up of superficial bladder tumours? J Urol 1986;136:32–34.
13. Abu-Yousef MM, Narayana AS, Brown RC, et al. Urinary bladder tumours studied by ultrasonography; part II: Staging. Radiology 1984;153:227–231.
14. Jorulf H, Lindstedt E. Urogenital schistosomiasis: CT evaluation. Radiology 1985;157:745–749.
15. Bouvier JF, Pascaud E, Mailhes F et al. Urachal cyst in the adult: ultrasound diagnosis. J Clin Ultrasound 1984;12:48–50.
16. Han SY, Wittan DM. Carcinoma of the urachus. AJR 1976;127:351–352.
17. Abu-Yousef MM; Narayana AS, Brown RC. Catheter induced cystitis: evaluation by cystosonography. Radiology 1984;151:471–473.
18. Kauzlaric D, Barmier E. Sonography of the emphysematous cystitis. J Ultrasound Med 1985;4:319–320.
19. Bergman A, Vermesh M, Ballard C et al. Role of ultrasound in urinary incontinence evaluation. Urology 1989;5:443–444.
20. Bergman A, McKenzie CJ, Richmond J et al. Transrectal ultrasound versus cystography in the evaluation of anatomical stress urinary incontinence. Br J Urol 1988;62:228–234.
21. Goldstein I, Krane RJ, Greenfield AJ, Padma-Nathan H. Vascular diseases of the penis: impotence and priapism. In: Pollack HM (ed): Clinical Urology; 1990:2231–2252.
22. Benson CB, Vickers MA. Sexual impotence caused by vascular disease. Diagnosis by duplex sonography. AJR 1989;153:1149.
23. Collins JP, Lewindowski BJ. Experience with ultracorporal injection of papaverine and duplex ultrasound scanning for assessment of arteriogenic impotence. Br J Urol 1987;59:84.
24. Benson CB, Vickers MA, Aruny J. Evaluation of impotence. Semin Ultrasound CT MR 1991;12:176–190.
25. McAninch JW, Laing FC, Jeffrey RB, Jr. Sonourethrography in the evaluation of urethral strictures: a preliminary report. J Urol 1988;139:294.
26. Gluck CD, Bundy AL, Fine C, Loughlin KR, Richie JP. Sonographic urethrogram: comparison to roentgenographic techniques in 22 patients. J Urol 1988;140:1404.
27. Chou YH, Tieu CM, Pan HB et al. High resolution realtime ultrasound in Peyronie's disease. J Ultrasound Med 1987;6:67.
28. Hamm B, Friedrich M, Kelami A. Ultrasound imaging in Peyronie's disease. Urology 1986;28:540.
29. Dierks PR, Hawkins H. Sonography and penile trauma. J Ultrasound Med 1983;2:417.
30. Yamashita T, Ogawa A. Ultrasound in penile cancer. Urol Radiol 1989;11:174.
31. Thomas RD, Dewbury KF. Ultrasound appearances of the rete testis.

Clin Radiol 1993;43:121.

32. Maxwell AJ, Mantora H. Sonographic appearance of epidermoid cysts of the testis. J Clin Ultrasound 1990;18:188.
33. Gronvall S, Brunner N, Jacobson GK, Holm HH. Ultrasound in the detection of testicular tumours. Int J Androl 1981;4:185.
34. Marth D, Scheideggar J, Studer UE. Ultrasonography of testicular tumours. Urol Int 1990;45:237.
35. Mudde AH, Haak A, Kruyt RH. Ultrasonic detection of occult Leydig cell tumours in two patients with gynaecomastia. Neth J Med 1987;31:72.
36. Nemcek AA, Fisher MR, Leschorn E, Garnett J. Mixed sex cord stromal tumour of the testis. Evaluation by ultrasonography and magnetic resonance imaging. Urol Radiol 1989;11:186.
37. Goodman JD, Carr L, Ostrobsky PD et al. Testicular lymphoma: sonographic findings. Urol Radiol 1985;7:25.
38. Lupetin AR, King W, III, Rich P, Lederman RB. Ultrasound diagnosis of testicular leukaemia. Radiology 1983;147:171.
39. Pienkos FJ, Jablokow VR. Secondary testicular tumours. Cancer 1972;30:481.
40. Frey P, Fliegel C, Herzog B. Testicular tumours in infancy and childhood – a review of 10 germ cell tumours and 10 non-germ cell tumours. Zeitschr Kinderchir 1990;45:229–234.
41. Broth G, Bullock WK, Morrow J. Epididymal tumours: 1. Report of 15 new cases including review of the literature. 2. Histochemical study of so-called adenomatoid tumours. J Urol 1986;100:530.
42. Beccia DJ, Krane RJ, Olsson CA. Clinical management of non testicular intrascrotal tumours. J Urol 1976;116:476.
43. Bird K. Rosenfield AT, Taylor KJW. Ultrasonography in testicular torsion. Radiology 1983;147:527.
44. Burks DD, Markey BJ, Burkhard TK et al. Suspected testicular torsion and ischaemia: evaluation with colour Doppler sonography. Radiology 1990;175:815.
45. See WA, Mack LA, Krieger JM. Scrotal ultrasonograhpy: a predictor of complicated epididymitis requiring orchidectomy. J Urol 1988;139:55.
46. Vick CW, Bird K, Rosenfield AT et al. Extratesticular haemorrhage associated with torsion of the spermatic cord: sonographic demonstration. Radiology 1986;158:401.
47. Mevorach RA, Lerner RM, Devoretsky PM, Rabinowitz R. Testicular abscess diagnosed by ultrasonography. J Urol 1986;136:1213.
48. Gonda RL, Jr, Karo JJ, Forte RA, O'Donnell KT. Diagnosis of subclinical varicocele in infertility. AJR 1987;148:71.
49. Albert NE. Testicular ultrasound for trauma. J Urol 1980;124:558.
50. Friedland GW, Chang P. The role of imaging in the management of the impalpable undescended testis. AJR 1988;151:1107.

CHAPTER 10

The Prostate, Seminal Vesicles, Rectum and Anal Canal

Archie Alexander, MD

Since the male population is aging, the number of cases of prostate cancer is likely to increase. Presently, prostate cancer has overtaken lung cancer as the number one cancer in US males (1). Heightened awareness by these individuals has brought many men to their physicians for a prostate evaluation. Traditional assessment has relied upon the digital rectal examination with palpable abnormalities digitally biopsied. Presently, endosonography (EUS) and serum prostate specific antigen determinations have enjoyed increasing utilization in this process (2–6). Even though EUS is primarily used in cancer detection, it has also played a role in the evaluation of cases of prostatitis complicated by abscess formation, benign prostatic hyperplasia and male infertility (7, 8).

Likewise, EUS has been one of the primary radiologic imaging modalities utilized to assess the rectum and in particular EUS has been utilized to locally stage rectal cancers although computed tomography and magnetic resonance imaging have also been used for this purpose (9–14). The role of EUS has broadened from rectal cancer evaluation to locating and guiding needles or catheters to drain deep pelvic abscesses that are considered unapproachable by the more traditional percutaneous routes (15). Also, EUS has been utilized to evaluate the anal sphincter complex in individuals complaining of incontinence (16).

The goal of this chapter is to acquaint those individuals unfamiliar with EUS and the various applications of this technology to the diagnosis and treatment of the more common disease processes of the prostate, rectum and anal canal. The salient anatomical features will be covered as they relate to interpretation of EUS images and interventional techniques such as sonographically guided prostate biopsies and transrectal drainages.

PROSTATE AND SEMINAL VESICLES

EUS anatomy and examination

The concept of zonal anatomy established by McNeil will serve as a framework for sonographic analysis of the prostate gland. The prostate gland is divided into a glandular portion (2/3 volume) and a non-glandular fibromuscular stroma (1/3 volume). The glandular prostate is further divided into the peripheral (outer) and central (inner) glands (17–18). Because of the confusion caused by the similarity in the terms *central gland and central zones*, central gland may be referred to as the inner gland. There are morphologic differences between the glands that are present within the different zones of the prostate which may be related to their embryologic origins (19).

The peripheral or outer gland is composed of a peripheral zone (70 % of cancers) and a central zone (10 % of cancers). The central or inner gland is made up of transitional zone (20 % of cancers) and periurethral glandular material which surround the prostatic urethra. The epithelial components of the glands within the peripheral and transition zones seem to originate from tissues of the urogenital sinus and those within the central zone have features in common with the seminal vesicles arising from the Wolffian ducts. These differences may have some relationship to the variation of cancer related to the various zones (17–20).

Ultrasonographically, the tissues of the peripheral gland have a stippled gray appearance in the young male. The anteriorly located hypoechoic fibromuscular stroma can be distinguished from the glandular portions of the prostate (Figure 1). On the other hand, it is often not possible to distinguish the peripheral and central zones ultrasonographically (21, 22). Likewise, the transition zone and periurethral glandular tissues which initially compose 5 % of the glandular volume may not be identified as distinct although this material may be less echogenic than the peripheral gland (Figure 2). The structures identified on EUS will vary depending on the level at which the image is obtained with the transition zone material no longer present below the verumonta-

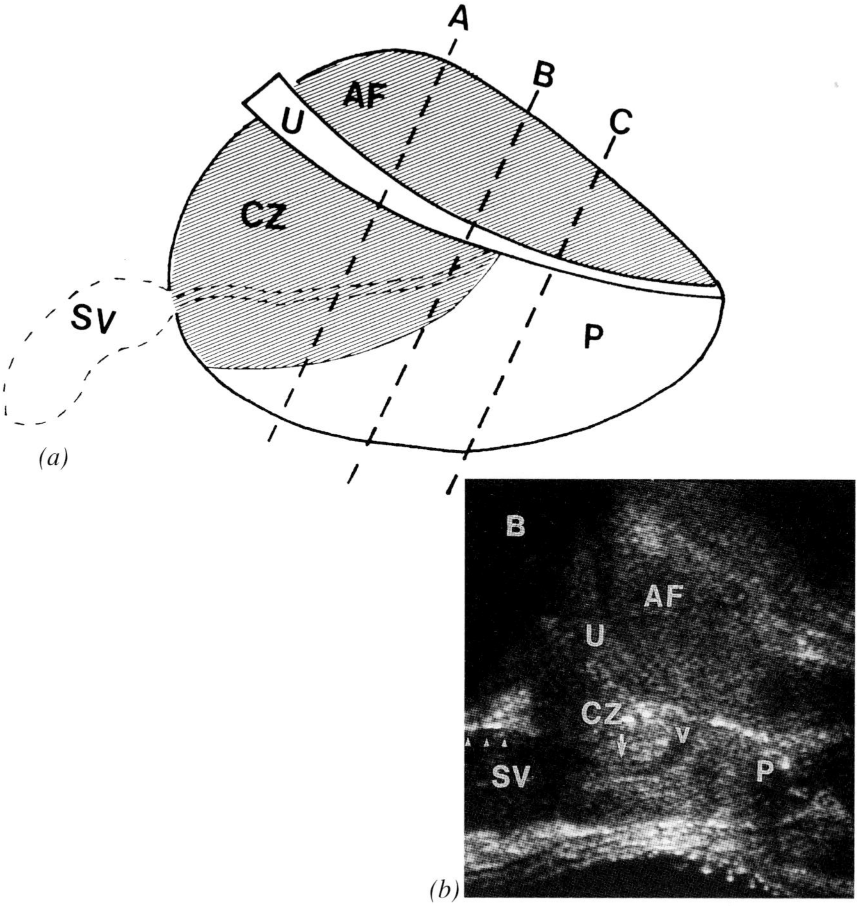

Figure 1
a. This schematic diagram of the prostate gland is drawn from a longitudinal section through the midline illustrating the zonal anatomy in a young male described by McNeal with transverse sections labeled at levels A, B, and C. Ideally, multiple transverse EUS images should be obtained at 5 mm increments to cover the entire gland from base to apex.
b. This sagittal EUS image is from the same level as in a. and depicts the sonographic features of the normal gland. The hypoechoic fibromuscular stroma (AF) lies anterior to the urethra (U) and posteriorly, the central (CZ) and peripheral (P) zones have a stippled grey echotexture with a very slight textural difference between the two zones. The more hypoechoic ejaculatory duct (arrow) is seen within the central zone (CZ) and inserts in the region of the verumontanum (v). A portion of the seminal vesicle (SV) is imaged behind the bladder (B) and superior to the base of the prostate. It has a relatively anechoic internal echotexture resulting from seminal fluid and its echogenic wall is also seen (arrowheads).

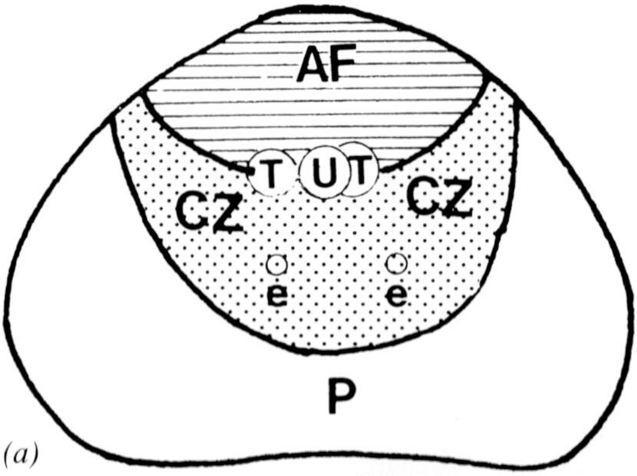

(a)

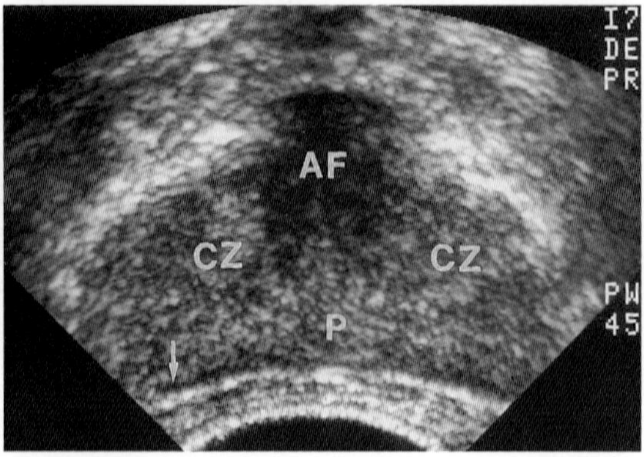

(b)

Figure 2

a. Diagram of prostatic tissues which are present in the transverse plane at level A. The central (inner) gland is composed of transition zone material (T) flanking either side of the urethra (U) and periurethral glandular material not shown here. The peripheral gland is formed by both central (CZ) and peripheral zones (P). The paired ejaculatory ducts (e) arise from a coalescence of epithelium from seminal vesicle (SV) and vas deferens (not shown), and they pass obliquely through the central zone to insert at the level of the verumontanum. The anterior fibromuscular stroma (AF) is nonglandular tissue which serves as a point of fixation.

b. Transverse EUS image which corresponds to level A. Figures 1 a and 2 a demonstrate the homogeneous stippled grey appearance of normal peripheral zone (P) and the adjacent central zone (CZ) which is similar in echogenicity and almost indistinguishable from the peripheral zone. The fibromuscular stroma (AF) is much less echogenic secondary to its smooth muscle and fibrous tissues. The hypoechoic capsule (arrows) is a pencil thin line unlike the adjacent hyperechoic periprostatic fat and fascia. The capsule may appear discontinuous at various points along the periphery of the prostate. The transition zones, urethra and ejaculatory ducts are not identified as discrete structures.

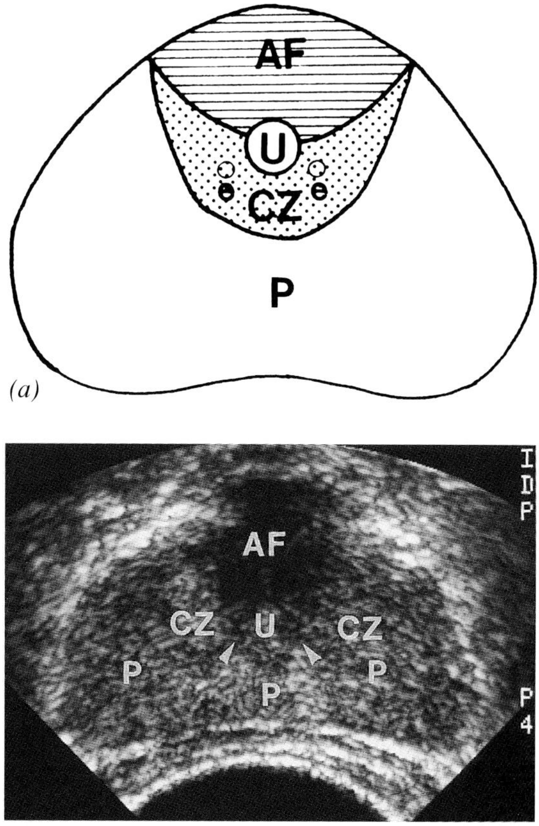

Figure 3
a. Section from level B just above the verumontanum that reveals the relative changes in the glandular constituents of the prostate gland with an increase in peripheral zone (P) material and a decrease in central zone (CZ) tissue and loss of the paired transition zones (T). The ejaculatory ducts (e) are medially directed and have not yet inserted onto the posterior surface of the verumontanum.
b. Transverse EUS image through level B illustrating echotextures of the various tissue components in a. with the peripheral zone (P), central zone (CZ), ejaculatory ducts (arrowheads), urethra (U) and anterior fibromuscular tissue (AF).

num (Figure 3). With aging, the sonographic features just described will be altered, especially since transition zone material undergoes hyperplasia (BPH). The inner gland soon occupies 95 % volume and its echotexture becomes more inhomogeneous and mixed. The peripheral and central zones become compressed, becoming more increased in echogenicity which may enhance or hide abnormalities for the unwary examiner (21, 22, 23). Toward the apex, the primary glandular tissue present is peripheral zone material (Figure 4).

The paired, epithelially lined ejaculatory ducts are considered as an extraprostatic space which courses obliquely through the central gland material from the base of the prostate to insert posteriorly on the urethra at the level of the verumontanum. These structures are formed by the coalescence of the seminal vesicles

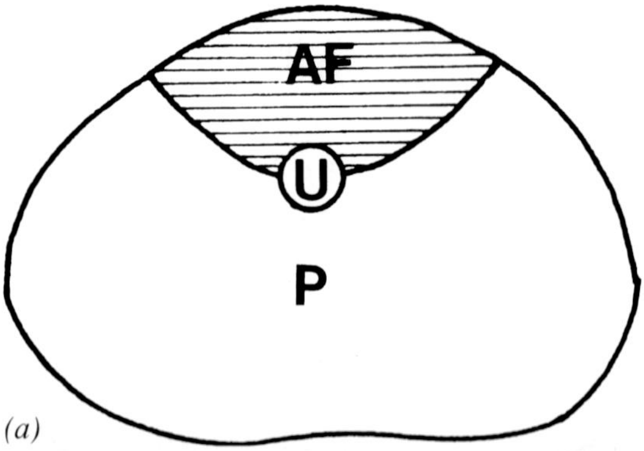

(a)

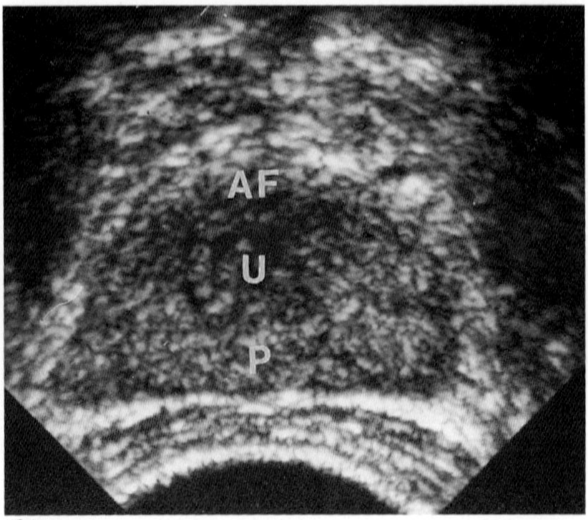

(b)

Figure 4
a. This diagram represents a transverse section at level C just cephalad to the prostatic apex and reveals that the remaining structures at this level include glandular tissue of the peripheral zone (P), urethra (U) and anterior fibromuscular stroma (AF).
b. This transverse EUS image presents sonographic features corresponding to level C (Figures 1 a and 4 a) with the three primary tissues of peripheral zone (P), urethra (U) and anterior fibromuscular stroma (AF).

with the ampullary portions of the vas deferens that lie posterior to the bladder and posterosuperior to the base of the prostate. The sonographic appearance of both of these structures is variable. Centrally, the seminal vesicles may be anechoic and fluid filled or hypoechoic with low level echoes. The vas deferens may have a similar feature (Figure 5). Both size and volume measurements are available but much variation exists so many investigators rely primarily on evaluation of symmetry (19, 20).

Patient preparation is usually unnecessary for a diagnostic EUS study of the prostate; however, an enema is needed in case a transrectal biopsy is to be performed. Scanning may be accomplished with the patient placed in the left lateral decubitus or dorsilithotomy positions. A variety of probe designs are now available with

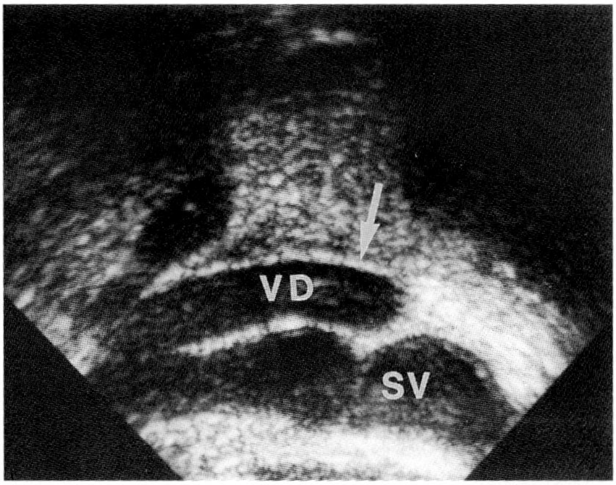

(a)

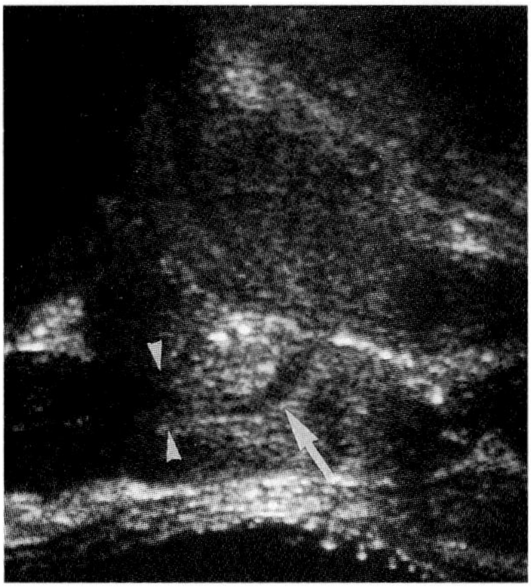
(b)

Figure 5
a. Transverse image through the region of the right seminal vesicle (SV) and vas deferens (VD) which are surrounded by bright fat (arrow). These structures join to form the epithelially lined ejaculatory duct (arrow) seen sagittally in b. This extra-prostatic space becomes beak-like (arrowheads) as it enters the gland and cancer can spread along the duct. Replacement of the beak-like appearance by a hypoechoic mass suggests invasion of the duct.

most manufacturers supplying endfire endorectal probes but sidefire probes are still routinely used. Endfire probes image the prostate, seminal vesicles and vas deferens in the coronal and sagittal planes. Sidefire probes image the prostate in the transverse and sagittal planes. Two orthogonal planes are required for lesion detection and verification (20) (Figure 6).

Measurements of the prostate are also obtained to calculate the glandular volume. The craniocaudad (CC) and anteroposterior dimensions (AP) are made from the largest dimensions at right angles to one another in the midline sagittal plane. The transverse measurement (W) is made in the transverse or coronal plane at the level with the widest diameter. A volume is calculated based on the mathematical formula for a prolate ellipse which reduces to

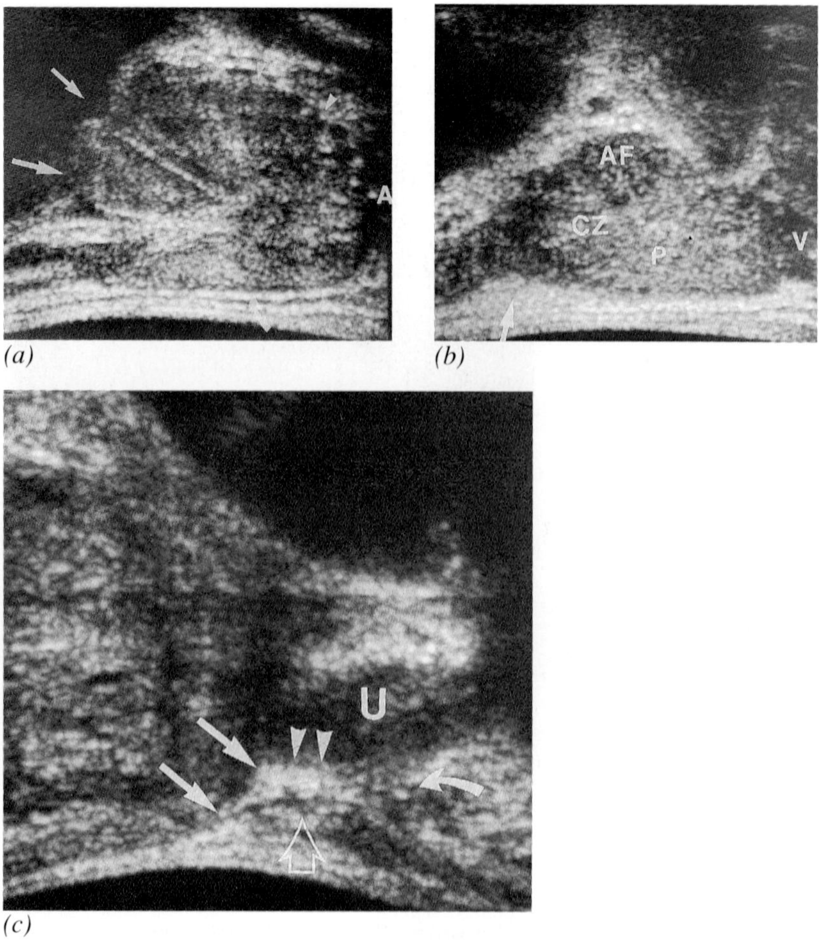

Figure 6 *Sagittal images are routinely acquired beginning in the midline (a), which shows the base (arrows), anterior (arrowheads), posterior (curved arrow) and apical (A) anatomic relationships to the prostate gland.*
b. is a sagittal image acquired approximately 20° lateral to the midline with the peripheral (P) and central (CZ) zones labeled. Note that the hypoechoic fibromuscular stroma (AF) lies anterior and portions of vessels (V) are seen near the prostatic apex. The "nipple" of periprostatic fat and fascia (arrow) is located at the posterior margin of the junction of the seminal vesicle with the base of the prostate. With the probe retracted slightly into the anal canal in c. the apex of the prostate gland (arrow) is imaged well and even the bulbomembranous portion of the urethra is seen. At the apex, the so-called trapezoid zone is formed by the posterior capsular margin of the apex (arrow), urethra (U), urethralis muscle (curved arrow) and rectal wall (open arrow). This represents a site of extracapsular spread of prostatic cancer.

Figure 7
a. Midline sagittal image of the prostate with the cranio-caudad (+) and antero-posterior (X) dimensions marked for measurements.
b. The width (+) is measured from the widest dimension obtained on the transverse image.

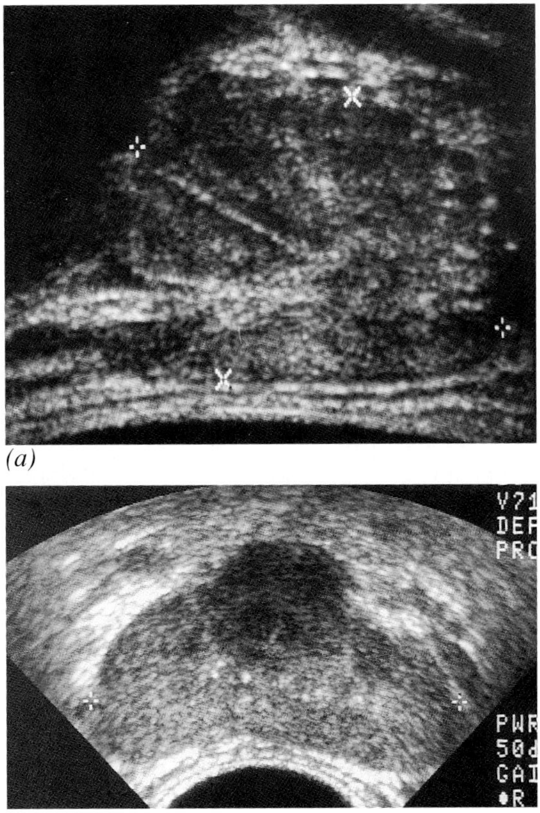

(a)

(b)

volume = 0.52 × CC × AP × W (in cm^3). This measurement can be converted into a weight in grams (gm) by multiplying by the specific gravity of tissue which is approximately 1 gm/cm^3 (24, 25) (Figure 7). Likewise, measurements for the seminal vesicles have been made with the maximal sagittal length as 7.5 cm and antero-posterior dimension as 1.9 cm. The seminal vesicle volume can be generated from planimetric measurements taken in the same fashion as those made for the prostate. Because of the wide variation in these measurements, it is often necessary to rely on a comparison of symmetry rather than an exact measurement (20).

EUS of prostate cancer

Most physicians utilize the Digital Rectal Examination (DRE) and Prostate Specific Antigen (PSA) for detection of cancer with the sensitivity of the PSA level better than the DRE. The PSA level is the measurement of a 34,000 dalton molecular weight serine protease liberated from both normal and abnormal prostate epithelium which can be detected by one of two methods: the monoclonal Tandem R and Tandem E (Hybritech, Inc., San Diego, CA) or the monoclonal-polyclonal IMX (Abbott Laboratories, Abbott Park, IL) with "normal" being 0 to 4 ng/ml. The polyclonal Pros-Check (Yang Laboratories, Bellevue, WA) method has a slightly lower range of normal (0–2.5 ng/ml) but sample values may be higher than those obtained with the Hybritech test. Problems arise with the sensitivity and specificity of the PSA level for values within 4.1 – 10 ng/ml because these levels may be due to benign prostatic hyperplasia, acute and chronic prostatitis, prostatic intraepithelial neoplasia, infarcts and the like. Also, individuals with normal PSA levels may have prostate cancer and some of these cancers can be clinically significant (26–29). Tumors associated with a normal PSA were either under 1 cm^3 or poorly differentiated cancers. To improve the specificity, investigators have developed additional parameters such as downwardly correcting the absolute PSA level to 3 ng/ml for biopsy, determining the acceleration of rise or calculating the PSA density. Endorectal Ultrasound (EUS) has been a part of this latter calculation, being needed to measure the volume of the prostate, while others have used lesion detection and biopsy guidance (9–31).

When the abnormal sonographic features of the prostate are considered, most focus on the appearance most indicative of can-

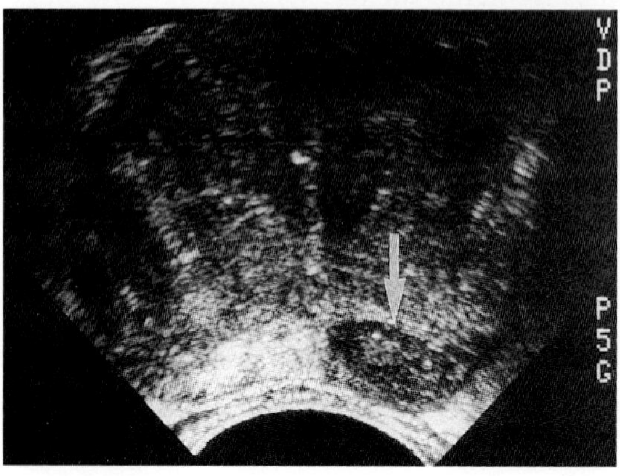

Figure 8 *A hypoechoic mass (arrow) occupies the posterolateral aspect of the prostate gland in this transverse EUS image from the mid-portion of the gland. It deforms the contour of the gland suggesting extracapsular extension (secondary feature).*

cer (32). Classically, most cancers are imaged as hypoechoic masses (70 %) (21, 32–35) (Figure 8). However, 30–40 % of cancers may not be imaged because they are equal in echogenicity to normal prostate (Figure 9). Rarely, a small percentage may be hyperechoic although many of these changes represent areas of BPH invaded by cancer (Figure 10). The situation is further complicated by the fact that many benign processes such as prostatitis, atrophy, fibrosis and hyperplastic nodules may have similar features so a differential diagnosis must be considered (21, 32–35).

To aid with differentiating these abnormalities, imagers look for secondary signs of cancers, i.e. alteration of the margin of the cap-

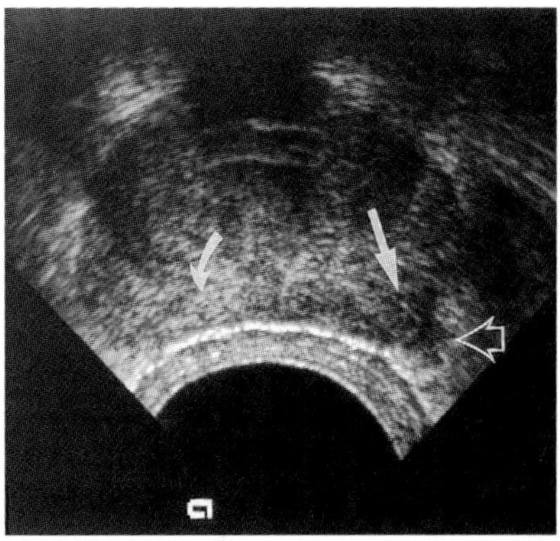

Figure 9 *In this transverse image of the prostate gland, both the hypoechoic (arrow) and isoechoic (curved arrow) appearances are present. The latter region of cancer was unsuspected sonographically but confirmed by multiple biopsies. The hypoechoic cancer also involves the left neurovascular bundle (open arrow).*

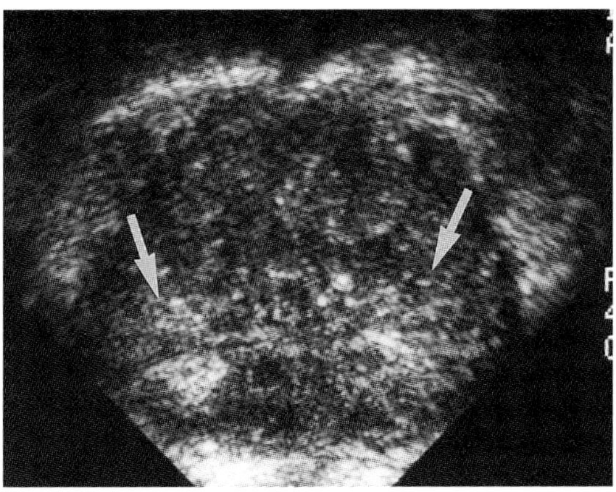

Figure 10 *The pure hyperechoic appearing cancer is less commonly imaged compared to the other presentations and when seen it is usually the comedo variety. Here, this very invasive cancer invades a region of benign prostatic hyperplasia accounting for the hyperehoic appearance (arrows). Features of extracapsular invasion are also present along the posterior capsular margin (irregular).*

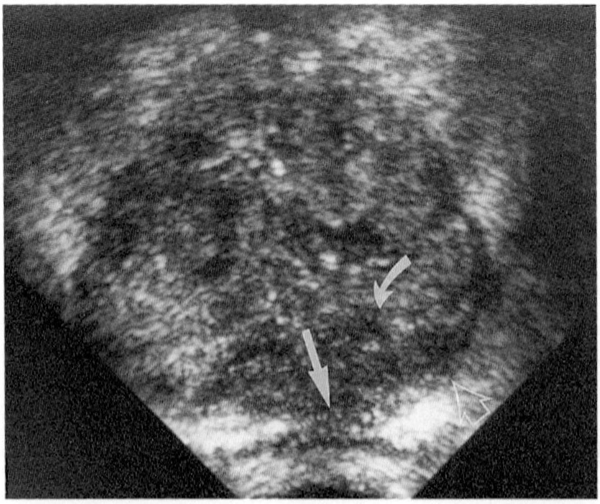

Figure 11 *All of the signs suggestive of extracapsular invasion are present in this transverse image including loss of the margin between the capsule and the periprostatic fat and fascia (arrow) as well as contour bulge (open arrow). The cancer also invades the inner gland based on the loss of the surgical capsule (curved arrow).*

sule indicated by a bulge or squaring of its normally convexly rounded margin (21–23). Loss of the so-called surgical capsule, the border of compressed glandular material separating hyperplastic tissue from peripheral gland, should arouse suspicion of an invasive cancer arising from the transition or central zones (Figure 11). Replacement of the ejaculatory duct complex may indicate a basal cancer which may have a spread from the apex or extend into the seminal vesicles (32–35).

Prostatic blood flow has been studied with duplex Doppler and color Doppler sonography (CDS) to improve lesion detection and discrimination (36–38). Early results with duplex imaging were less than optimal but results with CDS have been slightly more encouraging based on studies by Rifkin et al (37) and Kelly et al. (38) because blood flow was easier to image. Unfortunately, CDS has its limitations, some of which may be machine related. First, peripheral gland flow has been described as sparse with pericapsular and periurethral flow which may be related to the wall filter settings utilized (20). However, more prostatic flow has been demonstrated within the peripheral gland than initially described with units that allowed for lower levels for the pulse repetition frequency (PRF) and wall filter settings (20) (Figure 12). More importantly, prostate cancer has been shown to have increased flow secondary to the presence of tumor vascularity but overlap exists between increased flow associated with cancer and prostatitis (acute and chronic) (Figure 13).

Not every cancer will have sufficient flow to be detected by CDS (39, 40, 41). Tumor vessels may be acquired from pre-existing vessels recruited by the tumor for its blood supply or vessels which dilate to respond to the growing tumor. Tumor vessels may arise de novo from the tumor. The vessels are usually endothelially lined and surrounded by tumor cells. Lacking a muscular coat for support, the flow is usually of the low impedence (decreased resistance) type which is indicated by the pulsed Doppler tracings with high diastolic flow. Peak velocities may be elevated and arteriovenous flow patterns may also be present secondary to shunts. The presence of tumor neovascularity may be a predictor of the

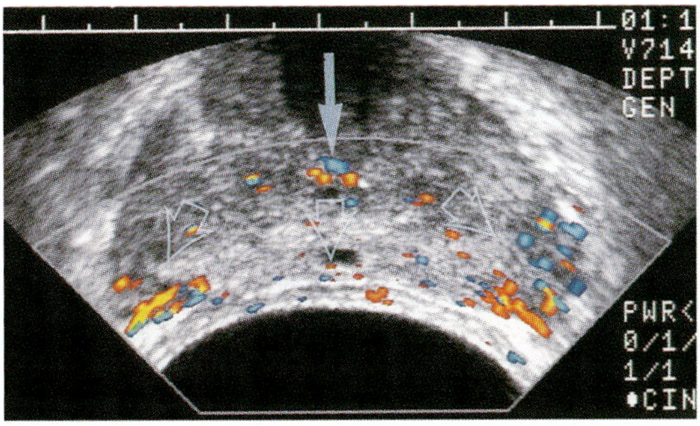

Figure 12 *Transverse image depicting color coded flow patterns of the normal prostate gland. The two principle arterial distributions to the gland arise from vessels entering at the bladder neck and traveling periurethrally (arrow) supplying the inner gland. The other enters posterolaterally and surrounds the capsular margin (open arrows) feeding much of the peripheral gland. Remember, the color coded flow demonstrated still depends on machine sensitivity with wall filter settings, pulse repetition frequency and color gain playing a very important role.*

Figure 13 *This transverse color coded flow image of the prostate gland reveals clustered color signal within a hypoechoic mass (arrow). Realize, acute as well as chronic prostatitis can have a similar appearance.*

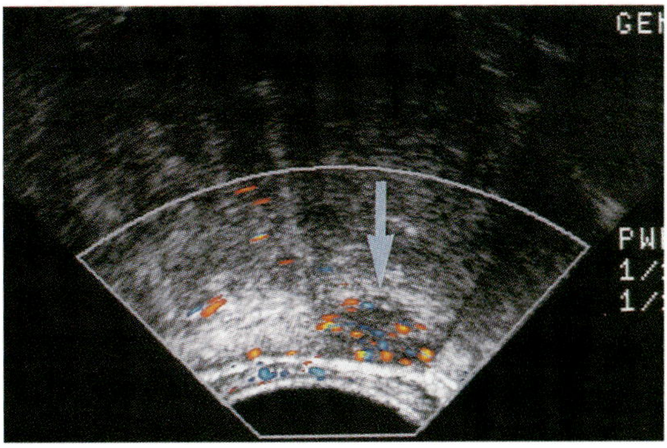

potential for bone metastasis which could identify a unique population of patients (39, 40, 41).

Prostate biopsy technique

Any physical or ultrasonographic finding arousing suspicion should be biopsied. Ultrasound may consist of transrectal or transperineal placement of needles into the prostate. Biopsy technique will vary and depends on the clinical situation. Certain patient factors should be considered when the decision for the best biopsy approach is made. These factors include patient mobility, location of the lesion, presence of large internal hemorrhoids and immune status of the patient (20). Both the transperineal and transrectal biop-

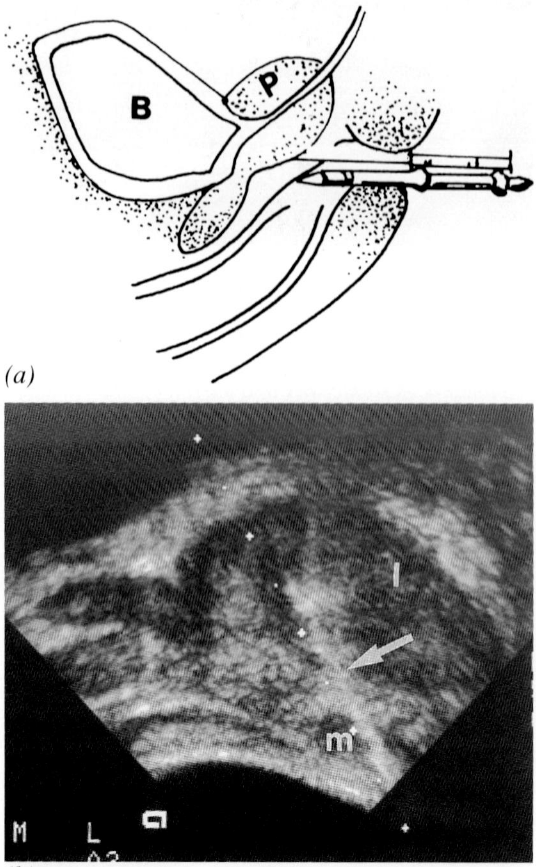

(a)

(b)

Figure 14
a. Schematic diagram indicates the desired positioning of the endorectal probe during a transrectal biopsy. The tip of the biopsy needle should be inserted through the rectal wall and then placed at the capsular margin to sample lesions adjacent to the capsule. b. Transrectal biopsy has been performed with hyperechoic tract of the needle (arrow) seen extending across the hypoechoic mass (m) as well as the inner gland (I). Note the path of the needle had covered approixmately 2 cm of the prostate gland.

sies have complications that occur following the procedure which include hematuria, hematochezea, hematospermia, and infection. The risk for hematochezea and infection are slightly higher following transrectal biopsies. Good aftercare instructions include signs of infection and urinary retention and a prescription for several days of post procedure antimicrobial coverage. Afterwards, a urine specimen should be taken to check for gross hematuria (20).

To achieve the best biopsy results, a pre-biopsy scan should be completed so lesions are detected and their location noted. For the transperineal biopsy, the patient should be in the dorsolithotomy position and his perineum sterilized, prepped and draped. Good local anesthesia should be given to the skin and underlying subcutaneous soft tissues. Then the transrectal probe is inserted into the rectum and the sterile transperineal guide attached to the probe. An important point to remember, the guide should be tight against the perineal skin surface. A 22 gauge 15 cm spinal needle is helpful for applying anesthetic at the capsule of the prostate prior to biopsy. Now the 18 gauge spring loaded trigger gun is in and advanced along the biopsy target indicated on the CRT screen (20).

Before initiating a transrectal biopsy, the patient should receive an oral antimicrobial coverage for urologic flora and the agent should provide rapid and adequate blood levels. The patient is also given a cleansing enema to clear the lower rectum of as much fecal debris as possible. The patient is positioned in the left lateral decubitous position and the properly prepared transrectal probe is inserted for the biopsy (Figure 14). As in the transperineal biopsy, a target grid is displayed on the screen to help guide the needle to the capsular margin of the gland. The tip of the needle is brought to the point of touching the capsule but not beyond (Figure 14). Remember, the typical core

Figure 15
A photograph taken at the tip of an 18 gauge needle freuqently used for biopsies of the prostate gland with exposed (arrow) and unexposed specimen notch in view.

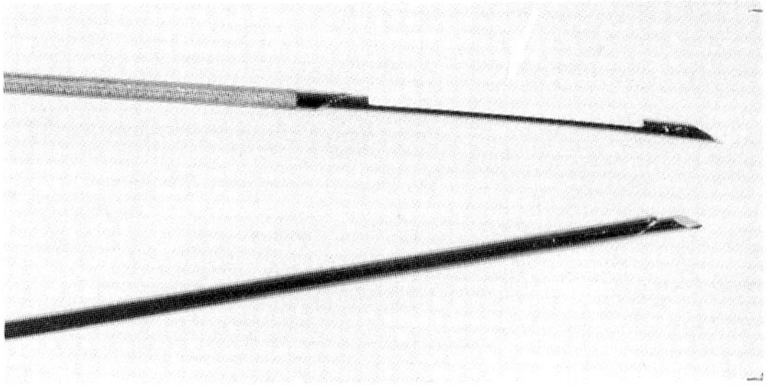

needle will have an inner cannula with a 17 mm specimen notch which upon firing will travel at least 2 cm (Figure 15). This distance should be kept in mind to avoid inadvertent passage of the needle through the gland into adjacent structures such as the blood vessels or urinary bladder. Once the needle is inserted into the rectum, probe movement should cease to avoid inadvertant laceration of rectum secondary to the exposed needle (Figure 16).

Benign prostatic hyperplasia

Benign prostatic hyperplasia (BPH) is rarely seen before the age of 40 but its incidence is steadily rising with approximately 50 % incidence in 50-year olds to nearly 85 % of males over 80 (42, 43). Some males remain asymptomatic while others may have it result in bladder outlet obstruction. Hyperplastic nodules initially form from the transition zone material above the level of the verumontanum. The proposed mechanisms for nodule formation include reversion of stromal cells to an embryonic state, nodular recruitment, and hormonal induction (42–45).

Hyperplastic tissue leads to alteration in the sonographic appearance of the normal prostate. Early on, discrete nodules may be imaged as regions of diminished echogenicity. As the process progresses, nodules may incrase in number and size becoming mixed in echotexture with regions of increased and decrased echogenicity and with further expansion, the adjacent peripheral gland becomes compressed (20, 46, 47). A hypoechoic margin is formed at the advancing margin of the hyperplastic tissues called the surgical capsule. In additon, regions of increased echogenicity lacking distal shadowing known as corpora amylacea (amorphouos, gel-like substance excreted from

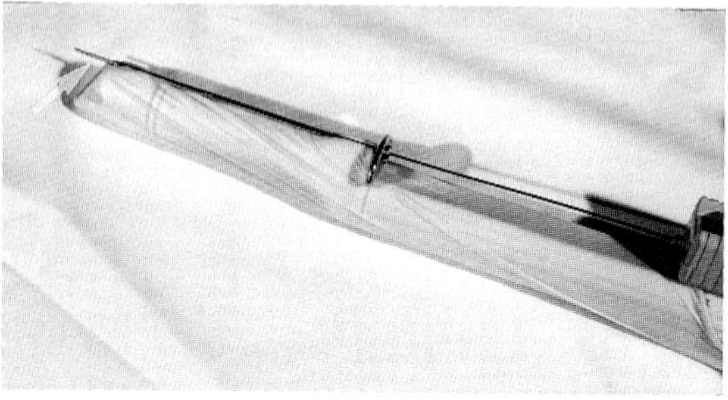

Figure 16 *In this photograph, the probe has been prepared for a transrectal bipsy with the biopsy needle inserted and the tip of the needle (arrow) is fully exposed even before it comes into view of the ultrasound beam.*

compressed acini) may become intermixed with the hyperplastic tissue (48). Deposits of hydroxic apatite are also echogenic but shadow unlike corpora amylacea and should not be confused with the midline shadow created by beam refraction artifact resulting from bending of the sound beam by two coalescing nodules (Figure 17). Another midline defect encountered is the anechoic void in the proximal prostatic urethra after hyperplastic tissue is removed during the transurethral resection (20, 48) (Figure 18).

Inflammation

Prostatitis may be bacterial or nonbacterial in origin and is a common problem (50). Unfortunately, referred abnormalities which may be nonprostate may produce the so-called pelvi-perineal pain (prostatodynia) (51). Both acute and chronic prostatitis are encountered with the acute form usually present with low back pain, fever, dysuria, and perineal pain. Offending agents include members of the enterobacteriaceae with E. coli and Pseudomonas with Enterococci and mixed infections less commonly encountered. If infection follows a transrectal or transperineal procedure then

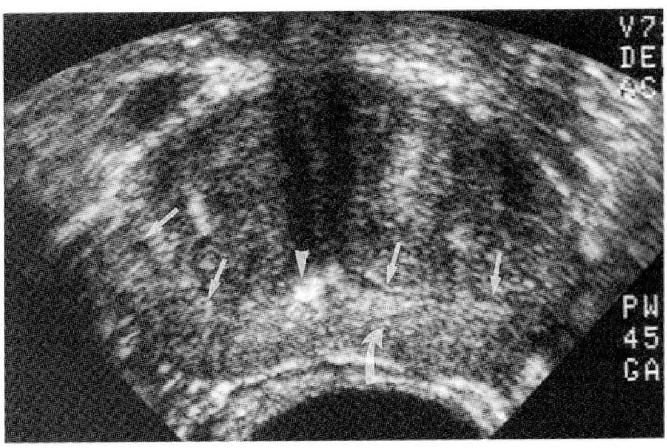

Figure 17 *A transverse image with many of the typical sonographic features of BPH. The amount of inner gland tissue is increased and there are both low and high level echoes. The expanding hyperplastic tissues compress the adjacent tissues of the peripheral gland with the boundary of the "surgical capsule" between them (arrows). The echogenicity of the peripheral zone may increase secondary to compression of the glandular interfaces (curved arrow). Corpora amylacea may become mixed with calcification which shadows (arrowhead) and usually resides along the posterior margins of the surgical capsule.*

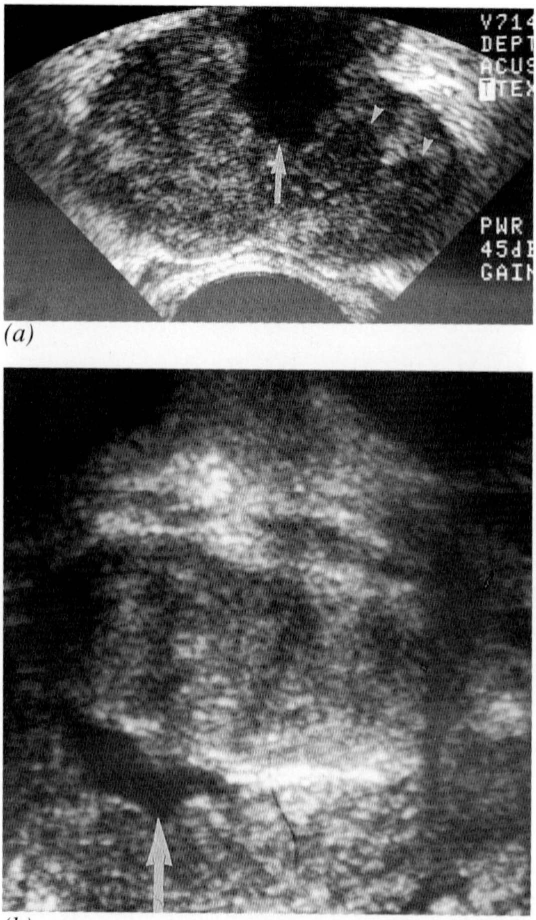

(a)

(b)

Figure 18
a. Transverse EUS image, and b. the companion sagittal image from a patient with symptomatic BPH treated by transurethral resection of the prostate gland. Notice the anechoic defect in the inner gland which is the surgically widened urethra (arrow). In a. there are two discrete hypoechoic nodules (arrowheads), which represent focal hyperplastic nodules.

anaerobic bacteria such as Bacteroides fragilis or Clostridium perfringens are most often responsible. Occasionally, granulomatous prostatitis may be present which is thought to represent a stage in the progressive resolution of acute bacterial prostatitis (50, 51).

Initially, three sonographic features of acute prostatitis were described by Griffiths et al. and included a sonolucent halo about periurethral tissue, diminished echogenicity within the peripheral zone associated with capsule indistinctness, and an increased sonolucency about the gland (52). However, no truly specific sonographic sign has been identified (Figure 19). A sonographically normal gland should exclude the diagnosis of acute bacterial prostatitis. In chronic prostatitis, single multiple calcifications are of-

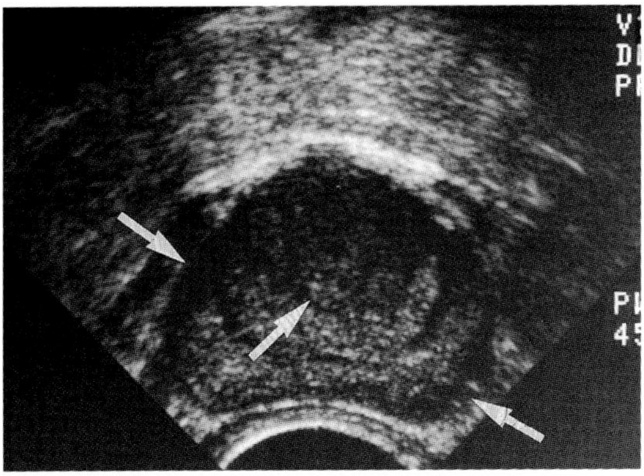

Figure 19 *This image shows both periurethral and pericapsular incrased lucency thought to represent prostatitis (arrows). The former finding may be due to artifact rather than being a true sonographic feature of acute prostatitis.*

ten present as a result of a dystrophic calcification following the extravasation of infected urine into the prostatic parenchyma (53, 54). Ultimately, bacteria entrapped within these calcifications are very difficult to irradicate by antimicrobial therapy. Occasionally, asymmetrically located patches of hypoechogenicity will be seen within the parenchyma and these most likely represent foci of inflammation (Figure 20). If a prostatic abscess develops, the patient may become acutely toxic and EUS will reveal a complex parenchymal collection with both cystic and solid elements resulting from cellular debris and necrotic material (55) (Figure 21).

Prostatic cysts

Congenital and acquired cysts of the prostate have been described with their clinical presentation depending on their origin, location and size. Acquired cysts are more common than the true congen-

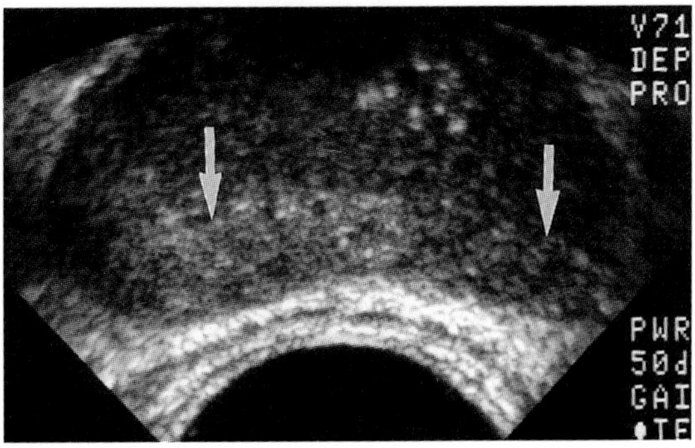

Figure 20 *This transverse image is from an asymptomatic patient suspected of having prostate cancer based on an elevated PSA level and abnormal echogenicity in the peripheral zone (arrows). Biopsy of this nonacute patient revealed multifocal acute and chronic prostatitis.*

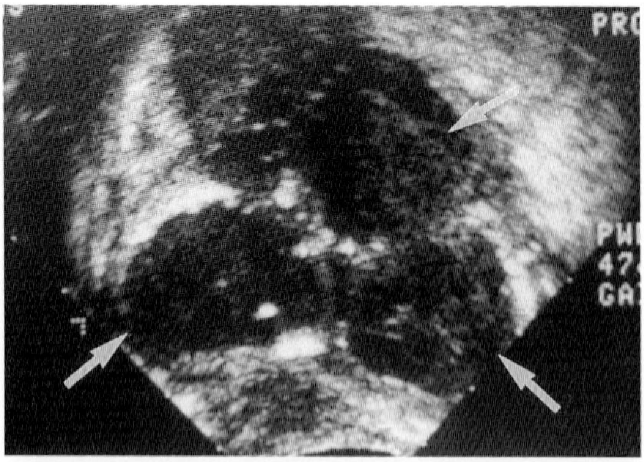

Figure 21 *An EUS image from an acutely toxic patient with severe prostatodynea reveals a complex multiloculated mass (arrows) occupying most of the gland which was aspirated, confirming the presence of a prostatic abscess.*

ital cyst. The most commonly encountered acquired cysts include the ejaculatory duct cyst, dilated prostatic ducts, and regions of cystic degeneration. Obstruction of the ejaculatory duct produces the ejaculatory duct cyst and the axis of dilatation follows the course of the ejaculatory duct (20, 56) (Figure 22).

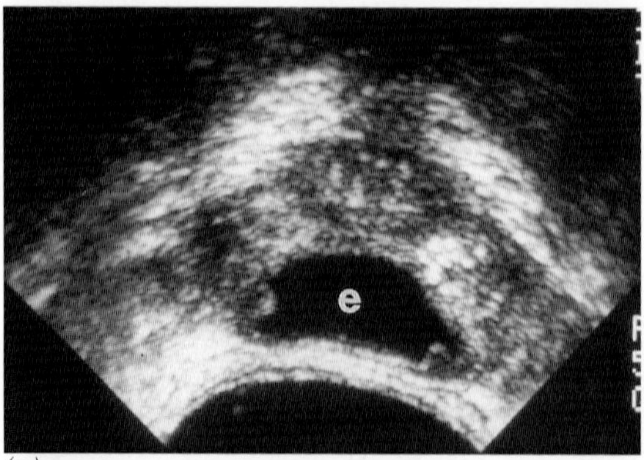

(a)

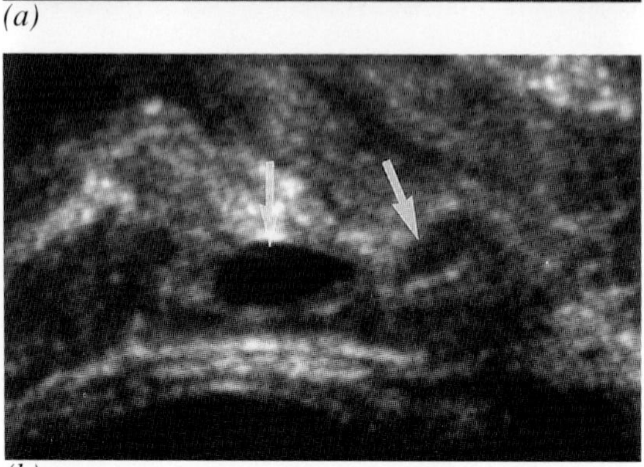

(b)

Figure 22
a. A markedly dilated ejaculatory duct (e) is seen indicating obstruction in a functionally infertile patient who underwent surgery to relieve the obstruction.
b. The follow-up sagittal image which shows that the duct is much less dilated (arrow).

The two most common congenital cysts are the Müllerian duct cyst and the utricle cyst which arises from the prostatic utricle. Even though their embryologic origins are different, they may have a similar appearance on EUS. Sonographically, the utricle cyst presents in the midline near the verumontanum and it is usually smaller than the Müllerian duct cyst. When large, it may be extremely difficult to make a distinction between these cysts. The utricle cyst, unlike the Müllerian duct cyst, is frequently associated with additional genitourinary abnormalities, such as hypospadia, incomplete testicular dissent or unilateral renal agenesis (20, 56) (Figure 23).

Abnormalities of the seminal vesicles

The seminal vesicles are paired hypoechoic structures easily imaged with EUS and usually of interest because of the increasing number of infertility cases. Absence of the seminal vesicles and vas deferens is indicated by the failure of the examiner to find them in their expected location. Bilateral absence of these structures is easily overlooked because symmetry is preserved (Figure 24). Seminal vesicle cysts may be encountered resulting from obstruction of the ejaculatory duct and they have been associated with ectopically inserting ureter (57, 58) (Figure 25).

Acute inflammation of the seminal vesicles or seminal vesiculitis may be clinically associated with acute prostatitis or present as an isolated event. The affected vesicle may become enlarged and its walls are often thickened. One or both vesicles can be involved and abscess formation can be a complicating event (57, 58) (Figure 26).

EUS OF THE RECTUM

Normal rectal anatomy

The histologic layers of the normal rectal wall are sonographically imaged as an alternating sequence of 5 to 7 hyperechoic-hypoechoic bands which are fed by the superior midline and inferior rectal arteries. The initial echo encountered is the hyperechoic band of the latex wall of the water filled condom as it abuts the distended rectum (60, 61, 62). The first hypoechoic layer of the

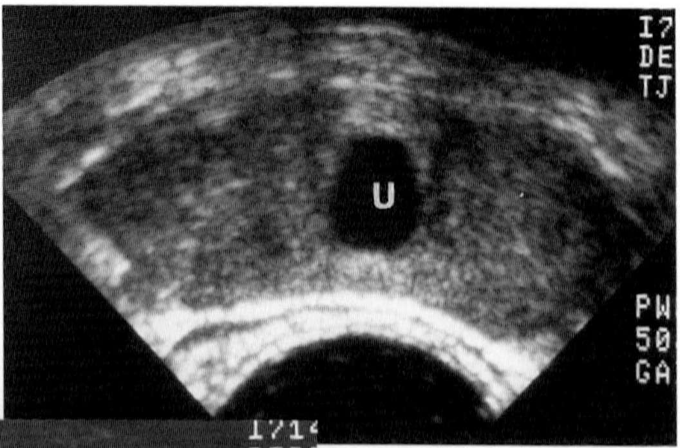

Figure 23 *The centrally anechoic utricular cyst (U) occupies the central portion of the gland and may be difficult to distinguish from Müllerian duct cyst.*

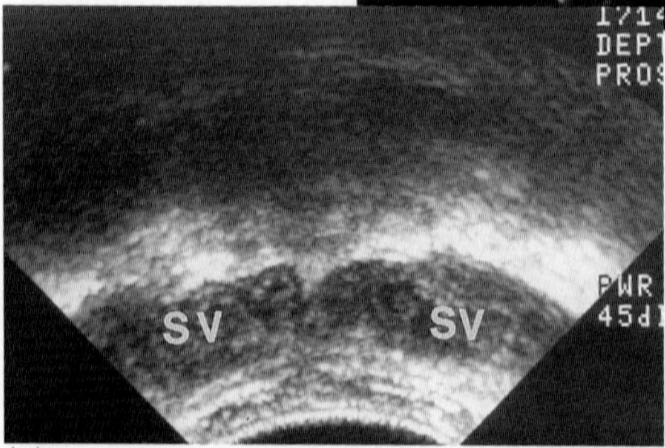

(a)

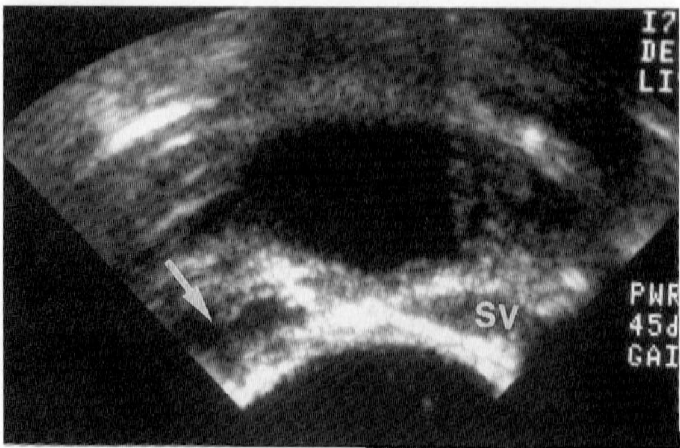

(b)

Figure 24
a. Transverse image of normally paired seminal vesicles (SV) which is compared to b., a transverse image at the same level revealing unilateral absence of the right seminal vesicle (arrow), while the left seminal vesicle (SV) is hypoplastic. The hypoechoic structure in its place is a prominent vein.

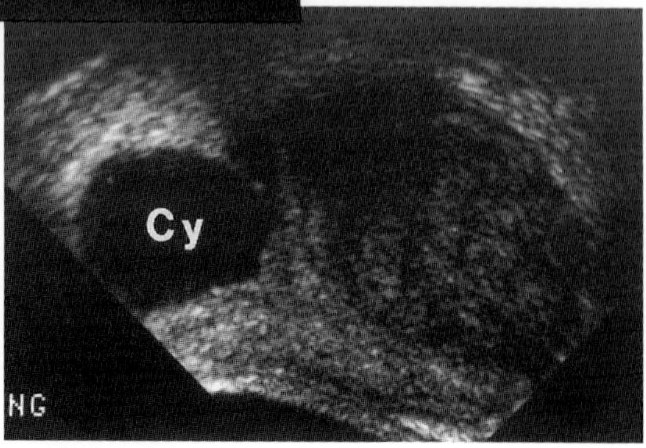

Figure 25 *This sagittal image illustrates the typical anechoic appearance of a seminal vesicle cyst (Cy) resulting from obstruction of the ejaculatory duct.*

Figure 26 *Transverse (a) and sagittal (b) images from a patient with seminal vesiculitis. Note the enlarged vesicle (arrow) which also contains internal echoes.*

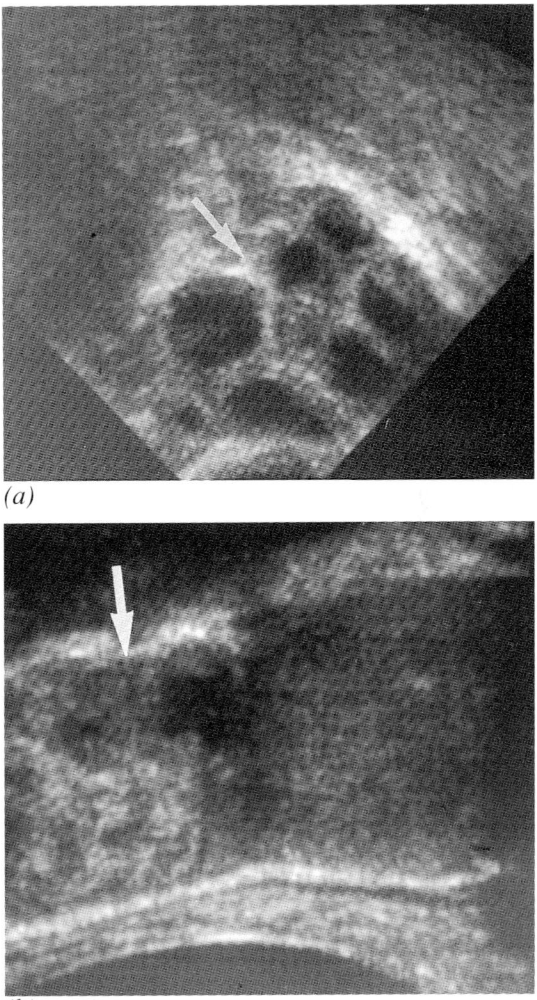

(a)

(b)

rectal wall represents the mucosa and probably the muscularis mucosa as well. The thickness of this latter layer is below the limit of resolution of the frequencies currently employed in endorectal probes. The second hyperechoic layer represents the submucosa and the third hypoechoic layer is the muscularis propria. The fifth layer is hyperecoic perirectal fact and not serosa since this layer is lacking as the peritoneum has made its reflection at the level of third sacral vertebrae. If a high frequency such as 7.5 MHz or 10 MHz is used, then the fourth layer may be imaged as alternating bands of hypoechoic inner circular muscle, hyperechoic connec-

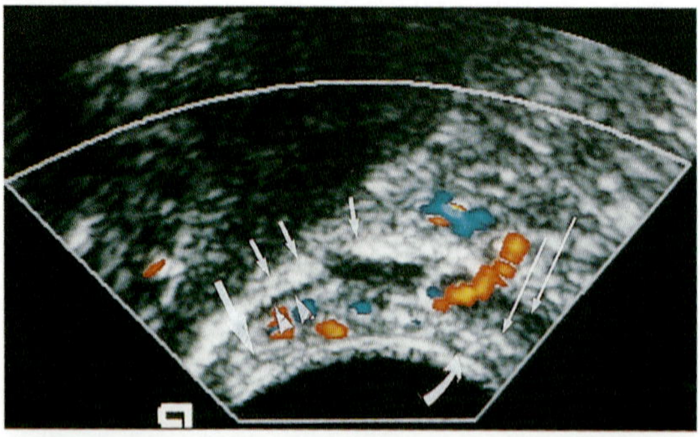

Figure 27 *This transverse image of the distended rectal wall illustrates the hypoechoic mucosa (curved arrow), hyperechoic submucosa (arrow), hypoechoic muscularis propria (arrowhead) and hyperechoic perirectal fat (short arrows) layers of the normal rectal wall. The muscularis propria may be imaged as three separate bands or layers which are the hypoechoic inner circular muscle (long stem arrows). A large perirectal feeding artery (orange) penetrates the rectal wall to form the submucosal arterial and venous plexuses (orange and blue).*

tive tissue and hypoechoic outer longitudinal muscle (9–14, 60–62) (Figure 27).

The principal arterial supply to the rectum comes from the superior rectal artery with the middle and the inferior rectal arteries furnishing a very limited portion of the mid to distal rectum (63). The perirectal branches surround the rectum entering the hypoechoic muscularis propria sending smaller branches into the adjacent hyperehcoic submucosa to form the submucosal arterial plexuses. Ultimately, the submucosal arterial plexuses give rise to tiny branches which will supply the muscularis mucosa and the hypoechoic mucosa (63, 64). Both high and low resistance vessels have been identified. The high resistant arterial waveforms (PI $\geq$ 2.1 $\pm$ 0.87) are thought to originate from muscle coated perirectal arteries and submucosal arteries (63, 64) (see Figure 27).

EUS staging of rectal cancer

The American Cancer Society expects nearly 42,000 new cases of rectal cancer to be discovered and that an estimated 7,000 patients will succumb to their disease (1). In order to improve outcomes, surgeons have tried to increase local control with adjuvant therapies

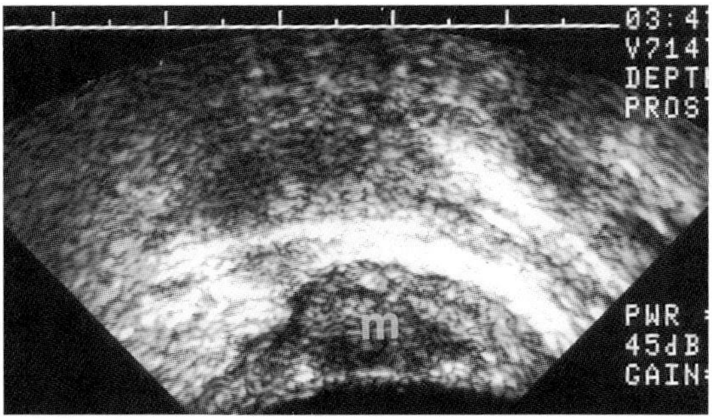

Figure 28 *An EUS image of a small hypoechoic mass (m) involving the mucosal and submucosal layers of the rectal wall.*

such as high dose preoperative radiation with or without chemotherapy and improved surgical techniques. To be successful, loco-regional staging is required with much of this information obtained by radiologic imaging (65, 66). Depending on the radiologic modality utilized, the accuracies for the determination of the level of mural invasion for rectal cancers have varied for EUS (63–93 %), computed tomography (33–70 %) and magnetic resonance imaging (79–89 %). Compared to the results achieved for mural staging, the accuracies for the detection of neoplastic lymph nodes have been somewhat less for endosonography (32–80 %), computed tomography (25–73 %) and magnetic resonance imaging (72 %) (67).

EUS wall staging (T) was based on discontinuity or loss of one or more of the 5 sonographic layers of the rectal wall. Lesions involving either the mucosal or submucosal layers were staged as T1 (Figure 28), those infiltrating the muscularis propria as T2 (Figure 29) and cancers invading the perirectal fat as T3 (Figure 30). T4 lesions extended from the perirectal fat into the pelvic side wall or adjacent solid pelvic organs (9–14, 68) (Figure 31). Color coded flow has been observed within these cancers and pulse wave Doppler has

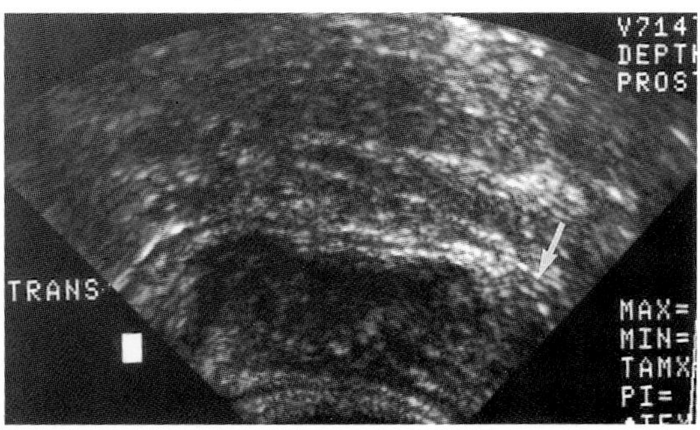

Figure 29 *An EUS image of a large hemicircumferential mass involving the mucosa, submucosa and muscularis propria layers of the rectal wall (arrow).*

identified both high and low resistance vessels (Figure 32). Vessels with waveforms of high central resistance (PI $\geq$ 1.36 $\pm$ 0.21) are thought to represent the perirectal artery feeding vessels and the lower resistant peripheral ones (PI $\geq$ 0.86 $\pm$ 0.14) are considered to be tumor vessels (63, 64). The EUS criteria for metastatic lymph nodes have relied on nodal size or alterations in nodal shape or echotexture. The upper limit for sonographically normal nodes has ranged from 5

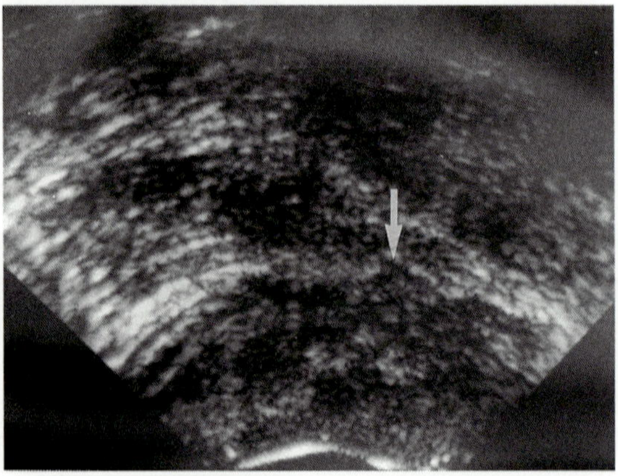

Figure 30 *A transverse image from patient with a cancer invading into the perirectal fat indicated by spiculation at the border between the musuclaris propria and the bright perirectal fat (arrow).*

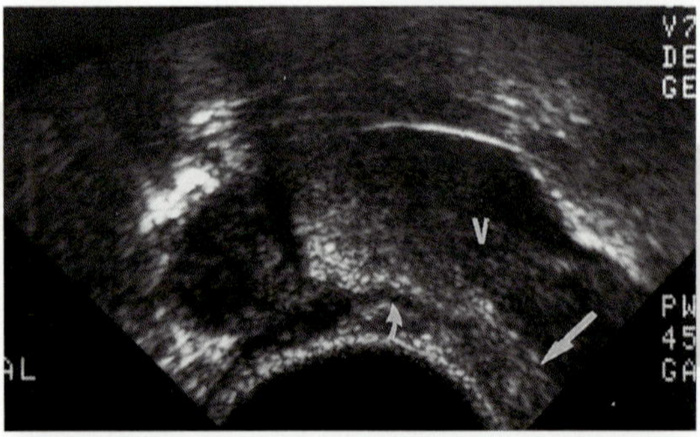

Figure 31 *This image is from a rectal cancer (arrow) that has invaded the vagina (V). Intact musuclaris propria (curved arrow) is present more laterally.*

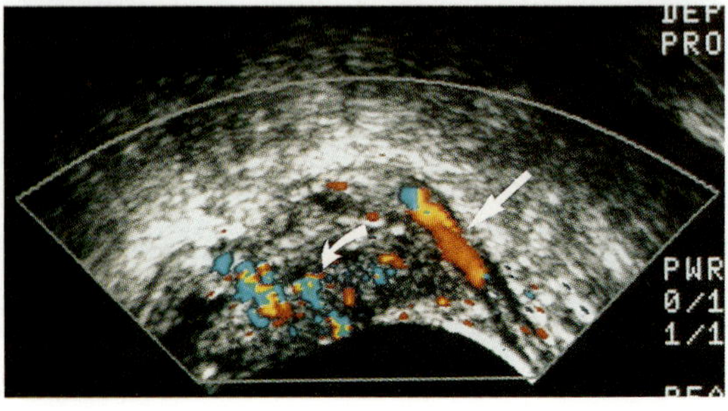

Figure 32 *A transverse color coded flow image from a T2 lesion with a high peripheral resistance. A perirectal feeding artery (arrow) is imaged in orange indicating flow into the mass. More centrally clustered flow is low resistance and would be consistent with tumor flow (curved arrow).*

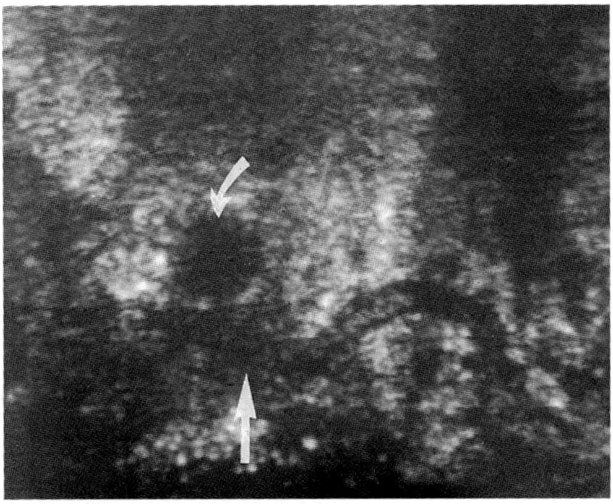

Figure 33 *This sagittal iamge reveals a hypoechoic metastatic perirectal lymph node (curved arrow) adjacent to an area of perirectal fat invasion (arrow).*

to 9 mm (69, 70). Nodes are also considered to be positive if they have a rounded instead of an oval shape or their internal echogenicity is hypoechoic or less commonly mixed (Figure 33). Nodes with a hyperechoic internal echogenicity are considered benign (69–71). Remember, rectal cancer and prostate cancer may rarely coexist in male patients and the unexpected rectal cancer should be sought on the digital examination (Figure 34).

EUS rectal interventions

EUS can play a role in guiding needles to sample perirectal lymph nodes as well as deep pelvic collections unapproachable by the more conventional percutaneous routes (15, 67, 70, 71). Since the needles or catheter must traverse the rectal wall, patients should be on the appropriate antimicrobial coverage. Like EUS guided biopsy of the prostate, patients may be placed preferably in the left lateral decubitus position, but the dorsilithotomy position may

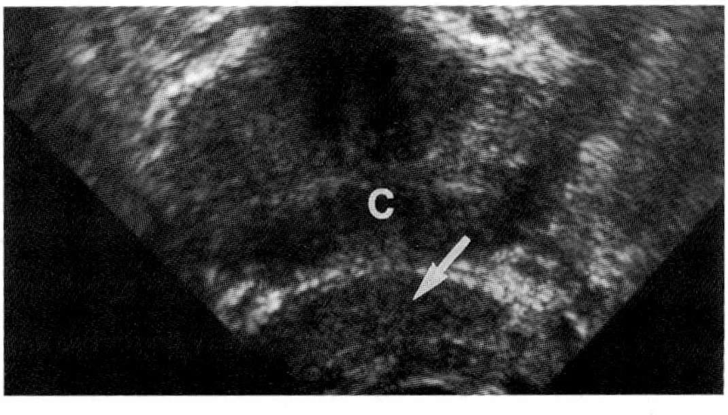

Figure 34 *A transverse image from a patient with cancers of the prostate gland (C) and rectum (arrow).*

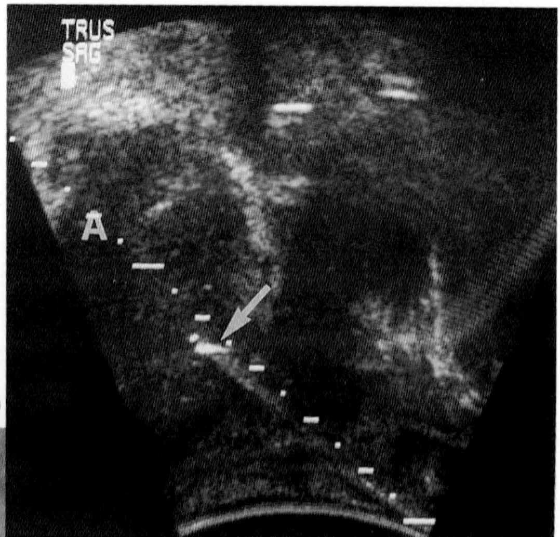

(a)

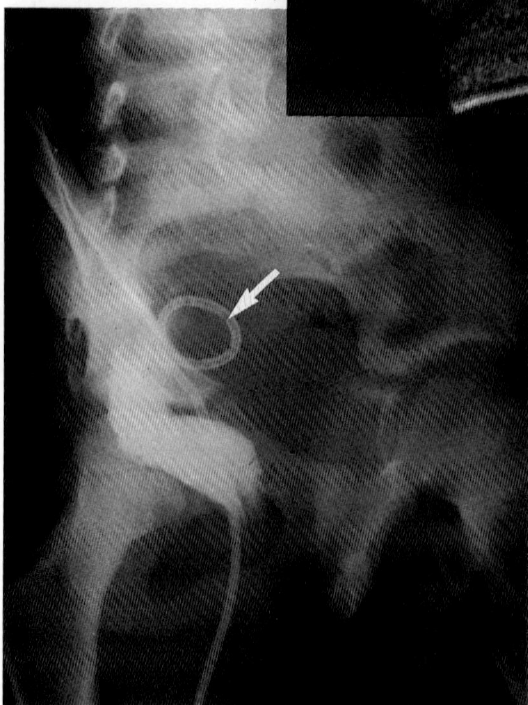

(b)

Figure 35 *a. Sagittal EUS image from a patient with deep pelvic abscess (A) following appendectomy which has been accessed by a needle (arrow) under EUS guidance.*
b. A fistulogram has been performed and reveals that the abscess has been drained and the self retaining catheter (arrow) is placed in good position.

be used when necessary. The patient should have a cleansing enema to remove as much of the rectal contents as possible. Although day time sedation may not be needed in cases for fine needle aspiration, it is a must for those individuals in which a drainage catheter will be placed. The probe should be covered with a sterile condom and then inserted into the rectal vault (15, 69, 70).

Needle size may vary from 22 gauge for nodal aspiration to 18 gauge in cases of perirectal abscess aspiration. Catheters should be of the self retaining variety and sized according to the viscosity of the collection to be drained with sizes usually ranging from 8 to 10 F. If the collection can be aspirated dry then catheter placement may not be needed (15).

For EUS catheter placement, the perirectal collection is localized with EUS and a needle is guided into it by EUS. Then a suitable guide wire is passed through the needle during EUS and the probe is removed. The tract is then sequentially dilated to allow placement of the catheter under fluoroscopic guidance (Figure 35). Duration of catheter placement may vary and is governed by persistence of drainage with removal following cessation of drainage and confirmation by contrast injection under fluoroscopic guidance. Once placed, catheters are well tolerated in both the pediatric and adult patients and they have not caused difficulties with defecation. Use of self retaining catheters markedly reduces the incidence of spontaneous expulsions. Bacterial superinfections have not been a problem but antimicrobial coverage is a must (15).

ANAL CANAL

Anal canal anatomy

The anal canal is the terminal 3 to 4 cm portion of intestinal tract with primary function to maintain fecal continence. The canal begins at the anorectal junction and extends caudally to end at the anal verge. It is surrounded by the anal sphincter complex which is formed by two primary muscles, the internal and external sphincters. The internal sphincter is the innermost muscle of the complex and is a continuation of circular smooth muscle from the muscularis propria of the rectum. The outermost, external sphincter is composed of a series of striated muscle bands arising from a downward extension of the puborectalis muscle (16).

Anal canal EUS

The anal sphincter complex and its surrounding structures have been imaged utilizing 5.0 to 7.5 MHz EUS probes positioned

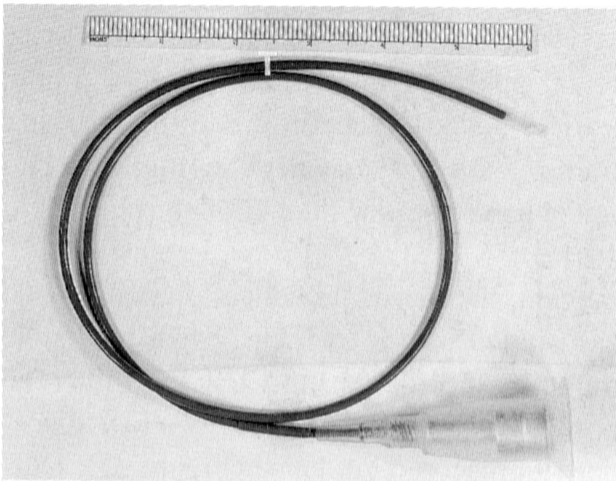

Figure 36
A photograph of the high frequency ultrasound catheter (T) that was inserted into the anal canal to obtain the transverse images in figures 37–39.

within the anal canal. The anatomical information obtained has provided a basis for assessment of anal canal abnormalities such as sphincter disruptions, fistulas and anal cancer (71–76). More recently, 12.5 MHz 9F catheter-based ultrasound probes have been placed into the anal canal to increase image resolution yielding better anatomic detail without the potential for distortion secondary to distention of the anal canal by the larger diameter endorectal probes (16) (Figure 36).

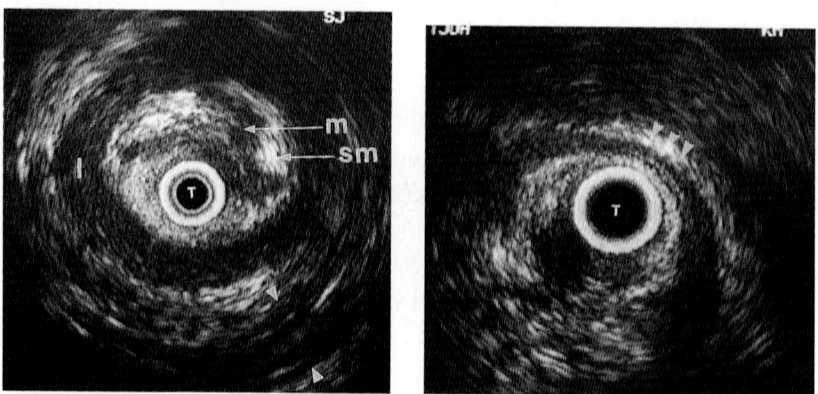

(a) *(b)*

Figure 37 *The hypoechoic mucosa (M) and hyperechoic submucosa (SM) are well seen with the high frequency ultrasound catheter (T). The hypoechoic smooth muscle of the internal sphincter (I) is imaged. Complete multiple rings of striated muscle of the external sphincter (arrowheads) are also present. The puborectalis muscle (arrowheads) is imaged.*

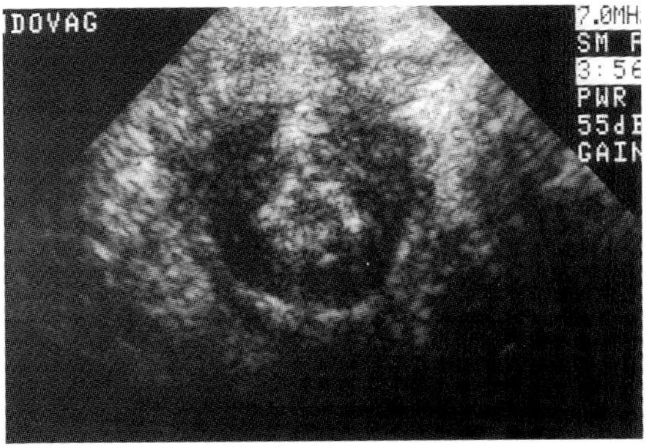

Figure 38 *A transverse image through the anal canal reveals a linear echogenic band (arrow) across the internal and external sphincters which is consistent with disruption.*

Most investigators have described the internal sphincter as a circular hypoechoic band which becomes more echogenic with age. With the more conventional EUS probes, the thickness of the internal sphincter has been measured in different series from 2 mm (range, 1–3 mm) up to 3.4 mm) (72–75). This muscle may become thinner with age. The mean thickness of the internal sphincter measures slightly larger with the endoluminal catheters at 3.5 mm ± 0.5 (2.6 to 4.3 mm) and unlike the echogenicity described for EUS studies, the muscle remains uniformly hypoechoic (72–75) Figure 37). In cases of sphincter disruption, the continuity of the muscles is lost (Figure 38) and in fistulas, a hypoechoic tract may be identified (Figure 39).

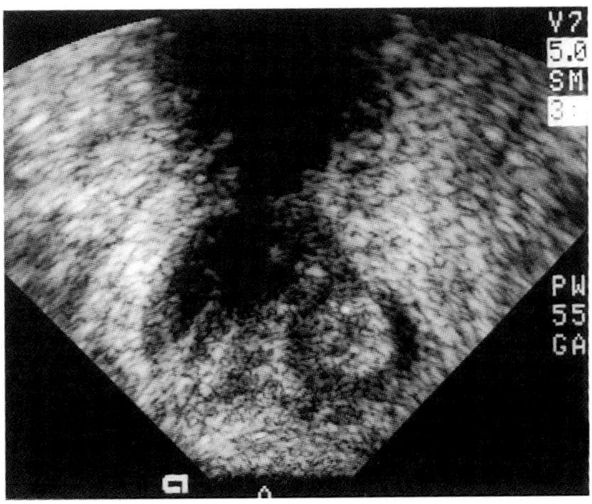

Figure 39 *This transverse image demonstrates a perirectal abscess (A) with a fistula tract (arrow) entering the canal at the anorectal junction.*

REFERENCES

1. Boring CC, Squires TS, Tong T et al. Cancer statistics. Ca-A Cancer. J Clin 1994;41:5–25.
2. Oesterling IF. Prostate specific antigen: a critical assessment of the most useful tumor marker for adenocarcinoma of the prostate. J Urol 1992;145:907–921.
3. Catalona WI, Richie JP, Ahmann FR et al. A multicenter evaluation of PSA and digital rectal examinations (DRE) for early detection of prostate cancer in 6,371 volunteers (Abstr). J Urol 1993;149 (suppl): 412A.
4. Labrie F, Dupont A, Suburu E. et al. Serum prostate-specific antigen as pre-screening test for prostate cancer. J Urol 1992;147:846–852.
5. Lee F, Littrup PJ, Torp-Pedersen ST et al. Prostate cancer: comparison of transrectal US and digital rectal examination for screening. Radiology 1988;168:389–394.
6. Cooper WH, Mosley BR, Rutherford CT et al. Prostate cancer: detection in a clinical urological practice by ultrasonography, digital rectal examination, and prostate-specific antigen. J Urol 1990;143:1146 –1154.
7. McClellan BL. Diagnostic imaging evaluation of benign prostatic hyperplasia. Radiol Clin N Am 1990;17:517–536.
8. Waterhouse RL, Resnick MI. The use of transrectal prostatic ultrasonography in the evaluation of patients with prostatic carcinoma. J Urol 1989;141:233–239.
9. Dershaw DD, Enker WF, Cohen AM et al. Transrectal ultrasonography of rectal carcinoma. Cancer 1990;66:2336–2340.
10. Boscaini M, Montori A. Transrectal ultrasonography: interpretation of normal intestinal wall structure for the preoperative staging of rectal cancer. Scand J Gastroenterol 1986;21 (suppl 123):87–98.
11. Heintz A, Bueb G, Frank K et al. Endoluminal ultrasonic examination of sessile polyps and early carcinomas of the rectum. Surg Endosc 1989;3:92–95.
12. Orrom WJ, Wong WD, Rothenberger DA et al. Endorectal ultrasound in the preoperative staging of rectal tumors. Dis Colon Rectum 1990;33:654–659.
13. Shanks B, Dershaw DD, Caravelli J et al. A prospective study of the accuracy of preoperative computed tomography staging of patients with biopsy-proven rectal carcinoma. Dis Colon Rectum 1990;33:285–290.
14. Rotte KH, Kluhs L, Kleinau H, Kriedemann E. Computed tomography and endosonography in the preoperative staging of rectal carcinoma. Europ J Radiol 1989;9:187–190.
15. Alexander AA, Eschelman DJ, Nazarian LN, Bonn J. Transrectal ultrasound drainage of deep pelvic abscesses. AJR 1994;62:1227–1230.
16. Alexander AA, Miller LS, Liu JB et al. High resolution endoluminal sonography of the anal sphincter complex. J Ultrasound Med 1994;13:281–284.

17. NcNeal JE. The prostate and prostatic urethra: a morphologic synthesis. J Urol 1972;107:1008–1016.
18. McNeal JE. Normal and pathologic anatomy of prostate. Urology (suppl XVII) 1981;11–16.
19. Shapiro E. Embryologic development of the prostate. Urol Clin N Am 1990;17:487–491.
20. Alexander AA, Goldberg BB. Prostate and seminal vesicles. In: Text Atlas of Urogenital Ultrasound. Martin Dunitz Inc., London, 1994:271–302.
21. Shinohara AK, Scardino PT, Carter C, Wheeler TM. Pathologic basis of the sonographic appearance of the normal and malignant prostate. Urol Clin N Am 1989;16:675–691.
22. Harada K, Tanahashi Y, Igari D et al. Clinical evaluation of inside echo patterns in gray scale prostatic echography. J Urol 1980;124:216.
23. Lee F, Gray JM, LcLeary RD et al. Transrectal ultrasound in the diagnosis of prostate cancer: location, echogenicity, histopathology and staging. Prostate 1985;1:117.
24. Littrup PJ, Kane RA, Williams CR et al. Determination of prostate volume with transrectal US for cancer screening. Part I. Comparison with prostate-specific antigen assays. Radiology 1991;178:537–542.
25. Littrup PJ, Williams CR, Eggelin TK, Kane RA. Determination of prostate volume with transrectal US for cancer screening. Part II. Accuracy of *in vitro* and *in vivo* techniques. Radiology 1991;179:49–53.
26. Walsh PC. Why make an early diagnosis of prostate cancer? J Urol 1992;147:853–854.
27. Brawer MK, Chetner MP, Beatie J et al. Screening for prostatic carcinoma with prostate specific antigen. J Urol 1992;147:841–845.
28. Smith F, Resnick MI. Prostate specific antigen: clinical applications and new developments: Kidney 1993;25:1–6.
29. Bretton PR, Evans WP, Borden JC, Castelanos RD. The use of prostate specific antigen density to improve the sensitivity of prostate specific antigen in detecting prostate carcinoma. Cancer 1994;74:2991–2995.
30. Colberg JW, Smith DS, Catalona WJ. Prevalence and pathological extent of prostate cancer in men with prostate specific antigen levels of 2.9 to 4.0 mg/ml. J Urol 1993;149:507–509.
31. Spencer JA, Alexander AA, Gomella L et al. Clinical and US findings in prostate cancer patients with normal prostate-specific antigen levels. Radiology 1993;189:389–393.
32. Stamey TA. Diagnosis of prostate cancer: a personal view. J Urol (editorial) 1992;147:830–832.
33. Rifkin MF, Choi H. Endorectal prostate ultrasound: implications of the small peripherally placed hypoechoic lesion. Radiology 1988;166:619–622.
34. Lee F, Torp-Pedersen S, Littrup PJ et al. Hypoechoic lesions of the prostate: clinical relevance of tumor size, digital rectal examination and prostate-specific antigen. Radiology 1989;170:29–32.

35. Shipohara K, Wheeler TM, Scardino PJ. The appearance of prostate cancer on transrectal ultrasonography correlation of imaging and pathological examinations. J Urol 1989;142:76–82.
36. Fornage BD. Transrectal duplex sonography of prostatic carcinoma: preliminary experience (abstr). Radiology 1989;173(P):81.
37. Rifkin MD, Sudakoff GS, Alexander AA. Prostate: techniques, results, and potential applications of color Doppler US scanning. Radiology 1993;186:509–513.
38. Kelly IMG, Lees WR, Rickards D. Prostate cancer and the role of color Doppler US. Radiology 1993;189:153–156.
39. Brawer MK, Deering RE, Brown M et al. Predictors of pathologic stage in prostatic carcinoma. The role of neovascularity. Cancer 1994;73:678–687.
40. Folkman J. Tumor angiogenesis: therapeutic implications. N Engl J Med 1971;285:1181–1186.
41. Folkman J, Cole P, Zimmerman S. Tumor behavior in isolated perfused organs: *in vitro* growth and metastasis of biopsy material in rabbit thyroid and canine intestinal segment. Ann Surg 1966;164:491–502.
42. Berry SJ, Coffey DS, Walsh PC et al. The development of human benign prostatic hyperplasia with age. J Urol 1984;132:474.
43. Barry MJ. Epidemiology and natural history of benign prostatic hyperplasia. Urol Clin N Am 1990;17:495–507.
44. McNeal J. Pathology of benign prostatic hyperplasia, insight into etiology. Urol Clin N Am 1990;17:477–487.
45. Coffey DS, Walsh PC. Clinical and experimental studies of benign prostatic hyperplasia. Urol Clin N Am 1990;17:461–475.
46. Jakobsen H, Torp-Pedersen S, Juul N. Ultrasonic evaluation of age related human prostatic growth and development of benign prostatic growth and development of benign prostatic hyperplasia. Scand J Urol Nephrol 1988;107 (suppl):107.
47. Greene DR, Egwa S, Hellerstein DK, Scardino PT. Sonographic measurements of transition zone of prostate in men with and without benign prostatic hyperplasia. Urology 1990;36:293–299.
48. Fornage BD, Ultrasound of the prostate. New York: John Wiley & Sons, 1988.
49. Fehr JL, Knonagel H. Importance of prostatic sonography in the evaluation of conservative therapy of prostatic hyperplasia. Urol Internat 1990;45:231–233.
50. Shaeffer AJ. Diagnosis and treatment of prostatic infections. Urology (suppl) 1990;36:13–17.
51. Drach GW, Fair WR, Meares EM et al. Classification of benign disease associated with prostatic pain: prostatitis or prostatopynia. J Urol (letter) 1978;120:266.

52. Griffiths GJ, Crooks AJR, Roberts EE et al. Ultrasonic appearance associated with prostatic inflammation: preliminary study. Clin Radiol 1984;35:343.
53. Doble A, Carter SC. Ultrasonographic findings in prostatitis. Urol Clin N Am 1989;16:763–772.
54. Meares EM, Jr. Infection stones of the prostate gland: laboratory diagnosis and clinical management. Urology 1974;4:560–565.
55. Cytron S, Weinberger M, Pitlik S, Servadio C. Value of transrectal ultrasonography for diagnosis and treatment of prostatic abscess. Urology 1988;32:454–458.
56. Ngheim HT, Kellman GM, Sandberg SA, Craig BM. Cystic lesions of the prostate. Radiographics 1990;10:635–650.
57. Colpi GM, Ballerini G, Zanollo A et al. Ultrasonography of the seminal vesicles in fertility. In: Bollack C, Clavert A (eds): Seminal vesicles and fertility: biology and pathology. Basel: S Charge, 1985:124–142.
58. Colpi GM, Zanollo CA, Ballerini G et al. Functional voiding disturbances of the ampullo-vesicular seminal tract: cause of male fertility. Acta Europ Fertilitatis 1987;18:165.
59. Hildebrandt U, Feifel G. Preoperative staging of rectal cancer by intrarectal ultrasound. Dis Colon Rectum 1985;28:42–46.
60. Shimizu S, Tada M, Kawai K. Use of endoscopic ultrasonography for the diagnosis of colorectal tumors. Endoscopy 1990;22:31–34.
61. Tio TL, Tytgat GNJ. Comparison of blind transrectal ultrasound with endoscopic transrectal ultrasonography in assessing rectal and perirectal diseases. Scand J Gastroenterol 1986;21 (suppl 123):104–111.
62. Gray H. Anatomy of the human body. In: Clemente CD (ed): Anatomy. A regional atlas of the human body. 3rd edition. Baltimore: Urban & Schwarzenberg, 1987.
63. Alexander AA, Liu JB, Palazzo JP et al. Endorectal color and duplex imaging of the normal rectal wall and rectal masses. J Ultrasound Med 1994;13:509–515.
64. Krook JE, Moertel CG, Gunderson LL et al. Effective surgical adjuvant therapy for high-risk rectal carcinoma. The New Engl J Med 1991;324:709–715.
65. Gall FP, Hermanek P. Cancer of the rectum: local excision. Surg Clin N Am 1988;68:353–368.
66. Alexander AA. The effects of endorectal ultrasound on the preoperative staging of rectal carcinoma. In: Milburn JJ (ed): Surgical Oncology Clinics of North America. Philadelphia: WB Saunders, vol. 1, July 1992; 39–56.
67. Hulsmans FJT, Tio TL, Fockens P et al. Assessment of tumor infiltration depth in rectal cancer with transrectal sonography: caution is necessary. Radiology 1994;190:715–720.

68. Tio TI, Tytgat NJ. Endoscopic ultrasonography in analysing periintestinal lymph node abnormality. Preliminary results of studies *in vitro* and *in vivo*. Scand J Gastroenterol 1986 (suppl 123);21:158–163.
69. Hildebrandt U, Klein T, Feifel G et al. Endosonography of pararectal lymph nodes. *In vitro* and *in vivo* evaluation. Dis Colon Rectum 1990;33:863–868.
70. Hulsmans FH, Bosma A, Mulder PJJ et al. Perirectal lymph nodes in rectal cancer: *in vitro* correlation of sonographic parameters and histopathologic findings. Radiology 1992;184:553–560.
71. Nielsen MB, Pedersen JF, Hauge C et al. Endosonography of the anal sphincter: findings in healthy volunteers. AJR 1991;157:1199–1202.
72. Law PJ, Kamm MA, Bartram CI. A comparison between electromyography and anal endosonography in mapping external anal sphincter defects. Dis Colon Rectum 1990;33:370–373.
73. Tjandra JJ, Milson JW, Stolfi VM et al. Endoluminal ultrasound defines anatomy of the anal canal and pelvic floor. Dis Colon Rectum 1992;35:465–470.
74. Burnett SJD, Bartram CI. Endosonographic variations in the normal internal anal sphincter. Int J Colorect Dis 1991;6:2–4.
75. Tio TL, Mulder JJ, Wijers OB et al. Endosonography of peri-anal and peri-colorectal fistula and/or abscess in Crohn's disease. Gastrointest Endosc 1990;36:331–336.
76. Law PJ, Talbot RW, Bartram CI, Northover JMA. Anal endosonography in the evaluation of perianal sepsis and fistula in ano. Br J Surg 1989;76:752–755.

CHAPTER 11

Gynecologic Ultrasound

Barbara S. Hertzberg, MD and James D. Bowie, MD

Ultrasonography plays an important role in the diagnosis and management of gynecologic problems. The advantages of ultrasound are manifold and include the ability to image in multiple scan planes, non-invasive nature, portability, lack of need for contrast administration or ionizing radiation, and relatively low price compared with similar cross-sectional imaging techniques. Ultrasound has long been considered the imaging procedure of choice for most clinical questions involving the female pelvis. The more recent introduction of the endovaginal scanning approach has even further improved diagnostic and imaging potential. This section reviews the use of ultrasonography in the evaluation of gynecologic problems, emphasizing scanning technique, sonographic anatomy, and commonly encountered pathology.

SCANNING APPROACH: TRANSABDOMINAL VS. ENDOVAGINAL SONOGRAPHY

The two ultrasound approaches used most commonly to image the female pelvis are transabdominal and endovaginal sonography. Both techniques have advantages and limitations, so they should be considered complementary procedures, with many cases necessitating a dual methodology (1–4).

The main advantage of endovaginal ultrasound is that the transducer is in close proximity to the pelvic organs, so higher imaging frequencies can be used. Consequently, endovaginal ultrasound affords far superior tissue characterisation, and display of detail unobtainable by the transabdominal approach. Additionally, the tran-

should be disinfected between uses. Prior to scanning, ultrasound gel is applied to the transducer head and the transducer is covered with a latex condom or other specially designed transducer covering. A lubricant such as KY jelly is applied over the protective covering. The transducer can be inserted by the patient, sonographer, or sonologist. Endovaginal scans are relatively contraindicated in patients who have never been sexually active, and may be difficult in the post-menopausal patient with atrophic vaginitis, particularly if sufficient lubrication is not applied to the transducer.

Endovaginal scanning is usually performed with the patient in a supine lithotomy position, either on a standard gynecologic examination table equipped with stirrups, or with the patient supine with a pillow or other bolster under her buttocks. The bolster elevates the hips off the scanning table, thereby allowing the transducer to be maneuvered to visualize the anterior portion of the pelvis without encountering the scanning table as an obstacle.

As with the transabdominal technique, it is easiest to orient to pelvic anatomy by beginning with sagittal images through the uterus. The transducer is subsequently angled laterally and medially to view the ovaries and remainder of the pelvis. At times, oblique images are needed to demonstrate pelvic anatomy and pathology to best advantage. If there is difficulty localizing the ovaries, it can be helpful to first identify the internal iliac vessels: the ovaries frequently lie directly anterior to these vessels. Images that are approximately coronal through the uterus and ovaries can be obtained by rotating the transducer 90° and angling it laterally and medially. The cervix is visualized by pulling the transducer slightly outward. Because endovaginal ultrasound does not provide the same overview of the pelvis that is afforded by transabdominal scanning, it is extremely important to angle and rotate the transducer sufficiently to image the entire pelvis.

Orientation of endovaginal images can be confusing to the inexperienced operator, as images are depicted in a different orientation than one becomes accustomed to using the transabdominal approach. With experience the new orientations become intuitive. By convention, the anatomy located closest to the transducer is displayed at the apex of the image, so in the case of an endovaginal scan, the most caudal portion of the pelvis is at the apex of the image (Figure 1 a, b).

Figure 1 *Schematic diagram of midline sagittal scan plane with endovaginal ultrasound (a). To conform to standard convention of displaying the image with structures located closest to the transducer at the apex of the image, the image has been rotated approximately 90° prior to display (b). Note that the cervix and lower uterus are near the top of the image.*

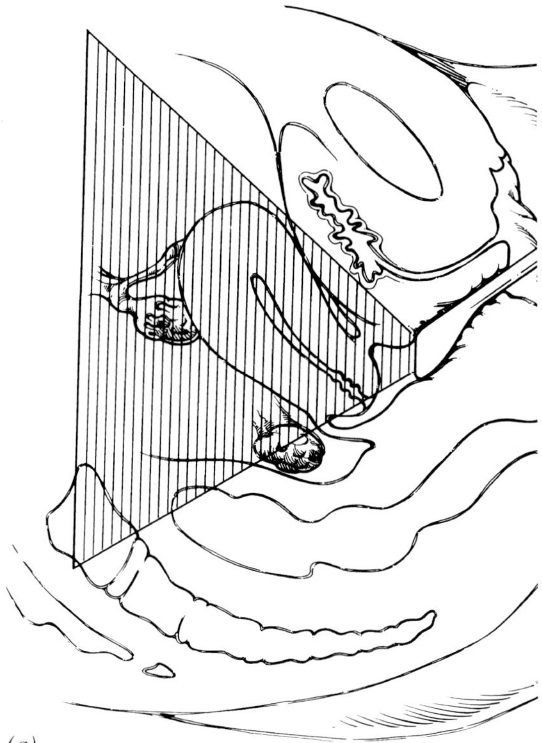

(a)

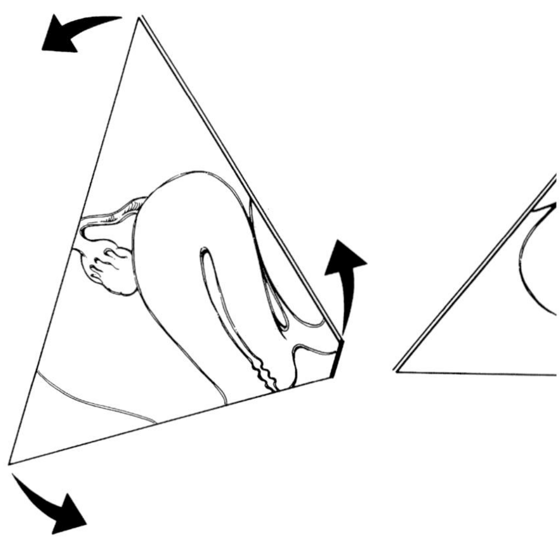

(b)

SONOGRAPHIC ANATOMY

It is critical to be familiar with the sonographic appearance of normal anatomic structures to properly perform and interpret ultrasound studies. This is particularly true of gynecologic ultrasound because cyclical changes during the menstrual cycle, and age related alterations in the size and configuration of pelvic organs result in a dynamic and changing appearance to pelvic sonoanatomy.

The normal uterus varies in size and shape depending on the patient's age (5, 6). Prior to menarche, the uterus measures under 4 cm in length, and the cervix is thick, long, and more prominent than the uterine fundus. Near puberty, the uterus begins to gradually increase in size and evolve in shape, such that the normal adult configuration is approximately pear-shaped, and the uterine fundus is about twice the size of the cervix. The normal length of the post-pubertal adult uterus is 6–8 cm in the nulliparous patient, although it often measures 1–2 cm more in multiparous individuals. After menopause, the uterus atrophies and the cervix becomes relatively more prominent compared with the fundus.

The uterus is usually a midline anteverted structure, but variations in uterine orientation are common. These anatomic variants include retroversion and/or tilting to the right or left, and are considered to be within the spectrum of normal. Such variants are important to recognize, however, because they can resemble pathologic processes. For example, the fundus of a retroverted uterus may exhibit a relatively hypoechoic appearance which simulates a fibroid.

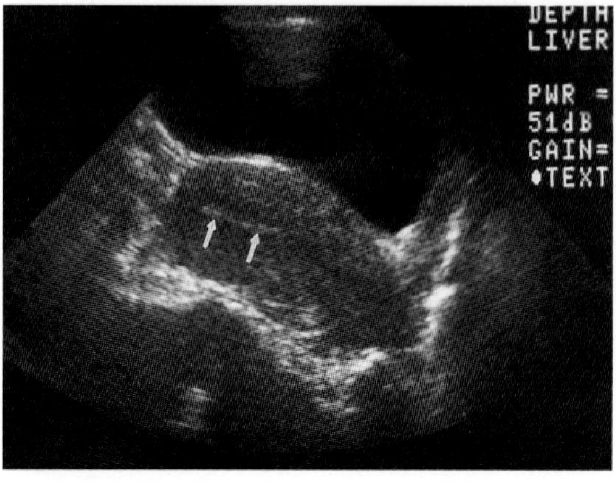

Figure 2 *Midline sagittal transabdominal ultrasound image of normal adult uterus reveals the endometrial stripe (arrows) early in the proliferative phase of the cycle.*

The uterus is localized based on its typical configuration and by identification of the hyperechoic central uterine echo or "endometrial stripe" (7) (Figure 2). Like uterine size, the central endometrial echo complex varies with patient age, but additionally shows considerable variation depending on the stage of the menstrual cycle (8–10). Early in the proliferative phase of the cycle, the endometrium is depicted as a thin echogenic stripe, but as this phase progresses, it thickens. Around the time of ovulation, the endometrium frequently exhibits a target or ring configuration (Figure 3), with a thin central echogenic line surrounded successively by a relatively echopenic zone (probably due to edema), another more echogenic zone, and sometimes a second hypoechoic zone due to the inner layer of surrounding myometrium. During the secretory phase of the cycle the endometrium becomes progressively more echogenic and thicker as endometrial glands enlarge and secrete mucin and glycogen. During the peak of the secretory phase the endometrium may measure 14 to 15 mm in width or more. The endometrial cavity has a variable appearance during menstruation, depending on the amount of fluid and clot trapped within the uterine cavity.

Endometrial thickness is optimally measured on a sagittal endovaginal image of the uterus. Coronal or transverse images can also be used, but are suboptimal because they frequently represent oblique scan planes which have the potential to overestimate endometrial thickness. Some investigators describe measurements of endometrial thickness in terms of a double layer (i.e. including both sides of opposing endometrium) whereas others use a single thickness measurement. All measurements discussed herein refer

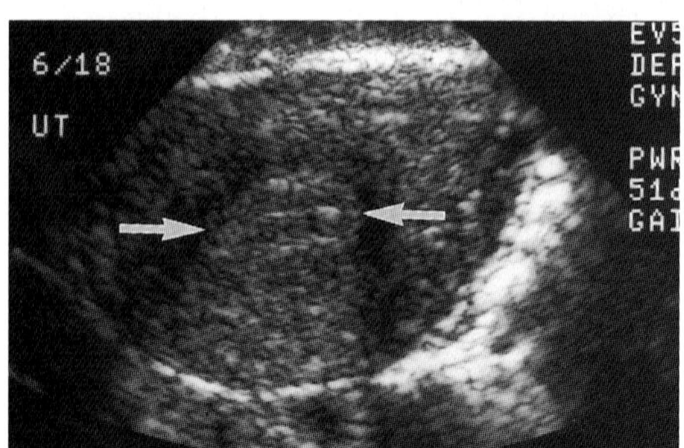

Figure 3 *Endovaginal ultrasound image of the uterus around the time of ovulation reveals "target" configuration (arrows) of the endometrial stripe.*

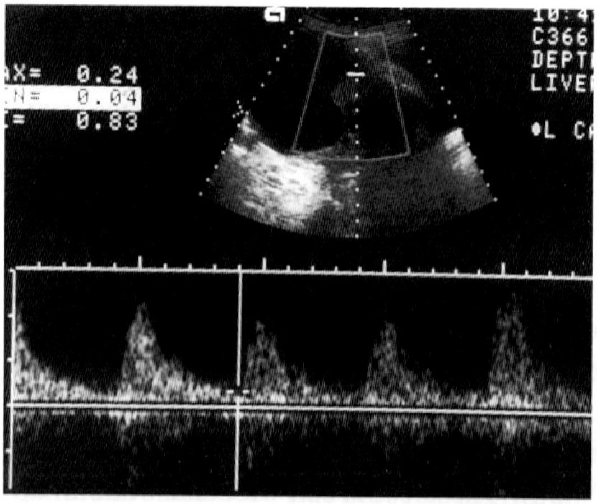

Figure 17 *Ultrasound with Doppler of a serous cystadenocarcinoma of the ovary. Although this tumor was malignant, only high resistance spectral waveforms could be detected within it.*

presence of high diastolic flow further strengthens the case for a malignant histology. Similarly, lack of high diastolic flow in a lesion whose morphology favors a benign tumor further strengthens the case for a benign process. It is, however, important to realize that some malignant tumors do not have evidence of high diastolic flow (Figure 17). Similarly, many benign conditions such as corpus luteal cysts, inflammatory masses, endometriomas, and exophytic fibroids can exhibit high diastolic flow (32).

Identification of a pelvic mass in a female does not necessarily implicate the gynecologic organs. Both the urinary tract and bowel are located in close proximity to the pelvic organs and pathology arising from these organ systems can simulate gynecologic disease. For example, a pelvic kidney can simulate the appearance of a solid pelvic mass but often exhibits a reniform appearance. Similarly, a bowel process such as an appendiceal abscess, a diverticular abscess, inflammatory bowel disease, or a tumor can present as a pelvic mass with clinical symptoms suggesting gynecologic pathology.

REFERENCES

1. DiSantis DJ, Scatarige JC, Kemp G et al. A prospective evaluation of transvaginal sonography for detection of ovarian disease. AJR 1993;161:91–94.
2. Sarti DA. Transvaginal sonography: a call for tempered enthusiasm. AJR 1993;161:95–96.

3. Nelson LH, Kremkau FW. Introduction to transvaginal imaging. Obstet Gynecol Clin N Am 1991;18:683–692.
4. Gratton D, Harrington C, Holt SC, Lyons EA. Normal pelvic anatomy using transvaginal scanning. Obstet Gynecol Clin N Am 1991;18:693–711.
5. Orsini LF, Salardi S, Pilu G et al. Pelvic organs in premenarcheal girls: real-time ultrasonography. Radiology 1984;153:113–116.
6. Nussbaum AR, Sanders RC, Jones MD. Neonatal uterine morphology as seen on real-time US. Radiology 1986;160:641–643.
7. Callen PW, DeMartini WJ, Filly RA. The central uterine cavity echo: a useful anatomic sign in the ultrasonographic evaluation of the female pelvis. Radiology 1979;131:187–190.
8. Forrest TS, Elyaderani MK, Muilenburg MI et al. Cyclic endometrial changes: US assessment with histologic correlation. Radiology 1988;167:233–237.
9. Fleischer AC, Kalemerisi GC, Entman SS. Sonographic depiction of the endometrium during normal cycles. Ultrasond Med Biol 1986;12:271–277.
10. Hall DA, Hann LE, Ferrucci JT Jr et al. Sonographic morphology of the normal menstrual cycle. Radiology 1979;133:185–188.
11. Mintz MC, Grumback K. Imaging of congenital uterine anomalies. Semin Ultrasound CT MR 1988;9:167–174.
12. Gross BH, Silver TM, Jaffe MH. Sonographic features of uterine leiomyomas: analysis of 41 proven cases. J Ultrasound Med 1983;2:401–406.
13. Baltarowich OH, Kurtz AB, Pennell RG et al. Pitfalls in the sonographic diagnosis of uterine fibroids. AJR 1988;151:725–728.
14. Bohlman ME, Ensor RE, Sanders RC. Sonographic findings in adenomyosis of the uterus. AJR 1987;148:765–766.
15. Siedler D, Laing FC, Jeffrey RB Jr, Wing VW. Uterine adenomyosis – a difficult sonographic diagnosis. J Ultrasound Med 1987;6:345–349.
16. Lin MC, Gosink BB, Wolf SI et al. Endometrial thickness after menopause: effect of hormone replacement. Radiology 1991;180:427–432.
17. Breckenridge JW, Kurtz AB, Ritchie WGM, Macht EL Jr. Postmenopausal uterine fluid collection: indicator of carcinoma. AJR 1982;139:529–534.
18. Fogel SR, Slasky BS. Sonography of nabothian cysts. AJR 1982;138:927–930.
19. Baltarowich OH, Kurtz AB, Pasto ME et al. The spectrum of sonographic findings in hemorrhagic ovarian cysts. AJR 1987;148:901–905.
20. Reynolds T, Hill MC, Glassman LM. Sonography of hemorrhagic ovarian cysts. J Clin Ultrasound 1986;14:449–453.
21. Athey PA, Diment DD. The spectrum of sonographic findings in endometriomas. J Ultrasound Med 1989;8:487–491.

22. Swayne LC, Love MB, Karasick SR. Pelvic inflammatory disease: sonographic-pathologic correlation. Radiology 1984;151:751–755.
23. Athey PA, Malone RS. Sonography of ovarian fibromas/thecomas. J Ultrasound Med 1987;6:431–436.
24. Moyle JW, Rochester D, Sider L et al. Sonography of ovarian tumors: predictability of tumor type. AJR 1983;141:985–991.
25. Herrmann UJ Jr, Locher GW, Goldhirsch A. Sonographic patterns of ovarian tumors: prediction of malignancy. Obstet Gynecol 1987;69:777–781.
26. Quinn SF, Erickson S, Black WC. Cystic ovarian teratomas: the sonographic appearance of the dermoid plug. Radiology 1985;155:477–478.
27. Sheth S, Fishman EK, Buck JL et al. The variable sonographic appearances of ovarian teratomas: correlation with CT. AJR 1988;151:331–334.
28. Wolf SI, Gosink BB, Feldesman MR et al. Prevalence of simple adnexal cysts in postmenopausal women. Radiology 1991;180:65–71.
29. Andolf E, Jörgensen C. Simple adnexal cysts diagnosed by ultrasound in postmenopausal women. J Clin Ultrasound 1988;16:301–303.
30. Goldstein SR, Subramanyam B, Snyder JR et al. The post-menopausal cystic adnexal mass: the potential role of ultrasound in conservative management. Obstet Gynecol 1989;73:8–10.
31. Kurjak A, Zalud I, Alfirevic Z. Evaluation of adnexal masses with transvaginal color ultrasound. J Ultrasound Med 1991;10:295–297.
32. Fleischer AC, Rodgers WH, Rao BK et al. Assessment of ovarian tumor vascularity with transvaginal color Doppler sonography. J Ultrasound Med 1991;10:563–568.

CHAPTER 12

Obstetrical Ultrasound: Normal Anatomy and Measurements

John P. McGahan, MD and Terry L. Coates, MD

For over 20 years ultrasound has provided a unique modality for evaluation of pregnancy and establishing gestational age. Transabdominal real-time ultrasound has produced exquisite detail of the fetus and a method of documenting fetal motion and viability. Most recently, high resolution endovaginal transducers have allowed improved real-time visualization of early pregnancy. High resolution real-time ultrasound allows a more accurate dating of menstrual age and documentation of fetal anatomy. This chapter will briefly review normal fetal anatomy, and present the more common methods utilized for establishing menstrual age.

MINIMUM STANDARDS

In an effort to provide some guidelines for obstetrical ultrasound, three organisations in the United States have tried to establish minimum standards for the obstetrical ultrasound examination. The American College of Obstetrics and Gynecology (ACOG) has published a technical bulletin regarding standards for the obstetrical ultrasound examination (1). This is similar to the guidelines previously published by the American College of Radiology (ACR) as guidelines for antenatal obstetrical ultrasound (2), and the American Institute of Ultrasound in Medicine (AIUM) has taken previous recommendations and published "Guidelines for the Performance of the Antepartum Obstetrical Ultrasound Examination" (3). These guidelines are presented as Appendix I in this chapter.

FETAL MEASUREMENTS

Accurate assessment of gestational age is one of the most important items needed for pregnancy management. Unfortunately, use of the last menstrual period as determination of gestational age is often not reliable because of early first trimester bleeding or problems with the patient recalling the exact day of her last menstrual period. As such, use of other criteria, including bimanual examination, have been utilized but are estimated to be in error by more than two weeks in most pregnancies (4). Unfortunately, other methods of establishing gestational age, such as fundal height, are even more inadequate (5). Furthermore, fundal height measurements are influenced by in utero factors, such as intrauterine growth retardation or polyhydramnios. Quickening is felt to be even more inacccurate than the previous methods. Therefore, ultrasound provides a potential for a more reliable method of establishing menstrual age.

First trimester

As established within the AIUM guidelines, two methods are routinely used to establish menstrual age in'the first trimester. These two methods are measurement of the gestational sac size and measurement of the crown rump length.

Gestational sac size

There was initial enthusiasm in measurement of the gestational sac diameter as a method of establishing gestational age (6) (Table I). These measurements are still used today. However, it is estimated that there may be up to two weeks error in establishing gestational age based on sac size (7). Part of the error is that gestational sac shape is variable depending on compression from surrounding structures, including the bladder. Therefore, measurement of the *mean sac diameter* is utilized. This method takes the length, height, and width of the sac and divides by three to establish the mean sac diameter (Figure 1).

More recently, gestational sac size has been used to establish if the sac contains a "fetus" or is "empty". Using transabdominal techniques, a *fetal pole* should be reliably identified when a mean sac diameter reaches 25 mm (8). A *yolk sac* should be identified earlier with transabdominal techniques when the mean sac diameter is 20 mm (8). Utilizing endovaginal technique, the embryo should be visualized approximately one week earlier. Utilizing endovaginal ultrasound, a *fetal pole* should be reliably identified when the mean sac diameter is 16 mm, and a *yolk sac* should be identified with a mean sac diameter of 8 mm (9) (Figures 1 and 2).

Table I. ***Gestational Sac Measurement Table.***

Mean Predicted Gestational Sac (cm)	Gestational Age (wk)	Mean Predicted Gestational Sac (cm)	Gestational Age (wk)
1.0	5.0	3.6	8.8
1.1	5.2	3.7	8.9
1.2	5.3	3.8	9.0
1.3	5.5	3.9	9.2
1.4	5.6	4.0	9.3
1.5	5.8	4.1	9.5
1.6	5.9	4.2	9.6
1.7	6.0	4.3	9.7
1.8	6.2	4.4	9.9
1.9	6.3	4.5	10.0
2.0	6.5	4.6	10.2
2.1	6.6	4.7	10.3
2.2	6.8	4.8	10.5
2.3	6.9	4.9	10.6
2.4	7.0	5.0	10.7
2.5	7.2	5.1	10.9
2.6	7.3	5.2	11.0
2.7	7.5	5.3	11.2
2.8	7.6	5.4	11.3
2.9	7.8	5.5	11.5
3.0	7.9	5.6	11.6
3.1	8.0	5.7	11.7
3.2	8.2	5.8	11.9
3.3	8.3	5.9	12.0
3.4	8.5	6.0	12.2
3.5	8.6		

$$\text{Gestation Age (weeks)} = \frac{\text{Gestation Sac (cm)} + 2.543}{0.702}$$

(Hellman LM, Kobayashi M, Fillisti L, et al: Growth and development of the human fetus prior to the twenthieth week of gestation. Am J Obstet Gynecol 1969; 103:784.)

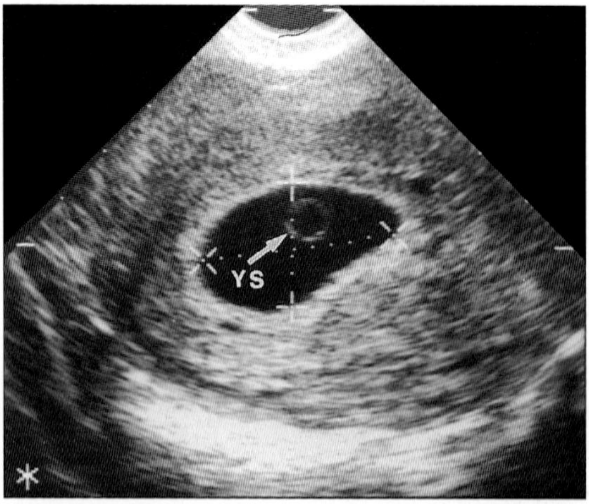

Figure 1 *Transvaginal ultrasound demonstrating two-dimensional measurement of the gestational sac (calipers). More centrally is noted a yolk sac (YS).*

Crown-rump Length

The ultrasound measurement of the crown-rump length was performed as early as 1973 by Robinson (10) (Table II). This measurement is considered the most accurate method of assessing gestational age (11). *Crown-rump length* is measured from the fetal head to the fetal buttocks (Figure 2). Crown-rump length measurement is accurate because there is little variability in the size of the crown-rump length between different pregnancies. Also, there is rapid change in the crown-rump length, and thus a measurement error will lead to a small error in establishing menstrual age. The growth of the crown-rump length is exponential up to 12 men-

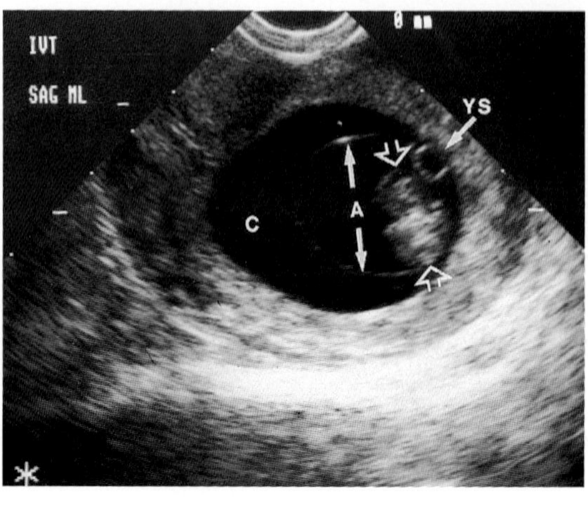

Figure 2 *Transvaginal ultrasound demonstrating crown-rump length (open arrows) and yolk sac (YS) in an early pregnancy. Note the amnion (A) which is surrounded by the chorionic cavity (C).*

strual weeks, and linear after that time. If a crown-rump length is identified, fetal cardiac activity is almost always identified. When a crown-rump length of 5 mm is seen and there is no fetal cardiac activity identified on high quality endovaginal ultrasound, this is reliable evidence of fetal demise (12).

Second/third trimester measurements

In general, measurements of the fetus become less reliable in establishing menstrual age in the second and third trimesters. However, fetal measurements performed in the late first or early second trimester may be nearly as accurate as crown-rump length in esti-

Table II. ***Predicted Menstrual Age (weeles) from Crown-to-Rump Length Measurements (cm).***

CRL (cm)	MA (wk)	CRL (cm)	MA (wk)	CRL (cm)	MA (wk)	CRL (cm)	MA (wk)	CRL (cm)	MA (wk)	CRL (cm)	MA (wk)
0.2	5.7	2.2	8.9	4.2	11.1	6.2	12.6	8.2	14.2	10.2	16.1
0.3	5.9	2.3	9.0	4.3	11.2	6.3	12.7	8.3	14.2	10.3	16.2
0.4	6.1	2.4	9.1	4 4	11.2	6.4	12.8	8.4	14.3	10.4	16.3
0.5	6.2	2.5	9.2	4.5	11.3	6.5	12.8	8.5	14.4	10.5	16.4
0.6	6.4	2.6	9.4	4.6	11.4	6.6	12.9	8.6	14.5	10.6	16.5
0.7	6.6	2.7	9.5	4.7	11.5	6.7	13.0	8.7	14.6	10.7	16.6
0.8	6.7	2.8	9.6	4.8	11.6	6.8	13.1	8.8	14.7	10.8	16.7
0.9	6.9	2.9	9.7	4.9	11.7	6.9	13.1	8.9	14.8	10.9	16.8
1.0	7.1	3.0	9.9	5.0	11.7	7.0	13.2	9.0	14.9	11.0	16.9
1.1	7.2	3.1	10.0	5.1	11.8	7.1	13.3	9.1	15.0	11.1	17.0
1.2	7.4	3.2	10.1	5.2	11.9	7.2	13.4	9.2	15.1	11.2	17.1
1.3	7.5	3.3	10 2	5.3	12.0	7.3	13.4	9.3	15.2	11.3	17.2
1.4	7.7	3.4	10.3	5.4	12.0	7.4	13.5	9.4	15.3	11.4	17.3
1.5	7.9	3.5	10.4	5.5	12.1	7.5	13.6	9.5	15.3	11.5	17 4
1.6	8.0	3.6	10.5	5.6	12.2	7.6	13.7	9.6	15.4	11.6	17.5
1.7	8.1	3.7	10.6	5.7	12.3	7.7	13.8	9.7	15.5	11.7	17.6
1.8	8.3	3.8	10.7	5.8	12.3	7.8	13.8	9.8	15.6	11.8	17.7
1.9	8.4	3.9	10.8	5.9	12.4	7.9	13.9	9.9	15.7	11.9	17.8
2.0	8.6	4.0	10.9	6.0	12.5	8.0	14.0	10.0	15.9	12.0	17.9
2.1	8.7	4.1	11.0	6.1	12.6	8.1	14.1	10.1	16.0	12 1	18.0

MA, menstrual age. The 95% confidence interval is 8% of the predicted age. (Hadlock FP, Shah YP, Kanon DJ, et al: Fetal crown-rump length: Re-evaluation of relation to menstrual age (15–18 weeks) with high-resolution real-time ultrasound. Radiology 1992; 182:501–5v5.)

mating menstrual age. This error may be as little as one week in earlier stages of pregnancy (13). However, this is not true later in pregnancy, especially in the third trimester. In this trimester, the fetal measurements vary considerably from pregnancy to pregnancy. This variability is due to both genetic factors and the in utero environment (nutrition) of the fetus. Therefore, establishing menstrual age in the third trimester is unreliable with estimates being inaccurate, at 2 standard deviations, by more than four weeks (13).

Biparietal diameter (BPD)

Initial studies by Campbell, as early as 1969, utilized the BPD as a measurement in establishing gestational age (14). Intracranial landmarks utilized for the BPD include visualization of the falx cerebri anteriorly and posteriorly, the cavum septi pellucidi anteriorly and the paired thalami in the midline with a Sylvian fissure noted laterally. The measurement of the BPD is made in the transverse axial plane from the outer margin of the near cranium (not including the scalp) to the inner margin of the far cranium (Figure 3) (Table III) (15).

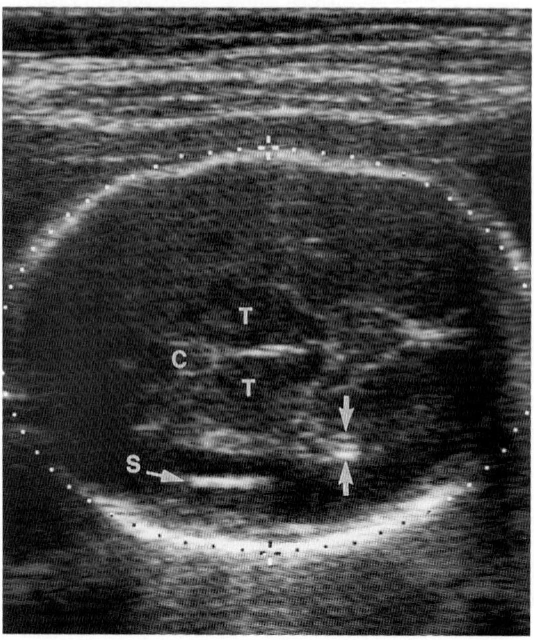

Figure 3 *Standard transaxial plane utilized for obtaining a BPD, including measurement of the downside ventricular atrium (arrows) and other anatomical features, including the thalami (T), cavum septi pellucidi (C) and the Sylvian fissure (S). HC includes outer perimeter of the skull (calipers), while the BPD is measured from the outer edge to the inner edge.*

Table III. ***Predicted Menstrual Ages* for Biparietal Diameter Values from 2 to 10 cm.***

BPD (cm)	Menstrual Age (wk)	BPD (cm)	Menstrual Age (wk)
2.0	12 2	6.1	25.0
2.1	12.5	6.2	25 3
2.2	12 8	6.3	25.7
2.3	13.1	6.4	26.1
2.4	13.3	6.5	26.4
2.5	13.6	6.6	26.8
2.6	13.9	6.7	27.2
2.7	14.2	6.8	27.6
2.8	14.5	6.9	28.0
2.9	14.7	7.0	28.3
3.0	15 0	7.1	28.7
3.1	15.3	7.2	29.1
3.2	15.6	7.3	29.5
3.3	15 9	7.4	29.9
3.4	16 2	7.5	30.4
3.5	16.5	7.6	30.8
3.6	16 8	7.7	31.2
3.7	17.1	7.8	31.6
3.8	17 4	7.9	32.0
3.9	17.7	8.0	32.5
4.0	18.0	8.1	32.9
4.1	18.3	8.2	33.3
4.2	18.6	8.3	33.8
4.3	18.9	8.4	34.2
4.4	19.2	8.5	34.7
4.5	19.5	8.6	35.1
4.6	19.9	8.7	35.6
4.7	20.2	8.8	36.1
4.8	20.5	8.9	36.5
4.9	20.8	9.0	37.0
5.0	21.2	9.1	37.5
5.1	21.5	9.2	38.0
5.2	21.8	9.3	38.5
5.3	22.2	9.4	38.9
5.4	22.5	9.5	39.4
5.5	22.8	9.6	39.9
5.6	23.2	9.7	40.5
5.7	23.5	9.8	41.0
5.8	23.9	9.9	41.5
5.9	24.2	10.0	42.0
6.0	24.6		

* Menstrual age = 6 8954 + 2 6345(BPD) + 0.08771(BPD)^3 ; (r^2 = 98 7%) (Hadlock FP. Deter L.R. Harrist RD. Park SK: Fetal biparietal diameter. A critical reevaluation of the relation to menstural age by means of realtime ultrasound. I Ultrasound Med 1992; I:97-104.)

Table V. ***Gestational Ages as Obtained from the Long Bones (in weeks + days).***

Bone Length (mm)	Femur Percentile			Humerus Percentile			Ulna Percentile			Tibia Percentile		
	5th	50th	95th	5th	50th	95th	5th	50th	95th	5th	50th	95th
10	10 + 3	12 + 4	14 + 6	9 + 6	12 + 4	15 + 2	10 + 1	13 + 1	16 + 1	10 + 4	13 + 3	16 + 2
11	10 + 5	12 + 6	15 + 1	10 + 1	12 + 6	15 + 4	10 + 4	13 + 4	16 + 4	10 + 6	13 + 5	16 + 4
12	11 + 1	13 + 2	15 + 4	10 + 3	13 + 1	15 + 6	10 + 6	13 + 6	16 + 6	11 + 1	14 + 1	17
13	11 + 3	13 + 4	15 + 6	10 + 6	13 + 4	16 + 1	11 + 1	14 + 1	17 + 2	11 + 4	14 + 3	17 + 2
14	11 + 5	13 + 6	16 + 1	11 + 1	13 + 6	16 + 4	11 + 4	14 + 4	17 + 5	11 + 6	14 + 6	17 + 5
15	12	14 + 1	16 + 3	11 + 3	14 + 1	16 + 6	11 + 6	15	18	12 + 1	15 + 1	18
16	12 + 3	14 + 4	16 + 6	11 + 6	14 + 4	17 + 2	12 + 2	15 + 3	18 + 3	12 + 4	15 + 4	18 + 3
17	12 + 5	14 + 6	17 + 1	12 + 1	14 + 6	17 + 4	12 + 5	15 + 5	18 + 6	13	15 + 6	18 + 6
18	13	15 + 1	17 + 3	12 + 4	15 + 1	18	13 + 1	16 + 1	19 + 1	13 + 2	16 + 1	19 + 1
19	13 + 3	15 + 4	17 + 6	12 + 6	15 + 4	18 + 2	13 + 4	16 + 4	19 + 4	13 + 5	16 + 4	19 + 4
20	13 + 5	15 + 6	18 + 1	13 + 1	15 + 6	18 + 5	13 + 6	16 + 6	20	14 + 1	17	19 + 6
21	14 + 1	16 + 2	18 + 4	13 + 4	16 + 2	19 + 1	14 + 2	17 + 2	20 + 3	14 + 4	17 + 3	20 + 2
72	14 + 3	16 + 4	18 + 6	13 + 6	16 + 5	19 + 3	14 + 5	17 + 5	20 + 6	14 + 6	17 + 6	20 + 5
23	14 + 5	16 + 6	19 + 1	14 + 2	17 + 1	19 + 6	15 + 1	18 + 1	21 + 1	15 + 1	18 + 1	21 + 1
24	15 + 1	17 + 2	19 + 4	14 + 5	17 + 3	20 + 1	15 + 4	18 + 4	21 + 4	15 + 4	18 + 4	21 + 3
25	15 + 3	17 + 4	19 + 6	15 + 1	17 + 6	20 + 4	16	19	22 + 1	16	18 + 6	21 + 6
26	15 + 6	18	20 + 1	15 + 4	18 + 1	21	16 + 3	19 + 3	22 + 4	16 + 3	19 + 2	22 + 1
27	16 + 1	18 + 2	20 + 4	15 + 6	18 + 4	21 + 3	16 + 6	19 + 6	22 + 6	16 + 6	19 + 5	22 + 4
28	16 + 4	18 + 5	20 + 6	16 + 2	19	21 + 6	17 + 2	20 + 2	23 + 3	17 + 1	20 + 1	23
29	16 + 6	19	21 + 1	16 + 5	19 + 3	22 + 1	17 + 5	20 + 6	23 + 6	17 + 4	20 + 4	23 + 4
30	17 + 1	19 + 3	21 + 4	17 + 1	19 + 6	22 + 4	18 + 1	21 + 1	24 + 2	18 + 1	21	23 + 6
31	17 + 4	19 + 6	22	17 + 4	20 + 2	23	18 + 4	21 + 5	24 + 6	18 + 4	21 + 3	24 + 2
32	17 + 6	20 + 1	22 + 2	18	20 + 5	23 + 4	19 + 1	22 + 1	25 + 1	18 + 6	21 + 6	24 + 5
33	18 + 2	20 + 4	22 + 5	18 + 3	21 + 1	23 + 6	19 + 4	22 + 5	25 + 5	19 + 2	22 + 1	25 + 1
34	18 + 5	20 + 6	23 + 1	18 + 6	21 + 4	24 + 2	20 + 1	23 + 1	26 + 1	19 + 5	22 + 4	25 + 4
35	19	21 + 1	23 + 3	19 + 2	22	24 + 6	20 + 4	34 + 4	26 + 5	20 + 1	23 + 1	26
36	19 + 3	21 + 4	23 + 6	19 + 5	22 + 4	25 + 1	21 + 1	24 + 1	27 + 1	20 + 4	23 + 4	26 + 3
37	19 + 6	22	24 + 1	20 + 1	22 + 6	25 + 5	21 + 4	24 + 4	27 + 5	21	23 + 6	26 + 6
38	20 + 1	22 + 3	24 + 4	20 + 4	23 + 3	26 + 1	22 + 1	25 + 1	28 + 1	21 + 4	24 + 3	27 + 2
39	20 + 4	22 + 5	24 + 6	21 + 1	23 + 6	26 + 4	22 + 4	25 + 4	28 + 5	21 + 6	24 + 6	27 + 5
40	20 + 6	23 + 1	25 + 2	21 + 4	24 + 2	27 + 1	23 + 1	26 + 1	29 + 1	22 + 3	25 + 2	28 + 1
41	21 + 2	23 + 4	25 + 5	22	24 + 6	27 + 4	23 + 4	26 + 5	29 + 5	22 + 6	25 + 5	28 + 4
42	21 + 5	23 + 6	26 + 1	22 + 4	25 + 2	28	24 + 1	27 + 1	30 + 2	23 + 2	26 + 1	29 + 1
43	22 + 1	24 + 2	26 + 4	23	25 + 5	28 + 4	24 + 5	27 + 5	30 + 6	23 + 5	26 + 4	29 + 4
44	22 + 4	24 + 5	26 + 6	23 + 4	26 + 1	29	25 + 1	28 + 2	31 + 2	24 + 1	27 + 1	30
45	22 + 6	25	27 + 1	24	26 + 5	29 + 4	25 + 6	28 + 6	31 + 6	24 + 4	27 + 4	30 + 4
46	23 + 1	25 + 3	27 + 4	24 + 4	27 + 1	30	26 + 2	29 + 3	32 + 3	25 + 1	28	30 + 6
47	23 + 4	25 + 6	28	25	27 + 5	30 + 4	26 + 6	29 + 6	33	25 + 4	28 + 4	31 + 3
48	24	26 + 1	28 + 3	25 + 4	28 + 1	31	27 + 3	30 + 4	33 + 4	26 + 1	29	31 + 6
49	24 + 3	26 + 4	28 + 6	26	28 + 6	31 + 4	28	31 + 1	34 + 4	26 + 4	29 + 3	32 + 3
50	24 + 6	27	29 + 1	26 + 4	29 + 2	32	28 + 4	31 + 4	34 + 5	27	29 + 6	32 + 6
51	25 + 1	27 + 3	29 + 4	27 + 1	29 + 6	32 + 4	29 + 1	32 + 1	35 + 2	27 + 4	30 + 3	33 + 2
52	25 + 4	27 + 6	30	27 + 4	30 + 2	33 + 1	29 + 5	32 + 6	35 + 6	28	30 + 6	33 + 6
53	26	28 + 1	30 + 3	28 + 1	30 + 6	33 + 4	30 + 2	33 + 3	36 + 3	28 + 4	31 + 3	34 + 2
54	26 + 3	28 + 4	30 + 6	28 + 5	31 + 3	34 + 1	30 + 6	34	37	29	31 + 6	34 + 6
55	26 + 6	29 + 1	31 + 2	29 + 1	32	34 + 5	31 + 4	34 + 4	37 + 5	29 + 4	32 + 3	35 + 2
56	27 + 2	29 + 4	31 + 5	29 + 6	32 + 4	35 + 2	32 + 1	35 + 1	38 + 2	30	32 + 6	35 + 6
57	27 + 5	29 + 6	32 + 1	30 + 2	33 + 1	35 + 6	32 + 6	35 + 6	38 + 6	30 + 4	33 + 3	36 + 2
58	28 + 1	30 + 2	32 + 4	30 + 6	33 + 4	36 + 3	33 + 3	36 + 3	39 + 4	31	33 + 5	36 + 6
59	28 + 4	30 + 5	32 + 6	31 + 3	34 + 1	36 + 6	34 + 34	37 + 1	40 + 1	31 + 4	34 + 3	37 + 2
60	28 + 6	31 + 1	33 + 2	32	34 + 6	37 + 4	+ 4	37 + 5	40 + 6	32	34 + 6	37 + 6
61	29 + 3	31 + 4	33 + 6	32 + 4	35 + 2	38 + 1	35 + 2	38 + 2	41 + 3	32 + 4	35 + 3	38 + 2
62	29 + 6	32	34 + 1	33 + 1	35 + 6	38 + 5	35 + 6	39	42	33	35 + 6	38 + 6
63	30 + 1	32 + 3	34 + 4	33 + 6	36 + 4	39 + 2	36 + 4	39 + 4	42 + 5	33 + 4	36 + 4	39 + 3
64	30 + 5	32 + 6	35 + 1	34 + 3	37 + 1	39 + 6	37 + 1	40 + 2	43 + 2	34 + 1	37	39 + 6
65	31 + 1	33 + 2	35 + 4	35	37 + 5	40 + 4				34 + 4	37 + 4	40 + 3
66	31 + 4	33 + 5	35 + 6	35 + 4	38 + 2	41 + 1				35 + 1	38	41
67	32	34 + 1	36 + 3	36 + 1	38 + 6	41 + 5				35 + 5	38 + 4	41 + 4
68	32 + 3	34 + 4	36 + 6	36 + 6	39 + 4	42 + 2				36 + 1	39 + 1	42
69	32 + 6	35	37 + 1	37 + 3	40 + 1	42 + 6				36 + 6	39 + 5	42 + 4
70	33 + 2	35 + 4	37 + 5									
71	33 + 5	35 + 6	38 + 1									
72	34 + 1	36 + 3	38 + 4									
73	34 + 4	36 + 6	39									
74	35 + 1	37 + 2	39 + 4									
75	35 + 4	37 + 5	39 + 6									
76	36	38 + 1	40 + 3									
77	36 + 3	38 + 4	40 + 6									
78	36 + 6	39 + 1	41 + 2									
79	37 + 2	39 + 4	41 + 5									
80	37 + 6	40	42 + 1									

(Jeanty P, Rodesch F, Delbeke D, Dumont JE: Estimation of gestational age from measurements of fetal long bones. J Ultrasound Med 1984; 3:75–79.)

taken to obtain the entire longitudinal rather than oblique plane of the femur. Table V lists femur and other long bone measurements.

Abdominal circumference

Measurement of the *abdominal circumference* is made from the axial plane at the level of the liver (Table VI) (19). The AIUM standards (3) utilized the junction of the umbilical vein with the

Table VI. ***Predicted Menstrual Age* for Abdominal Circumference Values.***

Abdominal Circumference (cm)	Menstrual Age (wk)	Abdominal Circumference (cm)	Menstrual Age (wk)
10.0	15.6	23.5	27.7
10.5	16.1	24.0	28.2
11.0	16.5	24.5	28.7
11.5	16.9	25.0	29.2
12.0	17.3	25.5	29.7
12.5	17.8	26.0	30.1
13.0	18.2	26.5	30.6
13.5	18.6	27.0	31.1
14.0	19.1	27.5	31.6
14.5	19.5	28.0	32.1
15.0	20.0	28.5	32.6
15.5	20.4	29.0	33.1
16.0	20.8	29.5	33.6
16.5	21.3	30.0	34.1
17.0	21.7	30.5	34.6
17.5	22.2	31.0	35.1
18.0	22.6	31.5	35.6
18.5	23.1	32.0	36.1
19.0	23.6	32.5	36.6
19.5	24.0	33.0	37.1
20.0	24.5	33.5	37.6
20.5	24.9	34.0	38.1
21.0	25.4	34.5	38.7
21.5	25.9	35.0	39.2
22.0	26.3	35.5	39.7
22.5	26.8	36.0	40.2
23.0	27.3	36.5	40.8

* Menstrual age = 7.6070 + 0.7645 (AC) + 0.00393 $(AC)^2$; r^2 = 97.8%; 1 SD = 1.2 weeks.

(Hadlock FP, Deter LR, Harrist RB, Park SK: Fetal aodominal circumference as a predictor of menstrual age. AJR 1982; 139:367–370.)

left portal vein as the proper level to obtain the abdominal circumference (Figure 5). The fetal stomach may often be identified on this level. The image of the abdomen should be as round as pos-

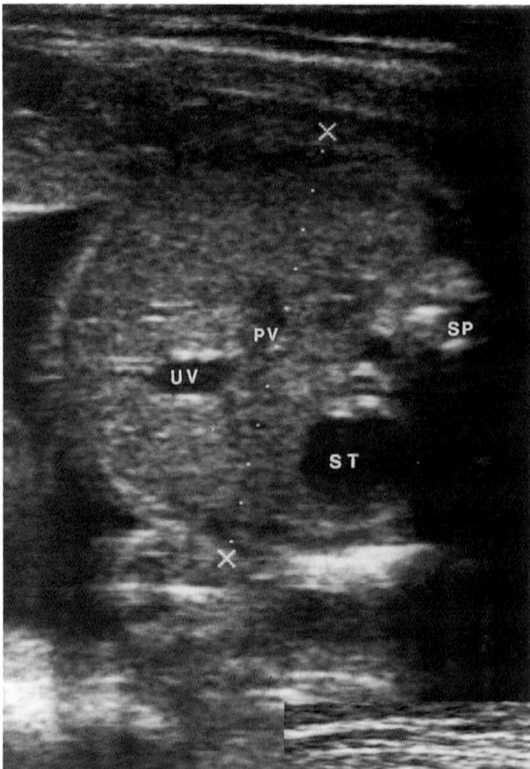

Figure 5 *Abdominal circumference of abdominal diameter is obtained at the junction of the umbilical vein (UV) with the left portal vein (PV). The circumference should be rounded. Also note other anatomical landmarks, such as the fetal stomach (ST) and spine (SP), may be identified on this view.*

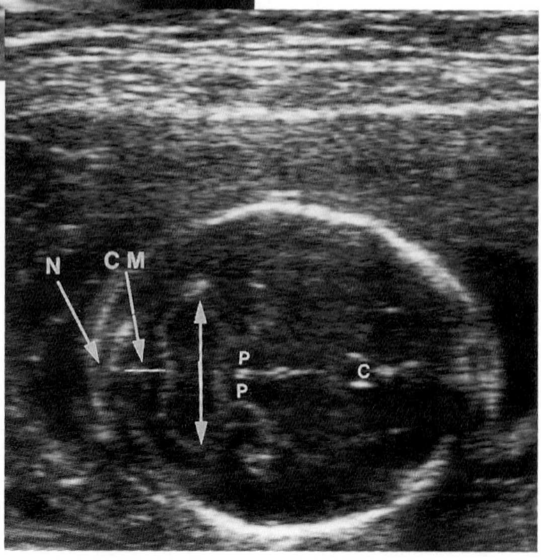

Figure 6 *Transaxial plane obtained through the cavum septi pellucidi (C) and the cerebellar peduncles (P) demonstrating measurement for the cerebellar diameter (arrows). Note that anterior to posterior measurement of the cisterna magna (CM) and nuchal thickness (N) may also be obtained on this view.*

sible. Oblique imaging of the abdomen will produce an oblong appearance and lead to over-estimation of the abdominal circumference, and thus an erroneous measurement.

Other measurements

There have been numerous other measurements for establishing menstrual age. These include, measurements of the cerebellar diameter (Figure 6) (Table VII) (20), orbital diameter (22), clavicular length (22), foot length (Table VIII) (23) (Figure 7), thigh circumference (24), and measurement of all other long bones (25) (Table V). Any of these measurements may be used for establishing men-

Table VII. ***Predicted Gestational Ages for Transverse Cerebellar Diameters of 14–56 mm.***

Cerebellum (mm)	Gestational Age (wk)	Cerebellum (mm)	Gestational Age (wk)
14	15.2	35	29.4
15	15.8	36	30.0
16	16.5	37	30.6
17	17.2	38	31.2
18	17.9	39	31.8
19	18.6	40	32.3
20	19.3	41	32.8
21	20.0	42	33.4
22	20.7	43	33.9
23	21.4	44	34.4
24	22.1	45	34.8
25	22.8	46	35.3
26	23.5	47	35.7
27	24.2	48	36.1
28	24.9	49	36.5
29	25.5	50	36.8
30	26.2	51	37.2
31	26.9	52	37.5
32	27.5	54	38.0
33	28.1	55	38.3
34	28.8	56	38.5

(Hill LM, Guzick D, Fries J, et al: The transverse cerebellar diameter in estimating gestational age in the large for gestational age fetus. Obstet Gynecol 1990; 75:981–985.)

strual age. Some of these have special significance. For instance, if the femur length is short then measurements of other long bones may be used to determine if the short femur is a measurement error or secondary to fetal dwarfism (Table V). Measurement of long bones is helpful to define dwarfism as rhizomelic (proximal), mesomelic (middle), or micromelic (generalized).

Table VIII. ***Comparison of Mean Postpartum and Ultrasonographic Foot Length with Streeter's Pathologic Data (1920).***

Gestation week	Ultrasonographic Foot Length (mm)
11	8
12	9
13	10
14	16
15	16
16	21
17	24
18	27
19	28
20	33
21	35
22	38
23	42
24	44
25	47
26	51
27	54
28	58
29	57
30	61
31	62
32	63
33	67
34	68
35	71
36	74
37	75
38	78
39	78
40	82

(Mercer BM, Sklar S, Shariatmader A, et al: Fetal foot length as a predictor of gestational age. Am J Obstet Gynecol 1987; 156: 350.)

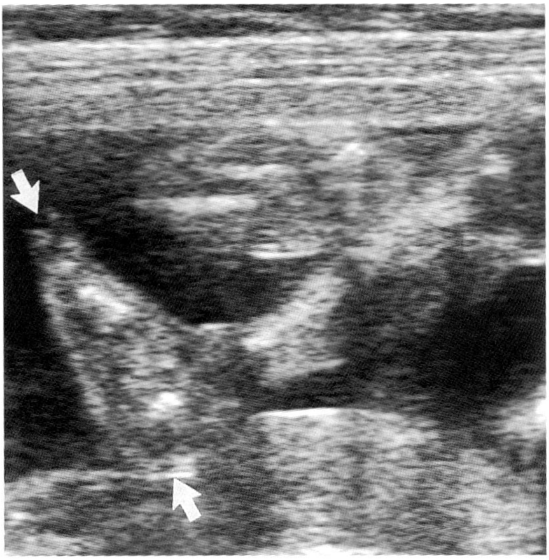

Figure 7 *Fetal foot length (arrows) may be obtained and correlated with either gestational age or compared to femur length.*

Ratios

While the AIUM standards only mention use of comparison of the head circumference to the abdominal circumference for detection of possible intrauterine growth retardation, other ratios may be useful (26) (Table IX). In general, one should pay close attention when one measurement parameter is substantially different than other measurements. For instance, if the femur length is much shorter than other measurements, one should consider the reason for an abnormally short femur length, such as an erroneous measurement or fetal dwarfism. The foot length is also useful in these cases, as foot length is rarely affected by dwarfism (23), and usually maintains a ratio of approximately 1:1 with the femur length. Ratios of other measurements may have significance. For instance, decreased size of the abdominal circumference as compared to other measurements may be an indicator of intrauterine growth retardation.

Fetal weight

Fetal weight can be established utilizing a number of different parameters, including use of composite measurements. Such formulas are now routinely programmed into most ultrasound units as

Table IX. ***Mean and Standard Deviation of Head Perimeter to Abdominal Perimeter Ratio as a Function of Gestational Age.***

	SD Above Mean			SD Below Mean				
Week No.	**+2**	**+1**	**Mean**	**–1**	**–2**	**–3**	**–4**	**–5**
20	1.43	1.34	1.25	1.16	1.07	0.98	0.89	0.8
21	1.42	1.33	1.24	1.15	1.06	0.97	0.88	0.79
22	1.41	1.32	1.23	1.14	1.05	0.96	0.87	0.78
23	1.4	1.31	1.22	1.13	1.04	0.95	0.86	0.78
24	1.39	1.3	1.21	1.12	1.03	0.94	0.86	0.77
25	1.38	1.29	1.2	1.11	1.02	0.94	0.85	0.76
26	1.37	1.28	1.19	1.1	1.02	0.93	0.84	0.75
27	1.36	1.27	1.18	1.1	1.01	0.92	0.83	0.74
28	1.35	1.26	1.17	1.09	1	0.91	0.82	0.73
29	1.34	1.25	1.17	1.08	0.99	0.9	0.81	0.72
30	1.33	1.25	1.16	1.07	0.98	0.89	0.8	0.71
31	1.33	1.24	1.15	1.06	0.97	0.88	0.79	0.7
32	1.32	1.23	1.14	1.05	0.96	0.87	0.78	0.69
33	1.31	1.22	1.13	1.04	0.95	0.86	0.77	0.68
34	1.3	1.21	1.12	1.03	0.94	0.85	0.76	0.68
35	1.29	1.2	1.11	1.02	0.93	0.84	0.76	0.67
36	1.28	1.19	1.1	1.01	0.92	0.84	0.75	0.66
37	1.27	1.18	1.09	1.00	0.92	0.83	0.74	0.65
38	1.26	1.17	1.08	1.00	0.91	0.82	0.73	0.64
39	1.25	1.16	1.08	0.99	0.90	0.81	0.72	0.63
40	1.24	1.16	1.07	0.98	0.89	0.80	0.71	0.62
41	1.24	1.15	1.06	0.97	0.88	0.79	0.70	0.61
42	1.23	1.14	1.05	0.96	0.87	0.78	0.69	0.60

(Chervenak FA, Jeanty P, Cantraine F, et al: The diagnosis of fetal microcephaly. Am J Obstet Gynecol 1984; 149:512–517.)

an obstetrical ultrasound calculation package. Table X lists a table for establishing fetal weight based upon the biparietal diameter and abdominal circumference as established by Shephard (27).

FETAL ANATOMY

Fetal anatomical survey as suggested by the AIUM is outlined for the first trimester in Table XI and for the second trimester in Table XII. Special comments can be made as to the utility of each of these anatomical landmarks.

Table X. *Estimated Fetal Weight (in grams) with BPD and AC*.*

BPD	AC (mm)												
(mm)	**155**	**160**	**165**	**170**	**175**	**180**	**185**	**190**	**195**	**200**	**205**	**210**	**215**
31	224	234	244	255	267	279	291	304	318	332	346	362	378
32	231	241	251	263	274	286	299	312	326	340	355	371	388
33	237	248	259	270	282	294	307	321	335	349	365	381	397
34	244	255	266	278	290	302	316	329	344	359	374	391	408
35	251	262	274	285	298	311	324	338	353	368	384	401	418
36	259	270	281	294	306	319	333	347	362	378	394	411	429
37	266	278	290	302	315	328	342	357	372	388	404	422	440
38	274	286	298	310	324	337	352	366	382	398	415	432	451
39	282	294	306	319	333	347	361	376	392	409	426	444	462
40	290	303	315	328	342	356	371	386	403	419	437	455	474
41	299	311	324	338	352	366	381	397	413	430	448	467	486
42	308	320	333	347	361	376	392	408	424	442	460	479	498
43	317	330	343	357	371	387	402	419	436	453	472	491	511
44	326	339	353	367	382	397	413	430	447	465	484	504	524
45	335	349	363	377	393	408	425	442	459	478	497	517	538
46	345	359	373	386	404	420	436	454	472	490	510	530	551
47	355	369	384	399	415	431	448	466	484	503	524	544	565
48	366	380	395	410	426	443	460	478	497	517	537	558	580
49	376	391	406	422	438	455	473	491	510	530	551	572	594
50	387	402	418	434	451	468	486	505	524	544	565	587	610
51	399	414	430	446	463	481	499	518	538	559	580	602	625
52	410	426	442	459	476	494	513	532	552	573	595	618	641
53	422	438	455	472	489	508	527	547	567	589	611	634	657
54	435	451	468	485	503	522	541	561	582	604	627	650	674
55	447	464	481	499	517	536	556	577	598	620	643	667	691
56	461	477	495	513	532	551	571	592	614	636	660	684	709
57	474	491	509	527	547	566	587	608	630	653	677	701	727
58	488	505	524	542	562	582	603	625	647	670	695	719	745
59	502	520	539	558	578	598	619	642	664	688	713	738	764
60	517	535	554	573	594	615	636	659	682	706	731	757	784
61	532	550	570	590	610	632	654	677	700	725	750	777	804
62	547	566	586	606	627	649	672	695	719	744	770	797	824
63	563	583	603	624	645	667	690	714	738	764	790	817	845
64	580	600	620	641	663	686	709	733	758	784	811	838	867
65	597	617	638	659	682	705	728	753	778	805	832	860	889
66	614	635	656	678	701	724	748	773	799	826	853	882	911
67	632	653	675	697	720	744	769	794	820	848	876	905	935
68	651	672	694	717	740	765	790	816	842	870	898	928	958
69	670	691	714	737	761	786	811	838	865	893	922	952	983
70	689	711	734	758	782	807	833	860	888	916	946	976	1,008
71	709	732	755	779	804	830	856	883	912	941	971	1,002	1,033
72	730	763	777	801	827	853	880	907	936	965	996	1,027	1,060
73	751	775	799	824	850	876	904	932	961	991	1,022	1,054	1,087
74	773	797	822	847	874	901	928	957	987	1,017	1,049	1,081	1,114
75	796	820	845	871	898	925	954	983	1,013	1,044	1,076	1,109	1,143
76	819	844	870	896	923	951	980	1,009	1,040	1,072	1,104	1,137	1,172
77	743	868	894	921	949	977	1,007	1,037	1,068	1,100	1,133	1,167	1,202
78	868	894	920	947	975	1,004	1,034	1,065	1,096	1,129	1,162	1,197	1,232
79	893	919	946	974	1,003	1,032	1,062	1,094	1,126	1,159	1,193	1,228	1,264
80	919	946	973	1,002	1,031	1,061	1,091	1,123	1,156	1,189	1,224	1,259	1,296
81	946	973	1,001	1,030	1,060	1,090	1,121	1,153	1,187	1,221	1,256	1,292	1,329
82	974	1,001	1,030	1,059	1,089	1,120	1,152	1,185	1,218	1,253	1,288	1,325	1,363
83	1,002	1,030	1,059	1,089	1,120	1,151	1,183	1,217	1,251	1,286	1,322	1,359	1,397
84	1,032	1,060	1,090	1,120	1,151	1,183	1,216	1,249	1,284	1,320	1,356	1,394	1,433
85	1,062	1,091	1,121	1,151	1,183	1,216	1,249	1,283	1,318	1,355	1,392	1,430	1,469
86	1,093	1,122	1,153	1,184	1,216	1,249	1,283	1,318	1,354	1,390	1,428	1,467	1,507
87	1,125	1,155	1,186	1,218	1,250	1,284	1,318	1,353	1,390	1,427	1,465	1,505	1,545
88	1,157	1,188	1,220	1,252	1,285	1,319	1,354	1,390	1,427	1,465	1,504	1,543	1,584
89	1,191	1,222	1,254	1,287	1,321	1,356	1,391	1,428	1,465	1,503	1,543	1,583	1,625
90	1,226	1,258	1,290	1,324	1,358	1,393	1,429	1,456	1,504	1,543	1,583	1,624	1,666
91	1,262	1,294	1,327	1,361	1,396	1,432	1,468	1,506	1,544	1,584	1,624	1,666	1,708
92	1,299	1,332	1,365	1,400	1,435	1,471	1,508	1,546	1,586	1,626	1,667	1,709	1,752
93	1,337	1,370	1,404	1,439	1,475	1,512	1,550	1,588	1,628	1,668	1,710	1,753	1,796
94	1,376	1,410	1,444	1,480	1,516	1,554	1,592	1,631	1,671	1,712	1,755	1,798	1,842
95	1,416	1,450	1,486	1,522	1,559	1,597	1,635	1,675	1,716	1,758	1,800	1,844	1,889
96	1,457	1,492	1,528	1,565	1,602	1,641	1,680	1,720	1,762	1,804	1,847	1,892	1,937
97	1,500	1,535	1,572	1,609	1,547	1,686	1,726	1,767	1,809	1,852	1,895	1,940	1,986
98	1,544	1,580	1,617	1,654	1,693	1,733	1,773	1,815	1,857	1,900	1,945	1,990	2,037
99	1,589	1,625	1,663	1,701	1,740	1,781	1,882	1,864	1,907	1,951	1,996	2,042	2,089
100	1,635	1,672	1,710	1,749	1,789	1,830	1,871	1,914	1,958	2,002	2,048	2,094	2,142

Table X. ***Estimated Fetal Weight (in grams) with BPD and AC*.***

BPD	AC (mm)												
(mm)	220	225	230	235	240	245	250	255	260	265	270	275	280
31	395	412	431	450	470	491	513	536	559	584	610	638	666
32	405	423	441	461	481	502	525	548	572	597	924	651	680
33	415	433	452	472	493	514	537	560	585	611	638	666	693
34	425	444	463	483	504	526	549	573	598	624	652	680	710
35	436	455	475	495	517	539	562	587	612	638	555	695	725
36	447	466	786	507	529	552	575	600	626	653	681	710	740
37	458	478	498	519	542	565	589	614	640	667	696	725	756
38	470	490	510	532	554	578	602	628	654	682	711	741	772
39	482	502	523	545	568	592	616	642	669	697	727	757	789
40	494	514	536	558	581	606	631	657	684	713	743	773	806
41	506	527	549	572	595	620	645	672	700	729	759	790	828
42	519	540	562	585	609	634	660	688	716	745	776	807	841
43	532	554	576	600	624	649	676	703	732	762	793	825	859
44	545	567	590	614	639	665	692	719	749	779	810	843	877
45	559	581	605	629	654	680	708	736	765	796	828	861	896
46	573	596	620	644	670	696	724	753	783	814	846	880	915
47	588	611	635	660	686	713	741	770	801	832	865	899	934
48	602	626	650	676	702	730	758	788	819	851	884	919	954
49	617	641	666	692	719	747	776	806	837	870	903	938	975
50	633	657	683	709	736	765	794	824	856	889	923	959	996
51	649	674	699	726	754	783	812	843	876	909	944	980	1,017
52	665	690	717	744	772	801	831	863	895	929	964	1,001	1,039
53	682	708	734	762	790	820	851	883	916	950	986	1,023	1,061
54	699	725	752	780	809	839	870	903	936	971	1,007	1,045	1,084
55	717	743	771	799	828	859	891	924	958	993	1,030	1,068	1,107
56	735	762	789	818	848	879	911	945	979	1,015	1,052	1,091	1,131
57	753	780	809	838	869	900	933	966	1,001	1,038	1,075	1,114	1,155
58	772	800	829	858	889	921	954	989	1,024	1,061	1,099	1,139	1,180
59	792	820	849	879	911	943	977	1,011	1,047	1,085	1,123	1,163	1,205
60	811	840	870	900	932	965	999	1,035	1,071	1,109	1,148	1,189	1,231
61	832	861	891	922	955	988	1,023	1,058	1,095	1,134	1,173	1,214	1,257
62	853	882	913	945	977	1,011	1,046	1,083	1,120	1,159	1,199	1,241	1,284
63	874	904	935	967	1,001	1,035	1,071	1,107	1,145	1,185	1,226	1,268	1,311
64	896	927	958	991	1,025	1,059	1,096	1,133	1,171	1,211	1,253	1,295	1,339
65	919	950	982	1,015	1,049	1,084	1,121	1,159	1,198	1,238	1,280	1,323	1,368
66	942	973	1,006	1,039	1,074	1,110	1,147	1,185	1,225	1,266	1,308	1,352	1,397
67	965	997	1,030	1,065	1,100	1,136	1,174	1,213	1,253	1,294	1,337	1,381	1,427
68	990	1,022	1,056	1,090	1,126	1,163	1,201	1,241	1,281	1,323	1,367	1,411	1,458
69	1,015	1,048	1,082	1,117	1,153	1,190	1,229	1,269	1,310	1,353	1,397	1,442	1,489
70	1,040	1,074	1,108	1,144	1,181	1,219	1,258	1,298	1,340	1,383	1,427	1,473	1,521
71	1,066	1,110	1,135	1,171	1,209	1,247	1,287	1,328	1,370	1,414	1,459	1,505	1,553
72	1,093	1,128	1,163	1,200	1,238	1,277	1,317	1,358	1,401	1,445	1,491	1,538	1,586
73	1,121	1,156	1,192	1,229	1,267	1,307	1,348	1,390	1,433	1,478	1,524	1,571	1,620
74	1,149	1,184	1,221	1,259	1,297	1,338	1,379	1,421	1,465	1,511	1,557	1,605	1,655
75	1,178	1,214	1,251	1,289	1,328	1,369	1,411	1,454	1,499	1,544	1,592	1,640	1,690
76	1,207	1,244	1,281	1,320	1,360	1,401	1,444	1,487	1,533	1,579	1,627	1,676	1,727
77	1,238	1,275	1,313	1,352	1,393	1,434	1,477	1,522	1,567	1,614	1,663	1,712	1,764
78	1,269	1,306	1,345	1,385	1,426	1,468	1,512	1,557	1,603	1,650	1,699	1,479	1,801
79	1,301	1,339	1,378	1,418	1,460	1,503	1,547	1,592	1,639	1,687	1,737	1,787	1,840
80	1,333	1,372	1,412	1,453	1,495	1,538	1,583	1,629	1,676	1,725	1,775	1,826	1,879
81	1,367	1,406	1,446	1,488	1,531	1,575	1,620	1,666	1,714	1,763	1,814	1,866	1,919
82	1,401	1,441	1,482	1,524	1,567	1,612	1,657	1,704	1,753	1,803	1,854	1,906	1,960
83	1,436	1,477	1,518	1,561	1,605	1,650	1,696	1,744	1,793	1,843	1,895	1,948	2,002
84	1,473	1,513	1,555	1,599	1,643	1,689	1,735	1,784	1,833	1,884	1,936	1,990	2,045
85	1,510	1,551	1,594	1,637	1,682	1,728	1,776	1,825	1,875	1,926	1,979	2,033	2,089
86	1,548	1,589	1,633	1,677	1,722	1,769	1,817	1,866	1,917	1,969	2,022	2,077	2,134
87	1,586	1,629	1,673	1,717	1,764	1,811	1,859	1,909	1,960	2,013	2,067	2,122	2,179
88	1,626	1,669	1,714	1,759	1,806	1,854	1,903	1,953	2,005	2,058	2,113	2,169	2,226
89	1,667	1,711	1,756	1,802	1,849	1,897	1,947	1,998	2,050	2,104	2,159	2,216	2,274
90	1,709	1,753	1,799	1,845	1,893	1,942	1,992	2,044	2,097	2,151	2,207	2,264	2,322
91	1,752	1,797	1,843	1,890	1,938	1,988	2,039	2,091	2,144	2,199	2,255	2,313	2,372
92	1,796	1,841	1,888	1,936	1,984	2,035	2,086	2,139	2,193	2,248	2,305	2,363	2,423
93	1,841	1,887	1,934	1,982	2,032	2,083	2,135	2,188	2,242	2,298	2,356	2,414	2,475
94	1,887	1,934	1,982	2,030	2,080	2,132	2,184	2,238	2,293	2,350	2,407	2,467	2,527
95	1,935	1,982	2,030	2,080	2,130	2,182	2,235	2,289	2,345	2,402	2,460	2,520	2,582
96	1,984	2,031	2,080	2,130	2,181	2,233	2,287	2,342	2,398	2,456	2,515	2,575	2,637
97	2,033	2,082	2,131	2,181	2,233	2,286	2,340	2,396	2,452	2,510	2,570	2,631	2,693
98	2,085	2,133	2,183	2,234	2,286	2,340	2,395	2,451	2,508	2,567	2,627	2,688	2,751
99	2,137	2,186	2,237	2,288	2,341	2,395	2,450	2,507	2,565	2,624	2,684	2,746	2,810
100	2,191	2,241	2,292	2,344	2,397	2,452	2,507	2,564	2,623	2,682	2,743	2,806	2,870

Table X. *Estimated Fetal Weight (in grams) with BPD and AC**.

BPD	AC (mm)												
(mm)	285	290	295	300	305	310	315	320	325	330	335	340	345
31	696	726	759	793	828	865	903	943	985	1,029	1,075	1,123	1,173
32	710	742	774	809	844	882	921	961	1,004	1,048	1,094	1,143	1,193
33	725	757	790	825	861	899	938	979	1,022	1,067	1,114	1,163	1,214
34	740	773	806	841	878	916	956	998	1,041	1,087	1,134	1,183	1,235
35	756	789	823	858	896	934	975	1,017	1,061	1,107	1,154	1,204	1,256
36	772	805	840	876	913	953	993	1,036	1,080	1,127	1,175	1,226	1,278
37	788	822	857	893	931	971	1,012	1,056	1,101	1,147	1,196	1,247	1,300
38	805	839	874	911	950	990	1,032	1,076	1,121	1,168	1,218	1,269	1,323
39	822	856	892	930	969	1,009	1,052	1,096	1,142	1,190	1,240	1,292	1,346
40	839	874	911	949	988	1,029	1,072	1,117	1,163	1,212	1,262	1,315	1,369
41	857	892	929	968	1,008	1,049	1,093	1,138	1,185	1,234	1,285	1,338	1,393
42	875	911	948	987	1,028	1,070	1,114	1,159	1,207	1,256	1,308	1,361	1,417
43	893	930	968	1,007	1,048	1,091	1,135	1,181	1,229	1,279	1,331	1,385	1,442
44	912	949	987	1,027	1,069	1,112	1,157	1,204	1,252	1,303	1,355	1,410	1,467
45	932	969	1,008	1,048	1,090	1,134	1,179	1,226	1,275	1,326	1,380	1,435	1,492
46	951	989	1,028	1,069	1,112	1,156	1,202	1,249	1,299	1,351	1,404	1,406	1,518
47	971	1,010	1,049	1,091	1,134	1,178	1,225	1,273	1,323	1,375	1,430	1,486	1,545
48	992	1,031	1,071	1,113	1,156	1,201	1,248	1,297	1,348	1,401	1,455	1,512	1,571
49	1,013	1,052	1,093	1,135	1,179	1,225	1,272	1,322	1,373	1,426	1,482	1,539	1,599
50	1,034	1,074	1,115	1,158	1,203	1,249	1,297	1,347	1,399	1,452	1,508	1,566	1,626
51	1,056	1,096	1,138	1,181	1,226	1,273	1,322	1,372	1,425	1,479	1,535	1,594	1,655
52	1,078	1,119	1,161	1,205	1,251	1,298	1,347	1,398	1,451	1,506	1,563	1,622	1,683
53	1,101	1,142	1,185	1,229	1,276	1,323	1,373	1,425	1,478	1,533	1,591	1,651	1,713
54	1,124	1,166	1,209	1,254	1,301	1,349	1,399	1,452	1,506	1,562	1,620	1,680	1,742
55	1,148	1,190	1,234	1,279	1,327	1,376	1,426	1,479	1,534	1,590	1,649	1,710	1,773
56	1,172	1,215	1,259	1,305	1,353	1,402	1,454	1,507	1,562	1,619	1,678	1,740	1,803
57	1,197	1,240	1,285	1,342	1,380	1,430	1,482	1,535	1,591	1,649	1,709	1,770	1,835
58	1,222	1,266	1,311	1,358	1,407	1,458	1,510	1,564	1,621	1,679	1,739	1,802	1,866
59	1,248	1,292	1,338	1,386	1,435	1,486	1,539	1,594	1,651	1,710	1,770	1,834	1,899
60	1,274	1,319	1,366	1,414	1,464	1,515	1,569	1,624	1,682	1,741	1,802	1,866	1,932
61	1,301	1,346	1,393	1,442	1,493	1,545	1,599	1,655	1,713	1,773	1,835	1,899	1,965
62	1,328	1,374	1,422	1,471	1,522	1,575	1,630	1,686	1,745	1,805	1,868	1,932	1,999
63	1,356	1,403	1,451	1,501	1,552	1,606	1,661	1,718	1,777	1,838	1,901	1,967	2,034
64	1,385	1,432	1,481	1,531	1,583	1,637	1,693	1,751	1,810	1,872	1,935	2,001	2,069
65	1,414	1,462	1,511	1,562	1,615	1,669	1,725	1,784	1,844	1,906	1,970	2,037	2,105
66	1,444	1,492	1,542	1,594	1,647	1,702	1,759	1,817	1,878	1,941	2,006	2,073	2,142
67	1,474	1,523	1,574	1,626	1,679	1,735	1,792	1,852	1,913	1,976	2,042	2,109	2,179
68	1,505	1,555	1,606	1,658	1,713	1,769	1,827	1,887	1,949	2,012	2,078	2,147	2,217
69	1,537	1,587	1,639	1,692	1,747	1,803	1,862	1,922	1,985	2,049	2,116	2,184	2,255
70	1,570	1,620	1,672	1,726	1,781	1,839	1,898	1,959	2,022	2,087	2,154	2,223	2,295
71	1,603	1,654	1,706	1,761	1,817	1,875	1,934	1,996	2,059	2,125	2,193	2,262	2,334
72	1,636	1,688	1,741	1,796	1,853	1,911	1,971	2,044	2,098	2,164	2,232	2,302	2,375
73	1,671	1,723	1,777	1,832	1,890	1,948	2,009	2,072	2,137	2,203	2,272	2,343	2,416
74	1,706	1,759	1,813	1,869	1,927	1,987	2,048	2,111	2,176	2,244	2,313	2,384	2,458
75	1,742	1,795	1,850	1,970	1,965	2,025	2,087	2,151	2,217	2,265	2,354	2,426	2,501
76	1,779	1,833	1,888	1,945	2,004	2,065	2,127	2,192	2,258	2,326	2,397	2,469	2,544
77	1,816	1,871	1,927	1,985	2,044	2,105	2,168	2,233	2,300	2,369	2,440	2,513	2,588
78	1,855	1,910	1,966	2,025	2,085	2,146	2,210	2,275	2,343	2,412	2,484	2,557	2,633
79	1,894	1,949	2,006	2,065	2,126	2,188	2,252	2,318	2,386	2,456	2,528	2,063	2,679
80	1,934	1,990	2,048	2,107	2,168	2,231	2,296	2,362	2,431	2,501	2,574	2,649	2,725
81	1,975	2,031	2,089	2,149	2,211	2,275	2,340	2,407	2,476	2,547	2,620	2,695	2,773
82	2,016	2,073	2,132	2,193	2,255	2,319	2,385	2,462	2,522	2,594	2,667	2,743	2,821
83	2,059	2,116	2,176	2,237	2,300	2,364	2,431	2,499	2,569	2,641	2,715	2,791	2,870
84	2,102	2,160	2,220	2,282	2,345	2,410	2,477	2,546	2,617	2,689	2,764	2,841	2,920
85	2,146	2,205	2,266	2,328	2,392	2,457	2,525	2,594	2,665	2,739	2,814	2,891	2,970
86	2,192	2,251	2,312	2,375	2,439	2,505	2,573	2,643	2,715	2,789	2,864	2,942	3,022
87	2,238	2,298	2,359	2,423	2,488	2,554	2,623	2,693	2,765	2,840	2,916	2,994	3,074
88	2,285	2,346	2,408	2,472	2,537	2,604	2,673	2,744	2,817	2,892	2,968	3,047	3,128
89	2,333	2,394	2,457	2,521	2,587	2,655	2,725	2,796	2,869	2,944	3,021	3,101	3,182
90	2,382	2,444	2,507	2,572	2,639	2,707	2,777	2,849	2,923	2,998	3,076	3,155	3,237
91	2,433	2,495	2,559	2,624	2,691	2,760	2,830	2,903	2,977	3,053	3,131	3,211	3,293
92	2,484	2,547	2,611	2,677	2,744	2,814	2,885	2,958	3,032	3,109	3,187	3,268	3,350
93	2,536	2,599	2,664	2,731	2,799	2,869	2,940	3,014	3,089	3,166	3,245	3,326	3,409
94	2,590	2,653	2,719	2,786	2,854	2,925	2,997	3,070	3,146	3,224	3,303	3,384	3,468
95	2,644	2,709	2,774	2,842	2,911	2,982	3,054	3,129	3,205	3,283	3,362	3,444	3,528
96	2,700	2,765	2,831	2,899	2,969	3,040	3,113	3,188	3,264	3,343	3,423	3,505	3,589
97	2,757	2,822	2,889	2,958	3,028	3,099	3,173	3,248	3,325	3,404	3,484	3,567	3,651
98	2,815	2,881	2,948	3,107	3,088	3,160	3,234	3,309	3,387	3,466	3,547	3,630	3,715
99	2,874	2,941	3,009	3,078	3,149	3,222	3,296	3,372	3,450	3,529	3,611	3,694	3,779
100	2,935	3,002	3,070	3,140	3,211	3,285	3,359	3,436	3,514	3,594	3,676	3,759	3,845

Table X. *Estimated Fetal Weight (in grams) with BPD and AC*[*]*.*

BPD	AC (mm)										
(mm)	350	355	360	365	370	375	380	385	390	395	400
31	1,225	1,279	1,336	1,396	1,458	1,523	1,591	1,661	1,735	1,812	1,893
32	1,246	1,301	1,258	1,418	1,481	1,546	1,615	1,686	1,761	1,838	1,920
33	1,267	1,323	1,381	1,441	1,504	1,570	1,639	1,711	1,786	1,865	1,946
34	1,289	1,345	1,403	1,464	1,528	1,595	1,664	1,737	1,812	1,891	1,973
35	1,311	1,367	1,426	1,488	1,552	1,619	1,689	1,762	1,839	1,918	2,001
36	1,333	1,390	1,450	1,512	1,577	1,645	1,715	1,789	1,865	1,945	2,029
37	1,356	1,413	1,474	1,536	1,603	1,670	1,741	1,815	1,893	1,973	2,057
38	1,379	1,437	1,498	1,561	1,627	1,696	1,768	1,842	1,920	2,001	2,086
39	1,402	1,461	1,523	1,586	1,653	1,722	1,794	1,870	1,948	2,030	2,115
40	1,426	1,486	1,548	1,612	1,679	1,749	1,822	1,898	1,977	2,059	2,145
41	1,451	1,511	1,573	1,638	1,706	1,776	1,849	1,926	2,005	2,088	2,174
42	1,475	1,536	1,599	1,664	1,733	1,804	1,878	1,954	2,035	2,118	2,205
43	1,500	1,562	1,625	1,691	1,760	1,832	1,906	1,984	2,064	2,148	2,236
44	1,526	1,588	1,652	1,718	1,788	1,860	1,935	2,013	2,094	2,179	2,267
45	1,552	1,614	1,679	1,746	1,816	1,889	1,964	2,043	2,125	2,210	2,298
46	1,579	1,641	1,706	1,774	1,845	1,918	1,994	2,073	2,156	2,241	2,330
47	1,605	1;669	1,734	1,803	1,874	1,948	2,024	2,104	2,187	2,273	2,363
48	1,633	1,697	1,763	1,832	1,904	1,976	2,055	2,136	2,219	2,306	2,396
49	1,661	1,725	1,792	1,861	1,934	2,009	2,086	2,167	2,251	2,339	2,429
50	1,689	1,754	1,821	1,891	1,964	2,040	2,118	2,200	2,284	2,372	2,463
51	1,718	1,783	1,851	1,922	1,995	2,071	2,150	2,232	2,317	2,406	2,498
52	1,747	1,813	1,882	1,953	2,027	2,103	2,183	2,266	2,351	2,440	2,532
53	1,777	1,843	1,913	1,984	2,059	2,136	2,216	2,299	2,386	2,475	2,568
54	1,807	1,874	1,944	2,016	2,091	2,169	2,250	2,333	2,420	2,510	2,604
55	1,838	1,906	1,976	2,049	2,124	2,203	2,284	2,368	2,456	2546	2,640
56	1,869	1,938	2,008	2,082	2,158	2,237	2,319	2,403	2,491	2,582	2,677
57	1,901	1.970	2,041	2,115	2,192	2,272	2,354	2,439	2,528	2,619	2,714
58	1,934	2,003	2,075	2,150	2,227	2,307	2,390	2,475	2,564	2,657	2,752
59	1,966	2,037	2,109	2,184	2,262	2,342	2,426	2,512	2,602	2,694	2,790
60	2,000	2,071	2,144	2,219	2,298	2,379	2,463	2,550	2,640	2,733	2,829
61	2,034	2,105	2,179	2,255	2,334	2,416	2,500	2,588	2,678	2,772	2,869
62	2,069	2,140	2,215	2,291	2,371	2,453	2,538	2,626	2,717	2,811	2,909
63	2,104	2,176	2,251	2,328	2,408	2,491	2,577	2,665	2,757	2,851	2,949
64	2,140	2,213	2,288	2,366	2,446	2,530	2,616	2,705	2,797	2,892	2,991
65	2,176	2,250	2,326	2,404	2,485	2,569	2,656	2,745	2,838	2,933	3,032
66	2,213	2,287	2,364	2,443	2,524	2,609	2,696	2,786	2,879	2,975	3,075
67	2,251	2,326	2,403	2,482	2,564	2,649	2,737	2,827	2,921	3,018	3,117
68	2,290	2,365	2,442	2,522	2,605	2,690	2,778	2,869	2,964	3,061	3,161
69	2,329	2,404	2,482	2,563	2,646	2,732	2,821	2,912	3,007	3,104	3,205
70	2,368	2,444	2,523	2,604	2,688	2,774	2,863	2,955	3,050	3,149	3,250
71	2,409	2,485	2,564	2,646	2,730	2,817	2,907	2,999	3,095	3,193	3,295
72	2,450	2,527	2,607	2,689	2,773	2,861	2,951	3,044	3,140	3,239	3,341
73	2,491	2,569	2,649	2,732	2,817	2,905	2,996	3,089	3,186	3,285	3,386
74	2,534	2,612	2,693	2,776	2,862	2,950	3,041	3,135	3,232	3,332	3.435
75	2,577	2,656	2,737	2,821	2,907	2,996	3,088	3,183	3,279	3,380	3,483
76	2,621	2,700	2,782	2,866	2,953	3,042	3,134	3,229	3,327	3,428	3,531
77	2,666	2,746	2,828	2,912	3,000	3,090	3,128	3,277	3,376	3,477	3,581
78	2,711	2,792	2,874	2,959	3,047	3,137	3,230	3,326	3,425	3,526	3,631
79	2,757	2,838	2,921	3,007	3,095	3,186	3,279	3,376	3,475	3,576	3,681
80	2,804	2,886	2,969	3,056	3,144	3,235	3,329	3,426	3,525	3,627	3,733
81	2,852	2,934	3,018	3,105	3,194	3,286	3,380	3,477	3,577	3,679	3,785
82	2,901	2,983	3,068	3,155	3,244	3,336	3,431	3,529	3,629	3,732	3,838
83	2,950	3,033	3,118	3,206	3,296	3,388	3,483	3,581	3,682	3,785	3,891
84	3,001	3,084	3,169	3,257	3,348	3,441	3,536	3,634	3,735	3,839	3,945
85	3,052	3,135	3,221	3,310	3,401	3,494	3,590	3,688	3,790	3,894	4,000
86	3,104	3,188	3,274	3,363	3,454	3,548	3,644	3,743	3,845	3,949	4,056
87	3,157	3,241	3,328	3,417	3,509	3,603	3,700	3,799	3,901	4,005	4,113
88	3,210	3,295	3,383	3,472	3,565	3,659	3,756	3,855	3,958	4,063	4,170
89	3,265	3,351	3,438	3,528	3,621	3,716	3,813	3,913	4,015	4,120	4,228
90	3,321	3,407	3,495	3,585	3,678	3,773	3,871	3,971	4,074	4,179	4,287
91	3,377	3,464	3,552	3,643	3,736	3,832	3,930	4,030	4,133	4,239	4,347
92	3,435	3,522	3,661	3,702	3,795	3,891	3,989	4,090	4,193	4,299	4,408
93	3,494	3,581	3,670	3,761	3,855	3,951	4,050	4,151	4,254	4,361	4,469
94	3,553	3,641	3,738	3,822	3,916	4,013	4,111	4,213	4,316	4,423	4,532
95	3,614	3,701	3,791	3,884	3,978	4,075	4,174	4,275	4,379	4,486	4,595
96	3,675	3,763	3,854	3,946	4,041	4,138	4,237	4,339	4,443	4,550	4,659
97	3,738	3,826	3,917	4,010	4,105	4,202	4,302	4,404	4,508	4,615	4,724
98	3,803	3,890	3,981	4,074	4,170	4,267	4,367	4,469	4,573	4,680	4,790
99	3,866	3,956	4,047	4,140	4,236	4,333	4,433	4,536	4,640	4,747	4,857
100	3,392	4,022	4,113	4,207	4,303	4,400	4,501	4,603	4,708	4,815	4,924

From: Shepard M.J., Richards V.A., Berkowitz R.L. et. al.: An evaluation of two equations for predicting fetal weight by ultrasound. Am. J. Obstet Gynecol 1982;142:47–54, with permission.

Cerebral ventricles

The anatomical region best suited for measurement of the fetal cerebral ventricles is the downside ventricular atrium. The ventricular atrium is best visualized on a standard transaxial plane taken through the region of the thalami. The ventriculoatrial measurement may remain fairly constant throughout pregnancy and the upper limit of normal has been established as 10 mm (28, 29) (Figure 3). Furthermore, if the medial wall of the fetal ventricle is separated from the choroid plexus by more than 3 mm, this may be a sign of ventriculomegaly (32).

Cisterna magna

While visualization of the cisterna magna is not included as a routine view in the AIUM guidelines, we feel strongly that it should be. By angling the transducer into the posterior fossa in a plane that includes the cavum septi pellucidi, the cerebral peduncles, and the cerebellar hemisphere, measurements of the normal posterior fossa may be made. Using this anatomical plane, the normal *cisterna magna* anterior to posterior measurement should be between 2 and 12 mm (31) (Figure 6). Increased size of the cisterna magna may be associated with such abnormalities as the Dandy-Walker malformation or its variants, while decreased size of the cisterna magna may be associated with Arnold-Chiari type 2 malformations (32, 33). Furthermore, the transverse diameter of the

Table XI. ***Guidelines for First Trimester Ultrasound (adapted from AIUM [3]).***

1.	Location of gestational sac Mean sac diameter recorded* – With embryo identified – Crown-rump length recorded (estimate of menstrual age)
2.	Presence or absence of fetal heart rate (fetal life)
3.	Documentation of fetal number.
4.	Evaluation of uterus (including cervix)
S	Evaluation of adenexa

* Author's comments.

cerebellar hemispheres increases by approximately 1 mm per menstrual week between 14 and 21 weeks (20) (Figure 6). Finally, this plane may be used to detect abnormalities of the fetal neck including *nuchal thickening* which may be associated with chromosomal abnormality. Measurement of the outer bony calvarium of the posterior fossa to the outer skin surface should be less than 6 mm (34).

Table XII. ***Guidelines for Second and Third Trimester Sonography (adapted from AIUM [3]).***

1. Presence or absence of fetal heart rate (fetal life) and rhythm
   - Fetal presentation
   - Documentation of fetal number (singleton vs. multiple pregnancies)
   - When multiple pregnancies, document:
     Placental number
     Sac number
     Comparison of fetal size
     Presence of membrane* (thick vs. thin)
     Fetal genitalia
2. Estimation of the amount of amniotic fluid
3. Placental location and relationship to cervical os
   - Placental appearance
4. Assessment of menstrual age
   A. Biparietal diameter (BPD)
      – include cavum septi pellucidi and the thalamus
   B. Head circumference (HC) using the BPD plane
   C. Femur length (FL)
   D. Abdominal circumference (AC) at the level of the junction of the umbilical vein and the portal sinus (HC/AC ratio may be recorded)
5. Fetal growth and weight assessment in third trimester.
6. Evaluation of uterus and evaluation of adnexa
7. Fetal anatomy
   - Cerebral ventricles
   - Cistema magna
   - Four-chamber view of the heart/thorax.
   - Spine
   - Stomach
   - Renal region
   - Urinary bladder
   - Umbilical cord insertion

* Author's comments

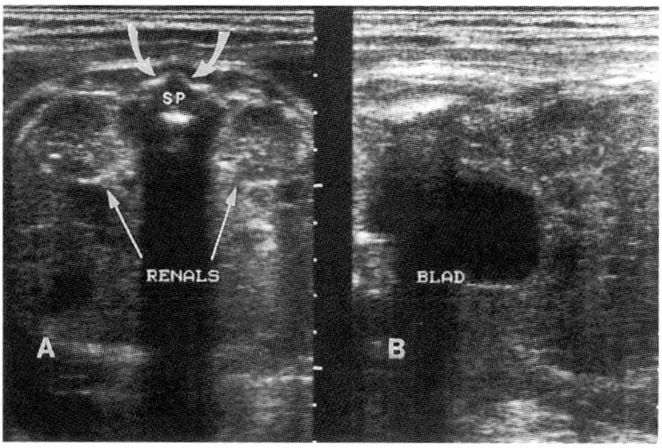

Figure 8
(a) Transverse view of the fetal abdomen showing the closed posterior elements of the fetal spine (curved arrows) and the two fetal kidneys (renals).
(b) Parasagittal view through the pelvis demonstrating the fetal bladder (Blad).

Spine

Transverse views of the fetal spine are helpful to demonstrate the closed posterior elements of the spine (Figure 8). Splaying of these posterior ossification elements is helpful to reliably diagnose an open neural tube defect (35). Sagittal images also may be used to observe the spinal cord and the bony spinal canal. Coronal views may be helpful to detect such abnormalities as hemivertebra (36).

Four-chamber heart

The four chamber view of the heart is helpful to detect not only major structural abnormalities of the heart, but also may be used as an anatomical marker for other intrathoracic abnormalities. On the transaxial plane, the apex of the heart is noted to point to the

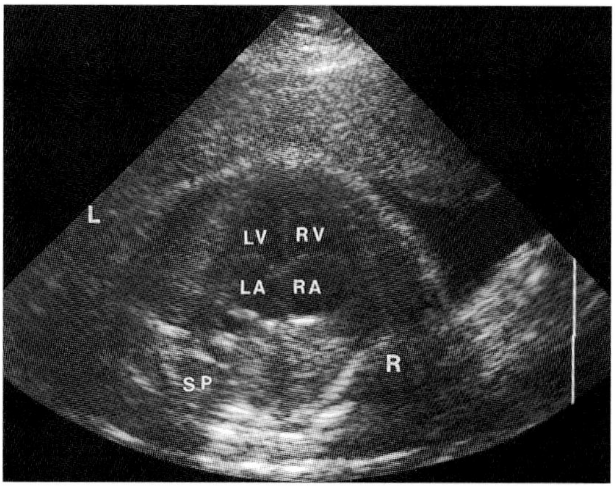

Figure 9 *Standard transaxial view of the thorax demonstrating normal four-chamber view of the heart with the left ventricle (LV), right ventricle (RV), left atrium (LA), and right atrium (RA) (L = left, R= right, SP=spine)*

left (Figure 9). The right ventricle is retrosternal and the left ventricle forms the left heart border. A thickened muscle (the moderator band) helps to identify the right ventricle. The right atrium is to the right side and blood is observed flowing through the foramen ovale from the right atrium into the more posteriorly located left atrium (37). Generally, the right ventricle and the left ventricle maintain a 1:1 ratio as identified sonographically during diastole at the atrial ventricular valve region. Identification of the ventricular size on the four-chamber view of the heart may be helpful to diagnose cardiac chamber hypoplasia (38). While the four-chamber view of the heart cannot be utilized to detect all anatomical cardiac malformations, it has been estimated to reliably detect approximately 65 % of structural abnormalities of the heart (39).

Renal region/bladder

Within the abdomen, the renal regions and bladder should be routinely visualized. The fetal kidneys appear as ovoid hypoechoic structures located in the paraspinal region (Figure 8). The kidneys increase in length throughout pregnancy with a length of approximately 2 cm at 20 weeks and increase to nearly 4 cm in length near

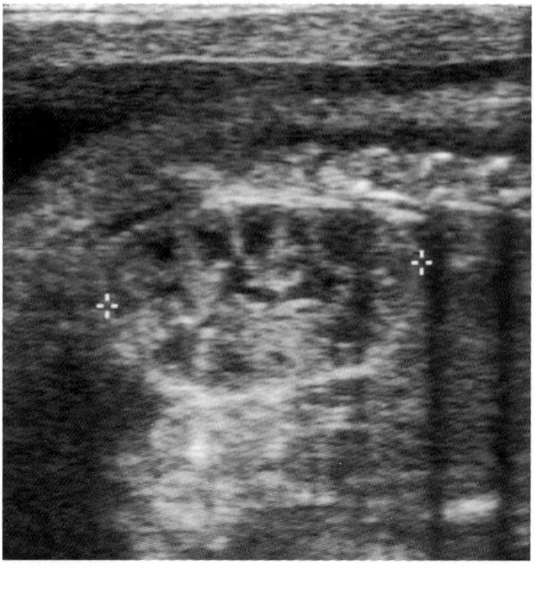

Figure 10 *Parasagittal view of the spine demonstrating the length of the fetal kidney between the calipers.*

term (40) (Figure 10). Identification of the fetal bladder is important, especially when the kidneys are difficult to visualize or there are bilateral fetal renal abnormalities (Figure 8). In the second and third trimester, identification of amniotic fluid volume is crucial to exclude oligohydramnios associated with bilateral renal pathology.

Stomach

Fetal swallowing occurs at approximately 14 weeks of gestational age (41). Thus, the fetal stomach should be visualized in all normal pregnancies (Figures 5, 11). Lack of visualization may indicate poor fetal swallowing or obstruction to the proximal stomach. In other situations where there is severe oligohydramnios, such as from premature rupture of membranes, there may be little amniotic fluid detected within the stomach. Later in pregnancy, stomach dilatation may be associated with outlet obstruction, including the classic "double bubble" abnormality associated with duodenal atresia (42).

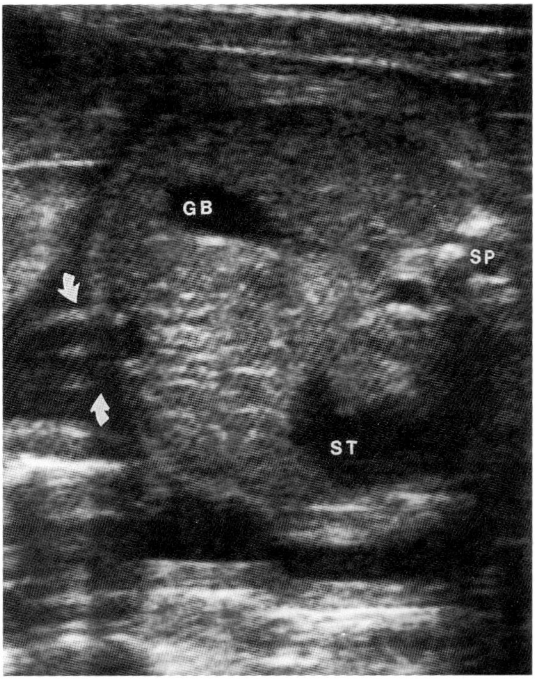

Figure 11
Transverse view of the abdomen showing cord insertion (arrows) with the gallbladder (GB), stomach (ST) and spine (SP).

Anterior abdominal wall

The umbilical cord enters the anterior abdominal wall where the umbilical vein flow cephalad into the liver and the two umbilical arteries are directed caudally, coursing around the fetal bladder. Cord insertion is helpful to identify the anterior abdominal wall for such defects as omphalocele or gastroschisis (35) (Figure 11).

OTHER OBSTETRICAL ANATOMY (TABLE XIII)

Fetal face

While not included in the AIUM guidelines (3), ultrasound may be used to visualize the fetal face. Most commonly, a coronal view through the nose and the lips is used to exclude cleft lip. Also, axial views of the orbits and sagittal views of the face have been advocated for cases in which a facial abnormality is suspected (3, 43).

Fetal heart – outflow tracts

The left ventricular outflow view may be used to observe the relationship of the aorta to the left ventricle. Likewise, the pulmonary artery can be observed exiting from the right ventricle utilizing the right ventricular outflow tract. While this is beyond the scope of this chapter, these are especially useful to detect outflow tract abnormalities, such as transposition of the great vessels or tetralogy of Fallot (39).

Genitalia

The parents "need to know" is usually reason for determination of fetal sex. Sex determination is correctly made in the majority of cases, but in up to 3 % of pregnancies fetal gender is inaccurate. This is probably secondary to the fact that labial hypertrophy may be misinterpreted as the scrotum (44).

Table XIII. ***Some Obstetrical Anatomy Not Included in AIUM Standards***

- Outflow tracts (heart)
- Face
- Limbs
- Genitalia
- Umbilical cord

Extremities

The AIUM guidelines only advocate views of the fetal femur length. More detailed visualization of the fetal limbs can be obtained throughout pregnancy. Transverse images through the radius/ulna or the tibia/fibula may be used to identify presence of the lower legs or forearms. Images of the hands and feet may be obtained, and unless specifically indicated are probably beyond the scope of the routine obstetrical ultrasound imaging.

Umbilical cord

While the AIUM standards do not recommend routine use of color Doppler or documentation of a three-vessel cord, others feel a transverse image of the cord is helpful. Documentation of the two arteries and single vein is helpful to identify a normal three-vessel cord, as a two vessel umbilical cord is associated with increased incidence of fetal anomalies (45).

REFERENCES

1. Hobbins J. Ultrasound in pregnancy. American College of Obstetricians and Gynecologists Technical Bulletin no. 116, Washington DC, 1988. American College of Obstetrics and Gynecology.
2. Americal College of Radiology: Guidelines for Performance of the Antepartum Obstetrical Examination, 1991. ACR, Reston, VA.
3. American Institute of Ultrasound in Medicine: Guidelines for Performance of the Antepartum Ultrasound Examination. J Ultrasound Med 1991;10:576–578.
4. Robinson HP. The Evaluation of Early Pregnancy and its Complications. Glasgow: University of Glasgow, 1978. Doctoral thesis.
5. Beazley JM, Underhill RA. Fallacy of the fundal height. Br Med J 1970;4:404–406.
6. Hellman LM, Kobayashi M, Fillisti L et al. Growth and development of the human fetus prior to the twentieth week of gestation. Am J Obstet Gyneocl 1969;103:789–800.
7. Kohorn EI, Kaufman M. Sonar in the first trimester of pregnancy. Obstet Gynecol 1974;44:473–483.
8. Nyberg DA, Laing FC, Filly RA. Threatened abortion: sonographic distinction of normal and abnormal gestation sacs. Radiology 1986;158:397–400.
9. Levi CS, Lyons EA, Lindsay DJ. Early diagnosis of nonviable pregnancy with endovaginal ultrasoud. Radiology 1988;167:383–385.
10. Robinson HP. Sonar measurement of the fetal crown-rump length as a

means of assessing maturity in the first trimester of pregnancy. Br Med J 1973;4:28–31.
11. Pedersen JF. Fetal crown-rump length measurement by ultrasound in normal pregnancy. Br J Obstet Gynecol 1982;89:929–930.
12. Levi CS, Lyons EA, Zheng XH et al. Endovaginal ultrasound: demonstration of cardiac activity in embroys of less than 5.0 mm in crown rump length. Radiology 1990;176:71–74.
13. Hadlock FP, Deter RL, Harrist RB, Park SK. Estimating fetal age: computer assisted analysis of multiple fetal growth parameters. Radiology 1984;152:497–501.
14. Campbell S. The prediction of fetal maturity by ultrasonic measurement of the biparietal diameter. J Obstet Gynaecol Br Commonw 1969;76:603–609.
15. Hadlock FP, Deter RL, Harrist RD, Park SK. Fetal biparietal diameter: a critical reevaluation of the relation to menstrual age by means of real-time ultrasound. J Ultrasound Med 1982;1:97–104.
16. Hadlock FP, Deter RL, Harrist RB, Park SK. Fetal head circumference: relation to menstrual age. AJR 1982;138:649–653.
17. Hadlock FP, Deter RL, Carpenter RJ, Park SK. Estimating fetal gestational age: effect of head shape on BPD. AJR 1981;137:83–85.
18. O'Brien GD, Queenan JT, Campbell S. Assessment of gestational age in the second trimester by realtime ultrasound measurement of the femur length. Am J Obstet Gynecol 1981;139:540-545.
19. Hadlock FP, Deter RL, Harrist RB, Park SK. Fetal abdominal circumference as a predictor of menstrual age. AJR 1982;139:367–370.
20. Hill LM, Guzick D, Fries J et al. The transverse cerebellar diameter in estimating gestational age in the large for gestational age fetus. Obstet Gynecol 1990;75:981–985.
21. Mayden KL, Tortora M, Berkowitz RL et al. Orbital diameters: a new parameter for prenatal diagnosis and dating. Am J Obstet Gynecol 1982;144:289–297.
22. Yarkoni S, Schmidt W, Jeanty P et al. Clavicular measurement: a new biometric parameter for fetal evaluation. J Ultrasound Med 1985;4:467–470.
23. Mercer BM, Sklar S, Shariatmader A et al. Fetal foot length as a predictor of gestational age. Am J Obstet Gynecol 1987;156:350-355.
24. Deter RL, Warda A, Rossavik IV et al. Fetal thigh circumference: a critical evaluation of its relationship to menstrual age. J Clin Ultrasound 1986;14:105–110.
25. Jeanty P, Ropesch F, Delbeke D, Dumon TJE. Estimation of gestational age from measurements of fetal long bones. J Ultrasound Med 1984;3:75–79.
26. Brons JT, Van der Harten JJ, Van Geijn HP et al. Ratios between growth parameters for the prenatal ultrasonographic diagnosis of skeletal dysplasias. Eur J Obstet Gynecol Reprod Biol 1990;34:37–46.
27. Shepard MJ, Richard VA, Berkowitz RL et al. An evaluation of two equations for predicting fetal weight by ultrasound. Am J Obstet Gynecol 1982;142:47–54.

28. Browning PB,Laorr A, McGahan JP et al. Ultrasound assessment of the ”upside” cerebral ventricle. Radiology 1994;192:337–341.
29. Cardoza JD, Goldstein RB, Filly RA. Exclusion of fetal ventriculomegaly with a single measurement. The width of the lateral ventricular atrium. Radiology 1988;169:711–714.
30. Hertzberg BS, Lile R, Foosaner DE et al. Choroid plexus-ventricular wall septation in fetuses with normal-sized cerebral ventricles at sonography: postnatal outcome. AJR 1994;163:405–410.
31. Mahony BS, Callen PW, Filly RA, Hoodick WK. The fetal cisterna magna. Radiology 1984;153:773–776.
32. Nicolaides KH, Campbell S, Gabbe SG, Guidetti R. Ultrasound screening for spina bifida: cranial and cerebellar signs. Lancet 1986;2:72–74.
33. Russ P, Pretorius D, Johnson M. Dandy-Walker syndrome: a review of 15 cases evaluated by prenatal sonography. Am J Obstet Gynecol 1989;161:401–406.
34. Crane JP, Gray DL. Sonographically measured nuchal skinfold thickness as a screening tool for Down syndrome: result of a prospective clinical trial. Obstet Gynecol 1991;77:533–536.
35. Lindfors KK, McGahan JP, Tennant F et al. Midtrimester screening for open neural tube defects: correlation of sonography with amniocentesis results. AJR 1987;149:141–145.
36. McGahan JP, Leeba JM, Lindfors KK. Prenatal sonographic diagnosis of VATER association. J Clin Ultrasound 1988;16:588–591.
37. McGahan JP. Sonography of the fetal heart: findings on the four-chamber view. AJR 1991;156:547–553.
38. McGahan JP, Choy M, Parrish MD, Brant WE. Sonographic spectrum of fetal cardiac hypoplasia. J Ultrasound Med 1991;10:539–546.
39. Bromley B, Estroff JA, Sanders SP et al. Fetal echocardiography accuracy: accuracy and limitations in a population at high and low risk for heart defects. Am J Obstet Gynecol 1992;166:1473–1481.
40. Bertagnoli L, Lalatta F, Gallicchio R et al. Quantitative characterization of growth of the fetal kidney. J Clin Ultrasound 1983;11:349–356.
41. Pretorius DH, Gosink BB, Clautice-Engle T et al: Sonographic evaluation of the fetal stomach: significance of nonvisualization. AJR 1988;151:987–989.
42. Romero R, Ghidine A, Costigan K et al. Prenatal diagnosis of duodenal atresia: does it make any difference? Obstet Gynecol 1988;71:739–741.
43. Coates TL, McGahan JP. Ultrasound of the fetal face. In: McGahan JP, Porto M (eds): Diagnostic Obstetrical Ultrasound. Philadelphia: JB Lippincott, 1994;207–238.
44. Elejalde BR, de Elejalde MM, Heitman T. Visualization of the fetal genitalia by ultrasonography: a review of the literature and analysis of its accuracy and ethical implications. J Ultrasound Med 1985;4:633–639.
45. Nyberg DA, Mahony BS, Luthy D, Kapur R. Single umbilical artery: prenatal detection of concurrent anomalies. J Ultrasound Med 1991;10:247–253.

APPENDIX 1

Guidelines for performance of the antepartum obstetrical ultrasound examination.

These guidelines have been developed for use by practitioners performing obstetrical ultrasound studies. A limited examination may be performed in clinical emergencies or if used as a follow-up to a complete examination. In some cases, an additional and/or specialized examination may be necessary. While it is not possible to detect all structural congenital anomalies with diagnostic ultrasound, adherence to the following guidelines will maximize the possibility of detecting many fetal abanormalities.

Equipment

These studies shold be conducted with real-time scanners, using an abdominal and/or vaginal approach. A transducer of appropriate frequency (3 MHz or higher abdominally, 5 MHz or higher vaginally) should be used. A static scanner (3 to 5 MHz) may be used but should not be the sole method of examination. The lowest possible ultrasonic exposure settings should be used to gain the necessary diagnostic information.

Comment: Real-time is necessary to reliably confirm the presence of fetal life through observation of cardiac activity, respiration and active movement. Real-time studies simplify evaluation of fetal anatomy, as well as the task of obtaining fetal measurements. The choice of frequency is a trade-off between beam penetration and resolution. With modern equipment, 3 to 5 MHz abdominal transducers allow sufficient penetration in nearly all patients, while providing adequate resolution. During early pregnancy, a 5 MHz abdominal or a 5–7 MHz vaginal transducer may provide adequate penetration and produce superior resolution.

Documentation

Adequate documentation of the study is essential for high quality patient care. This should include a permanent record of the ultrasound images, incorporating whenever possible the measurement parameters and anatomical findings proposed in the following sections of this document. Images should be appropriately labeled with the examination date, patient identification, and, if appropriate, image orientation. A written report of the ultrasound findings should be included in the patient's medical record regardless of where the study is performed.

GUIDELINES FOR FIRST TRIMESTER SONOGRAPHY

Overall comment: Scanning in the first trimester may be performed either abdominally or vaginally. If an abdominal scan is performed and fails to provide definitive information concerning any of the following guidelines, a vaginal scan should be performed whenever possible.

1. The location of the gestational sac should be documented. The embryo should be identified and the crown-rump length recorded.
   Comment: The crown-rump length is an accurate indicator of fetal age. Comparison should be made to standard tables. If the embryo is not identified, characteristics of the gestational sac including mean diameter of the anechoic space to determine fetal age and analysis of the hyperechoic rim should be noted. During the late first trimester, biparietal diameter and other fetal measurements may also be used to establish fetal age.
2. Presence or absence of fetal life should be reported.
   Comment: Real-time observation is critical in this diagnosis. It should be noted that fetal cardiac activity may not be visible prior to seven weeks abdominally and frequently at least one week earlier vaginally as determined by crown-rump length. Thus, confirmation of fetal life may require follow-up evaluation.
3. Fetal number should be documented
   Comment: Multiple pregnancies should be reported only in those instances where multiple embroys are seen. Due to variability in fusion between the amnion and chorion, the appearance of more than one sac-like structure in early pregnancy is often noted and may be confused with multiple gestation or amniotic band.

4. Evaluation of the uterus (including cervix) and adnexal structures should be performed.
   Comment: This will allow recognization of incidental findings of potential clincial significance. The presence, location, and size of myomas and adnexal masses should be recorded.

GUIDELINES FOR SECOND AND THIRD TRIMESTER SONOGRAPHY

1. Fetal life, number and presentation should be documented.
   Comment: Abnormal heart rate and/or rhythm shold be reported. Multiple pregnancies require the reporting of additional information: placental number, sac number, comparison of fetal size, and when visualized, fetal genitalia and presence or absence of an interposed membrane.
2. An estimate of the amount of amniotic fluid (increased, decreased, normal) should be reported.
   Comment: While this evaluation is subjective, there is little difficulty in regognizing the extremes of amniotic fluid volume. Physiologic variation with stage of pregnancy must be taken into account.
3. The placental location, appearance, and its relationship to the internal cervical os should be recorded.
   Comment: It is recognized that placental position early in pregnancy may not correlate well with its location at the time of delivery.
4. Assessment of gestational age should be accomplished using combination of biparietal diameter (or head circumference), and femur length. Fetal growth and weight (as opposed to age) should be assessed in the third trimester and requires the addition of abdominal diameters or circumferences. If previous studies have been performed, an estimate of the appropriateness of interval change should be given.
   Comment: Third trimester measurements may not accurately reflect gestational age. Initial determination of gestational age should therefore be performed prior to the third trimester whenever possible. If one or more previous studies have been performed, the gestational age at the time of the current ex-

amination should be based on the earliest examination that permits measurement of crown-rump length, biparietal diameter, head circumference and/or femur length by the equation: current fetal age = initial embryo/fetal age + number of weeks from its first study. The current measurements should be compared with norms for the gestational age based on standard tables. If previous studies have been performed, interval change in the measurements should be assessed.

4A. Biparietal diameter at a standard reference level (which should include the cavum septi pellucidi, and the thalamus) should be measured and recorded.
Comment: If the fetal head is dolichocephalic or brachycephalic, the biparietal diameter alone may be misleading. On occasion, the computation of the cephalic index, a ratio of the biparietal diameter to fronto-occipital diameter, is needed to make this determination. In such situations, the head circumference or corrected biparietal diameter is required.

4B. Head circumference is measured at the same level as the biparietal diameter.

4C. Femur length should be measured routinely and recorded after the 14th week of gestation.
Comment: As with biparietal diameter, considerable biological variation is present late in pregnancy.

4D. Abdominal circumference should be determined at the level of the junction of the umbilical vein and portal sinus.
Comment: Abdominal circumference measurement may allow detection of growth retardation and macrosomia – conditions of the late second and third trimester. Comparison of the abdominal circumference with the head circumference should be made. If the abdominal measurement is below or above that expected for a stated gestation, it is recommended that circumferences of the head and body be measured and the head circumference/abdominal circumference ratio be reported. The use of circumferences is also suggested in those instances where the shape of either the head or body is different from that normally encountered.

5. Evaluation of the uterus and adnexal structures should be performed.

Comment; This will allow recognition of incidental findings of potential clinical significance. The presence, location, and size of myomas and adnexal masses should be recorded.

6. The study should include, but not necessarily be limited to, the following fetal anatomy: cerebral ventricles, four-chamber view of the heart (including its position within the thorax), spine, stomach, urinary bladder, umbilical cord insertion site on the anterior abdominal wall, and renal region.
   Comment: It is recognized that not all malformations of the above-mentioned organ systems (such as the spine) can be detected using ultrasonography. Nevertheless, a careful anatomical survey may allow diagnosis of certain birth defects which would otherwise go unrecognized. Suspected abnormalities may require a specialized evaluation.

From the American Institute of Ultrasound in Medicine: Guidelines for Performance of Antenatal Obstetrical Ultrasound Examinations.

CHAPTER 13

Fetal Abnormalities

Sturla H. Eik-Nes, MD PhD, Harm-Gerd Blaas, MD, Eva Tegnander, CNM

With the advanced use of ultrasound in obstetrics in large populations, the detection rate of fetal developmental disorders has increased (1). Such information might have direct impact on the pregnancy care system in some cases, the information might help improve the obstetrical neonatal care in other cases. The knowledge of the presence of a malformation might contribute to changing the day of delivery, mode of delivery, location of delivery and ensure that a perinatal team be ready at delivery.

Screening for malformations

Most of the available information about the detection rate of malformations is derived from studies on selected populations, making it difficult to find out how efficient the screening programs really are. Studies on large non-selected populations with regular risk are important to facilitate a quality assurance of the efficiency of a systematic ultrasound examination in pregnancy.

In the city of Trondheim there is one obstetrical department only, and all the women planning to deliver at this institution have their general 18 week routine fetal examination performed there by trained midwives (1, 2). From 1987–1993, all the detected fetal developmental disorders at the routine fetal examination, as well as those detected later based on a clinical indication or accidentally, were registered prospectively. After birth, the pediatric examination was carried out, and all developmental disorders detected in the first week of life were registered.

A total of 19,087 were born in the study period. The incidence of developmental disorders in the population was 2.9 %. Forty per cent of the disorders were detected antenatally. When minor disorders, such as isolated lip/palate defects, foot deformities and minor heart defects (small VSD and ASD) were excluded, the overall detection rate increased from 60 % in 1987 to 80 % in 1993. Forty-nine per cent of the disorders were karyotyped antenatally and 27 % of the karyotyped fetuses had an abnormal karyotype.

In 35 % of the cases where an abnormality was found, the parents elected to terminate the pregnancy; 5 % died during observation later in pregnancy. The rest were born alive, but an additional 5 % of the total died during the neonatal period, 17 % of the total were operated upon in the neonatal period, while 38 % were treated in the neonatal department. Only 3.5 per 1,000 women who had a routine examination terminated their pregnancy as a consequence of the examination; most of these fetuses had lethal disorders.

Of those aborted 63 % were characterised as having a lethal malformation, 17 % came into a category where it was difficult to know whether or not the newborn would have died. In 19 % of the aborted cases a serious handicap was present. This indicates the conservative attitude of the Norwegian women on the abortion issue.

At present, a significant portion of the developmental disorders can be diagnosed antenatally with ultrasound. The detection rate has been increasing slightly over time, probably as a result of the improved quality of the machines and the improved skill of the operators.

CEREBRAL MALFORMATIONS

Spine and neural tube defects

About one third of all congenital malformations affect the central nervous system. Grossly, the great variety of CNS defects can be classified by their clinical appearance as hydrocephalus, hydrocephalus-like conditions, and brain substance deficiency syndromes. It should be considered that the etiology and pathogenesis may be identical in malformations of different classes; for instance the maldevelopment of the neural tube may lead to brain deficiency such as anencephaly or to spina bifida and hydrocephalus.

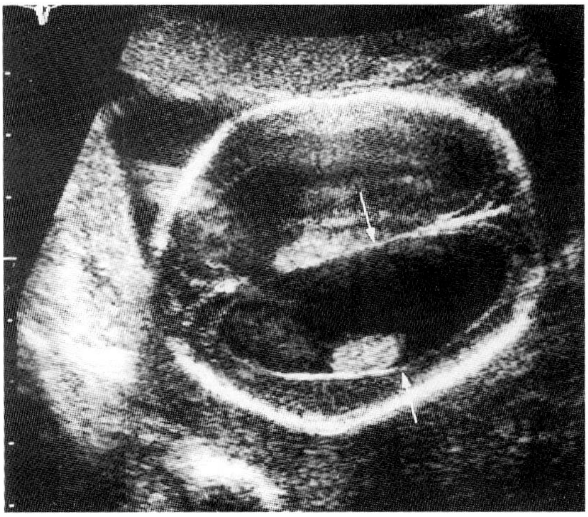

Figure 1 *Horizontal section through the lateral ventricles in a 19-week-old fetus with hydrocephalus. The diameter of the lateral ventricle (arrows) was 20 mm. The echogenic choroid plexus lies on the lateral wall.*

Hydrocephalus

Hydrocephalus (Figure 1) is a condition with increased cerebral spinal fluid pressure and/or amount in the ventricular system (3). Associated CNS-defects can be found in 50–60 % of the cases of hydrocephalus (3, 4). Defects in other organ systems in addition to the hydrocephalus increases the probability for chromosomal aberration as the fundamental cause. The transverse diameter of the lateral ventricles below 10 mm and 11 mm is considered to be normal as measured on the ultrasound image. A ventriculomegaly between 10 mm and 15 mm is highly indicative of abnormal development, while a diameter of more than 15 mm is considered to be pathologic.

Meningomyelocele

Meningomyelocele (Figure 2) is found in 30 % of all cases of hydrocephalus, and is a frequent malformation caused by the defective closure of the neural tube (5). The etiology and pathogenesis of neural tube defects are heterogeneous. Impaired interaction between the notochord and the neuroectoderm, extreme curvature of the caudal region of the embryo, and other pathogenic mechanisms have been discussed. A decreased recurrence risk of neural tube defects (NTD) in subsequent pregnancies has been demonstrated as an effect of folic acid given to the pregnant mother-to-be.

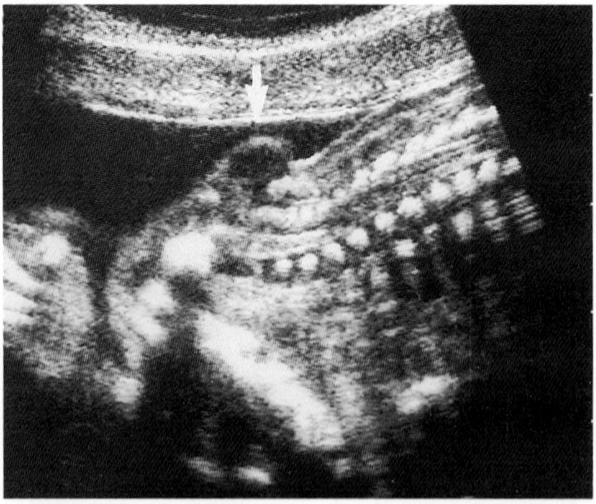

Figure 2 *Sagittal section through the spine in a 19-week-old fetus with sacral myelomeningocele (arrow).*

NTD

The three main types of NTD are anencephaly (substantial brain deficiency), encephalocele and spina bifida. They usually occur sporadically, but certain connections with geographic and socioeconomic factors have been demonstrated.

Anencephaly

The non-closure of the rostral neuropore leads to anencephaly (1:1,000, female:male = 4:1) (5). The cranium, the cerebral hemispheres and part of the brain stem are absent.

Acrania

In acrania the calvarium is absent, and more or less unstructured brain tissue lies open. Usually, amniotic adhesions are the etiologic factor, but in some cases the cause may be NTD.

Encephalocele

Encephalocele (1:2,000 – 1:10,000) involves a cranial defect with herniation of meninges or cerebral tissue, usually in the occipital region (5). When found anteriorly or asymmetrically, amniotic rupture sequence should be suspected. Occipital encephalocele is a typical association found in Meckel-Gruber syndrome.

Spina bifida

In 74 % of the cases with spina bifida in Trondheim, hydrocephalus was associated. The diagnosis of spina bifida is made by looking at the head in the BPD section: the "lemon shape" of the skull and the "banana sign" of the cerebellum. Herniation of the caudal brain structures through the foramen magnum is called Arnold Chiari malformation. Type II is characterized by herniation of the medulla oblongata and fourth ventricle and is usually found in spina bifida. There are three types of spina bifida: myelomeningocele (> 90 %) is characterized by a dysraphic defect of the spine including the neural elements. In meningocele, only the meninges are herniated through the dysraphic defect, while in spina bifida occulta (2 – 3 %) the incomplete vertebral arch is closed by an intact skin surface. We found 15 % of the chromosomal aberrations in spina bifida.

Iniencephaly, craniorachischisis

Inincephaly is a rare special form of NTD with mainly an occipital (Greek = inion) defect. Rachischisis characterizes the complete non-closure of the spinal tube, and in cranio-rachischisis there is additional involvement of the head (= anencephaly + rachischisis).

Aqueductal stenosis

Aqueductal stenosis (Figure 3) is one of the most common causes (17 %) of hydrocephalus. It may be x-linked or autosomal recessive congenital, but is usually the sequele after hemorrhage, infection, or has a heterogeneous cause. Typically the aqueductal stenosis is not associated with additional malformations or chromosomal aberrations. Increasing dilatation of the third and especially the lateral ventricles is observed. Most fetuses survive, but about half of the patients will develop serious a handicap.

Agenesis of the corpus callosum

This condition may be partial or complete. It can be seen as an isolated defect, but is commonly found as part of syndromes. Iso-

common, but often additional gastrointestinal abnormalities can be found. If the content of the bowel is echogenic, cystic fibrosis must be considered. The ultrasound appearance is characterized by increasing visibility of bowel dilatation (Figure 13) showing peristalsis. If bowel dilatation is more than 17 mm and mural thickness more than 3 mm, obstruction should be suspected. Colonic and jejunoileal atresia are difficult to distinguish from each other prenatally.

Anal obstruction

This anomaly has a prevalence of 1:5,000 (12, 13), and is found more often in males than in females. Associated anomalies are common such as rectourethral fistula, VACTERL association, syndromes and chromosomal aberrations. In Trondheim 16 of 18 prenatally evaluated fetuses with anal atresia had associated anomalies; 1 had a trisomy 18. Only 2 of these 18 fetuses survived. Polyhydramnios was found in 2 cases (13 %), while oligohydramnios was found in 6 cases (33 %). The prenatal diagnosis is usually difficult because anal atresia often does not show significant dilatation of the bowel proximal to the obstruction. Increased fluid in the distal bowel and rectum should lead to the suspicion of a recto-vesical fistula, especially when intraluminar calcifications are present.

Echogenic bowel

Echogenic bowel is a condition "created" by prenatal ultrasound. It describes the strikingly high echogenicity of bowel occasionally found in conditions like cystic fibrosis, chromosomal aberrations and IUGR (12). Echogenic bowel is characterized by the bowel showing identical or even greater brightness than the iliac bone. Possible causes of this phenomenon are dense bowel content because of delayed passage, decreased bowel motility, abnormal meconium as found in cystic fibrosis, or ischemia of the bowel. Echogenic bowel is a normal finding before 20 weeks of gestation (Figure 14) and will usually dissolve later.

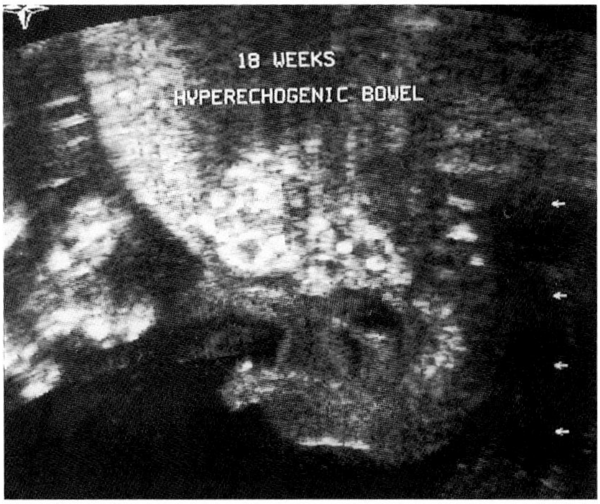

Figure 14 *Sagittal section (transvaginal approach) through the lower abdomen in an 18-week-old male fetus. The bowel is echogenic. The fetus developed normally and proved to be healthy at birth.*

Meconium peritonitis

Gastrointestinal anomalies in the fetus such as intestinal obstruction, meconium ileus, volvulus, intussusception, gastroschisis or Meckel's diverticulum may lead to meconium peritonitis, which is a sterile chemical peritonitis caused by bowel perforation (12). Bowel dilatation, fetal ascites, abdominal calcifications and polyhydramnios are typical ultrasound findings. The possible association with cystic fibrosis is well known. The management should be expectant.

Intraabdominal masses, diseases of the liver, spleen and pancreas

Fetal intraabdominal masses are mainly cystic structures of various origins, but also echogenic and solid tumors can be found. Apart from genitourinary anomalies, dilated bowel, enteric duplications, mesenteric, omental, hepatic, choledochal, splenic or pancreatic cysts must be considered when a cystic structure is present. Usually expectant management is wise, but a transabdominal puncture may be performed on a cyst of considerable size. Hemangioma, hamartomas, hemangioendothelioma and other rare neoplasms may be found prenatally. In sacrococcygeal teratoma a considerable part of the tumor often grows intraabdominally. Sacrococcygeal teratoma may cause heart failure with hydrops due to its extensive size or to arterio-venous shunts, or it may cause compression of the genitourinary system leading to hydro-(urino-) metrocolpos in females. Some metabolic diseases of the hepatosplenic entity may be suspected prenatally when alterations of the echogenicity and size of these organs associated with ascites are found. Hepatic calcifications may be idiopathic, but may be due to intrauterine infections, ischemic processes or tumors.

Situs anomalies

Situs anomalies should be thoroughly evaluated when the situs of the thorax is discordant to the situs of the abdomen. This is the case when the stomach is found on the opposite side of the heart, or when both the heart and the stomach are found on the right side of the fetus. Complex anomalies of the heart, the vasculatory system and the intraabdominal organs should be expected.

Abdominal wall defects

Embryology

At four and a half weeks the embryonic disc starts to fold and develop a cylindrical body. At about six completed weeks the body stalk, coelom and vitelline duct are ensheathed by amnion to form the umbilical cord. The ventral migration of the hypaxial mesoderm derivates leads to the definitive development of the ventral

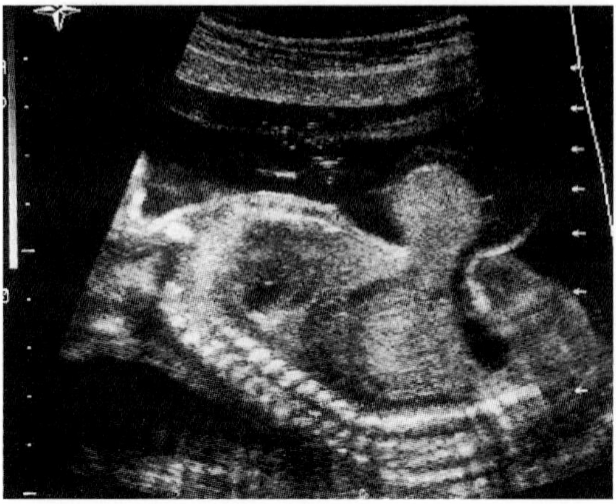

Figure 15 *Sagittal section through the body in a 22-week old feus with an epigastric omphalocele containing the fetal liver. The umbilical cord insertion was located at the lower border of the omphalocele to the right.*

wall in the following weeks. When the embryo has a CRL of 11 mm – 14 mm (7–6 to 8–1 weeks) the primary intestinal loop projects into the umbilical cord. This physiological herniation starts as a result of traction from the vitelline duct, and continues to approximately 11–4 weeks (CRL 48 mm) while the elongated and coiled intestine rotates counterclockwise 90 degrees. When returning into the abdomen, the intestine rotates an additional 180 degrees. Disturbance of this complicated development leads to specific malformations, which can be categorized in cranial, medial, caudal and complex defects.

Cranial defects

Ectopia cordis

This is a rare condition with poor prognosis. The heart lies partially or completely extrathoracic. In 95 % of the cases this defect is found thoracally or thoraco-abdominally (14).

Pentalogy of Cantrell

This condition is rare, and its prognosis is poor. The condition comprises 1/ epigastric omphalocele, 2/ diaphragmatic defect, 3/ pericardial defect, 4/ ectopia cordis, and 5/ heart defect (as Tetralogy og Fallot). Additional defects such as anencephaly, hydrocephaly and cleft lip and palate have been described.

Epigastric omphalocele

Epigastric omphalocele is a supraumbilical midline defect with the cord at its caudal border (Figure 15). It is covered by an amnioperitoneal membrane and usually both the liver and the bowel are located inside. Associated defects including chromosomal defects can be found, but isolated epigastric omphaloceles are usually not associated with chromosomal abnormalities. Isolated, the condition carries a good prognosis.

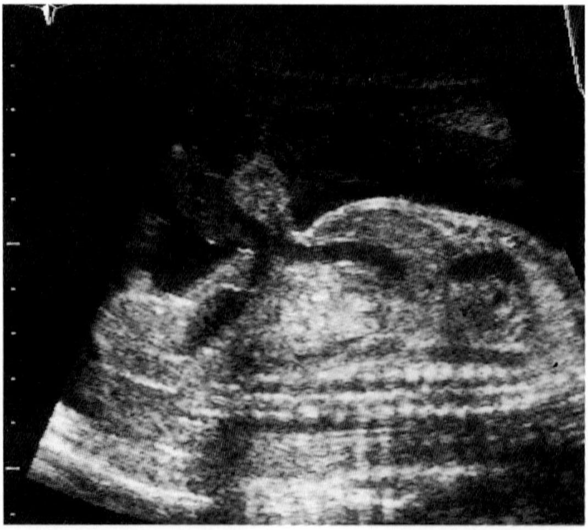

Figure 16 *Sagittal section through the body in a 22-week-old fetus with a small medial omphalocele containing only bowel. This fetus had trisomy 21.*

Medial defects

Medial omphalocele

A medial omphalocele is a central wall defect with the umbilical cord insertion in its center. It contains mainly bowel, but in large defects the liver is herniated, too. Independent of the size of the defect (Figure 16) there is a very high association with chromosomal disorders, and other sonographically detectable malformations. The prevalence of omphaloceles is generally about 1:4,000, with a ratio of about 2:3 between epigastric and medial omphaloceles.

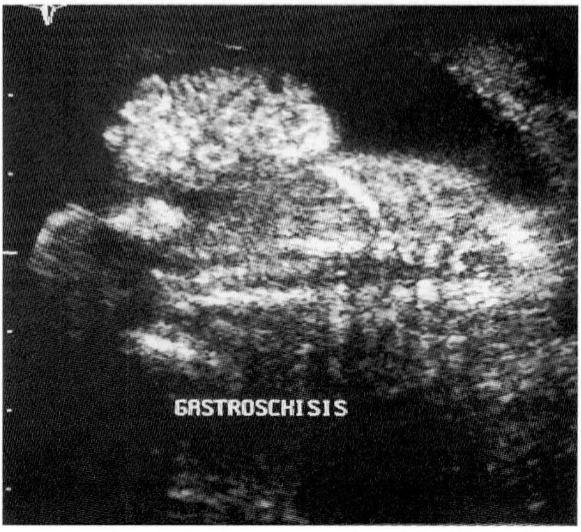

Figure 17 *Coronal section through the body of a 17-week-old fetus with gastroschisis, the bowel located lateral to the fetal abdomen. The thorax to the right.*

Gastroschisis

A gastroschisis is a specific entity, where a right-sided paraumbilical wall defect not covered by a membrane is found. Part of the bowel is located extracorporally in the amniotic fluid (Figure 17). Except for possible mechanical impairment of the bowel development, associated malformations and chromosomal disorders are not found (15, 16). The prognosis after surgical repair is good (Trondheim: 22 of 23 prenatally detected cases of gastroschises survived).

Caudal defects

Bladder exstrophy

In bladder exstrophy the ventral wall of the bladder is open. Diastasis of the symphysis and bifid genitalia belong to this condition. The prevalence is 1:30,000 (16). It may be associated with other malformations.

Cloacal exstrophy

The prevalence of cloacal exstrophy is 1:200,000 (16). This caudal folding defect carries a poor prognosis because of the serious organic changes: omphalocele, bladder exstrophy, rectal exstrophy, anal malformation, and unidentifiable genitalia. There are usually other serious associated malformations.

Complex defects

Amniotic rupture sequence

This is a malformation sequence where rupture of the amniotic membrane early during embryogenesis can lead to serious mutilizing defects of the embryonic body.

Limb-body-wall complex

Defective body folding leads to the limb-body-wall complex (LBWC), which is a lethal entity. There is no isolated umbilical cord, but an open connection of abdominal content, lying in the extraembryonic coelom, to the placenta. Usually, there are only two, sometimes three, umbilical vessels in the wall of the defect. The pelvic girdle is often defective, and associated malformations of the CNS, the spine and the limbs are usual. In our series of 18 LBWC no chromosomal disorder was found. Often amniotic adhesions are associated.

Genitourinary anomalies

The detectable fetal genitourinary anomalies are cystic and obstructive lesions, renal agenesis and polycystic diseases of the kidneys. Genitourinary tumors in the fetus are rare. Once a defect is detected, a thorough examination of the fetus and the assessment of the amniotic fluid amount is necessary. Oligohydramnios is a predictor of poor outcome, while normal amniotic fluid amount usually predicts a good prognosis. Associated anomalies have to be excluded. Chromosomal aberrations are described in 3 % of these cases in isolated renal abnormalities and up to 34 % in renal abnormalities associated with other structural defects (17). Combinations of genitourinary anomalies are common. Different classification systems have been proposed depending on the choice of criteria. Table III gives a systematic overview of main genitourinary anomalies visible with ultrasound.

Obstructive lesions

Obstructions of the urinary tract show large variations, depending on the degree and the location of the lesion. In the proximal obstruction the renal pelvis is dilated, and the calyces are plump. Lower obstructions of the ureter affect the proximal tract, e.g. dilatation of the upper ureter and the renal pelvis. If the bladder outflow is obstructed, as may be the case in posterior urethral valves (PUV, Figure 18), distension of the bladder, of both ureters and renal pelvis will occur. Either hydronephroses (Figure 19) and/or dysplastic kidneys can be found. In the 80's an enthusiastic attitude favored draining the distended urinary bladder in PUV. But the results were disappointing because irreversible damage of the kidneys was present in most cases already at the time of the drainage (18). Today the generally accepted management of obstructive lesions of the fetal urinary tract is to be exptectant.

The sonographic examination of the urinary tract points at the kidneys and the ureters (renal parenchyma, its thickness, echogenicity and presence of cystic lesions, degree of upper tract dilatation, unilaterality or bilaterality, ureteral dilatation), the bladder and the urethra (bladder size, wall thickness, key-hole phenome-

Table III ***Genitourinary anomalies and main sequeles detectable by ultrasound***

	Side predilection	Ultrasound
Obstructive lesions		
Ureteropelvic junction	Unilateral/bilateral	Hydronephrosis
Distal ureter	Unilateral/bilateral	Hydronephrosis-ureter
Posterior urethral valves (PUV)/urethral atresia	Bilateral	Hydronephrosis-ureter & dilated bladder
Cystic lesions		
Macroscopic cysts		
Multicystic dysplasia	Unilateral/bilateral	Variable renal cysts & abnormal stroma
Renal cysts, urinoma	Unilateral/bilateral	Solitary cysts
Ureterocele	Unilateral/bilateral	Cyst in the urinary bladder
Ovarian cyst	Unilateral/bilateral	Cyst in the lower abdomen; if septated, or if sediment: torsion
Microscopic cysts		
Polycystic kidney disease	Bilateral	"White" enlarged kidneys
Renal tubular dysgenesis	Bilateral	"White" enlarged kidneys
Renal agenesis	Unilateral/bilateral	Adrenal gland lies along the posterior wall/spine
Double kidneys/ureter	Unilateral/bilateral	Occasionally hydronephrosis-ureter, ureterocele
Tumors (rare)	Unilateral/bilateral	Neoplasm in the renal parenchyma
Genital anomalies		Abnormal shape of fetal gender

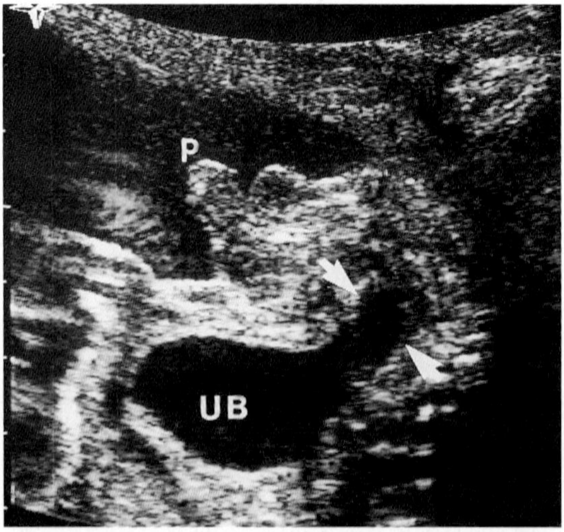

Figure 18 *Dilated urinary bladder (UB) and bladder neck (arrows) in a fetus with urethral stenosis (sagittal section). There is sufficient amniotic fluid indicating that the obstruction is not complete. P = penis.*

non). The evaluation of the amniotic fluid amount, of extrarenal fluid collections, of other anatomic abnormalities, of the gender and of the fetal growth should be included.

Cystic lesions

The embryonic development of the urinary tract is complicated and relatively often maldevelopment of the metanephros or the ureteric bud result in different anomalies. Early obstruction to the

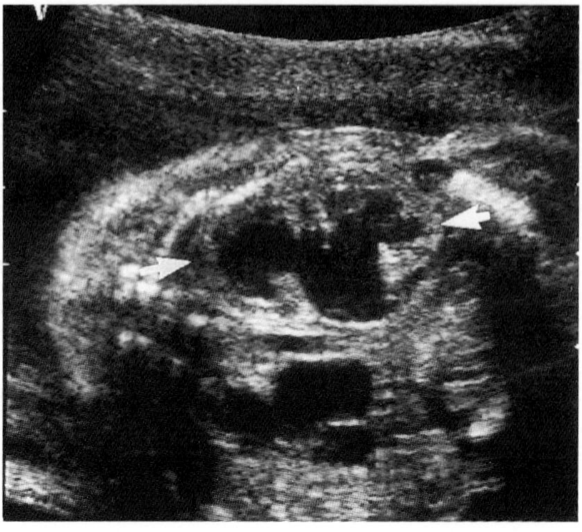

Figure 19 *Coronal section of the kidneys of the same fetus as in Figure 18. The left kidney (arrows) is hydronephrotic with dilated renal pelvis, plump calyces and reduced renal parenchyma.*

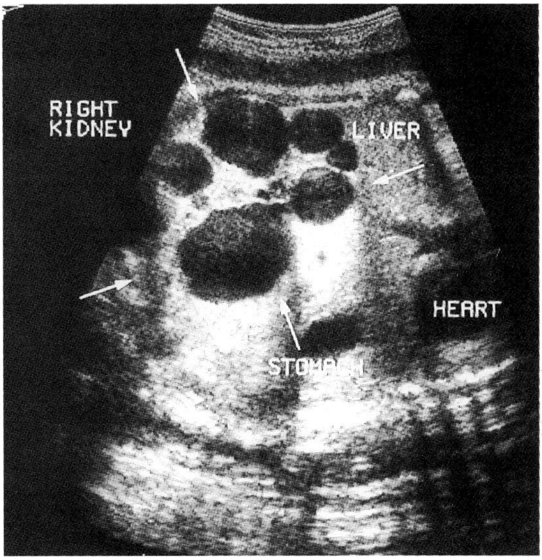

Figure 20 *Large cystic dysplastic kidney in a 31-week old fetus. The contralateral kidney was normal.*

urinary outlet will result in cystic degenerative lesions of the early kidney. The size and number of cysts in the dysplastic kidneys may vary (Figure 20). If both kidneys are cystic dysplastic no amniotic fluid will be found, and the prognosis is poor. Solitary cystic lesions, especially the unilateral ones, carry a good prognosis if a normal amount of amniotic fluid indicates a reasonable kidney function.

Infantile polycystic kidney disease is an autosomal recessive condition with a prevalence of 1:6,000 to 1:16,000 (19). Dilatation of renal collecting tubules is accompanied by liver cysts. Four different subtypes and a dominant type are described. The early form is detectable prenatally, usually between 16 to 24 weeks. Characteristic are large bright kidneys (Figure 21) and decreasing urine production resulting in oligohydramnios and non-visualization of the bladder. Other congenital renal diseases may present a similar sonographic appearance, such as in renal tubular dysgenesis, where the kidneys progrediently enlarge. Here, the urine production may even be increased.

In females, ovarian cysts may occasionally occur in the third trimester. Large simple ovarian cysts with a diameter of more than 4–5 cm may be punctured to prevent torsion and loss of the ovary. Septation or sediment in ovarian cysts is a sign of torsion.

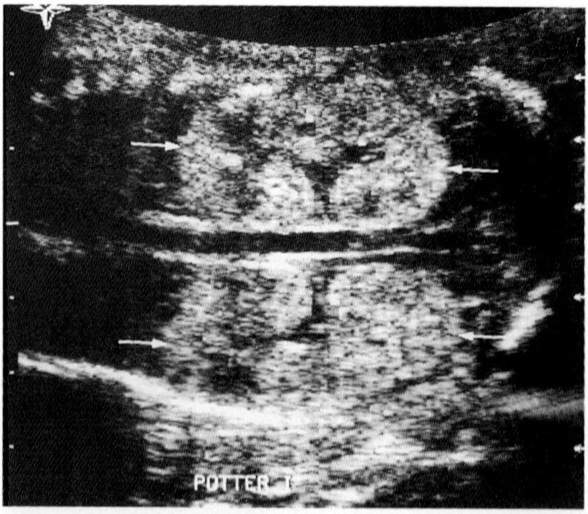

Figure 21 *Large bright kidneys in a 22-week-old fetus with the autosomal recessive polycystic infantile kidney disease.*

Renal agenesis

Bilateral agenesis of the kidneys (Potter syndrome) is uniformly fatal, whereas unilateral agenesis is compatible with life in the presence of a normal contralateral kidney. Sonographic anhydramnios, non visualization of the urinary bladder and absence of the kidneys are found. Pathognomonic is the position of the adrenal glands which lie along the posterior wall and the spine.

Double kidneys/ureter

Double kidneys and ureters are often accompanied by a defective outlet of the upper ureter into the lower bladder wall resulting in a cystic expansion in the fetal bladder. Hydroureter or hydronephrosis may be present.

Skeletal defects

A large number of different disorders can cause local or general abnormal shape and size of the skeleton. The specter ranges from the absence of a single finger to the grotesque torsion of the fetal skeleton due to amniotic adhesions. There may be reduced growth of one limb due to vascular compromise, or general dwarfism caused by a serious congenital dysplasia of the bone comprising the normal development and growth of such bones as the calvari-

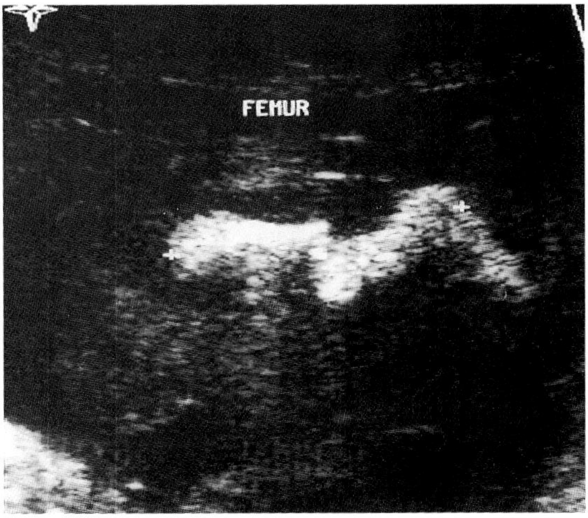

Figure 22 *The fractured femur of a 19-week-old fetus with osteogenesis imperfecta IIa, a lethal condition.*

um, the girdle of the shoulder and pelvis, the long bones of the limbs, the ribs and the vertebrae.

The classification of skeletal disorders is difficult (20). An International Nomenclature for Skeletal Dysplasias was proposed in Paris in 1977 and revised in 1984. The diseases were subdivided into five different groups: 1/ osteochondrodysplasias (abnormalities of cartilage and/or bone growth and development); 2/ dysostoses (malformations of individual bones singly or in combination); 3/ idiopathic osteolysis (disorders associated with multifocal resorption of bone); 4/ skeletal disorders associated with chromosomal aberrations; and 5/ primary metabolic disorders.

Skeletal dysplasias are a heterogeneous group of rare bone dysplasias resulting in abnormal growth and shape of the fetal skeleton. Table IV shows the approximate birth prevalence of some dysplasias (21).

Approach to the diagnosis of skeletal dysplasia

Numerous nomograms with the normal growth and size of the fetal skeleton are available and may be used as the basis for evaluating the abnormal growth in fetal dysplasia. The length, shape and echogenicity of all long bones as well as the ribs (Figure 23) should be registered. In lethal dysplasias, the disproportion of the small chest to the normal abdomen is typically found. Hands and

Table IV

Dysplasia	Birth prevalence
Lethal	
Thanatophoric dysplasia	1/ 10,000
Achondrogenesis	1/ 40,000
Osteogenesis imperfecta, type II (Figure 22)	1/ 60,000
Congenital hypophosphatasia	1/ 100,000
Chondrodysplasia punctata, rhizomelic type	1/ 110,000
Others	1/ > 200,000
Non-lethal	
Heterozygous achondroplasia	1/ 30,000
Osteogenesis imperfecta, type I	1/ 30,000
Asphyxiating thoracic dysplasia	1/ 70,000
Others	1/ > 200,000
TOTAL	**1/ 4,000**

feet should be examined to exclude polydactyly and missing fingers. Several skeletal disorders are associated with defects of the membraneous ossification affecting the calvarium. Thus, the skull bones should be examined. Important, too, is the evaluation of the face, since some dysplasias are associated with hypotelorism, facial cleft or micrognathia. Further, the thoracal, intraabdominal and genitourinary organs should be evaluated. A detailed description of the different skeletal dysplasias and their prenatal diagnosis is beyond the scope of this chapter.

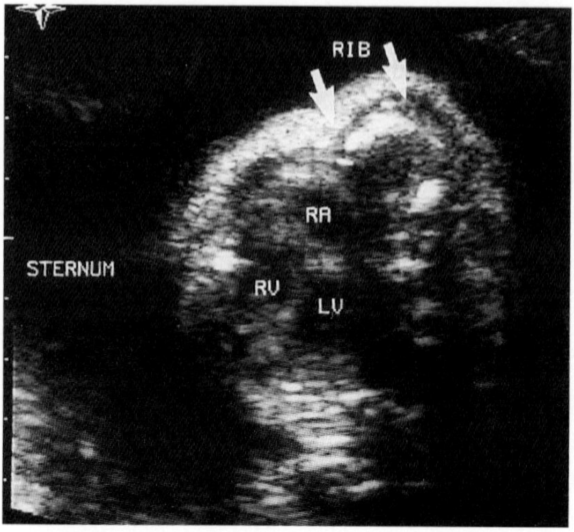

Figure 23 *Horizontal section through the thorax of a 29-week-old fetus with short-rib-polydactyly syndrome, type II. The extremely short ribs (arrows) and the heart with the right atrium (RA), right ventricle (RV) and left ventricle (LV) can be identified.*

REFERENCES

1. Tegnander E, Eik-Nes SH, Linker DT. Prenatal detection of heart defects at the routine fetal examination at 18 weeks in a non-selected population. Ultrasound Obstet Gynecol 1995;5:372–380.
2. Tegnander E, Eik-Nes SH, Linker DT. Incorporating the four-chamber view of the fetal heart into the second-trimester routine fetal examination. Ultrasound Obstet Gynecol 1994;4:24–28.
3. Nyberg DA, Pretorius DH. Cerebral malformations. In: Nyberg DA, Mahoney BS, Pretorius DH (eds): Diagnostic Ultrasound of Fetal Anomalies. St Louis: Mosby Year Book, 1990:83–145.
4. Paidas MJ, Cohen A. Disorders of the central nervous system. Semin Perinatology 1994;18:266–282.
5. Nyberg DA, Mack LA. The spine and neural tube defects. In: Nyberg DA, Mahoney BS, Pretorius DH (eds). Diagnostic Ultrasound of Fetal Anomalies. St Louis: Mosby Year Book 1990:146–202.
6. Hilpert PL, Pretorius DH. The thorax. In: Nyberg DA, Mahoney BS, Pretorius DH (eds): Diagnostic Ultrasound of Fetal Anomalies. St Louis: Mosby Year book 1990:262–299.
7. Romero R, Pilu G, Jeanty P, Ghidini A, Hobbins JC (ed). Prenatal Diagnosis of Congenital Anomalies. Norwalk: Appleton & Lange, 1988.
8. Allan L (ed). Manual of Fetal Echocardiography. Lancaster: MTP Press Ltd, 1986.
9. Reed KL, Anderson CF, Shenker L (eds). Fetal Echocardiography: an Atlas. New York: Alan R. Liss, Inc., 1988.
10. DeVore GR. The aortic and pulmonary outflow tract screening examination in the human fetus. J Ultrasound Med 1992;11:345–348.
11. Nyberg DA, Emerson DS. Cardiac malformations. In: Nyberg DA, Mahoney BS, Pretorius DH (eds). Diagnostic Ultrasound of Fetal Anomalies. St Louis: Mosby Year Book, 1990:300–341
12. Robertson FM, Crombleholme TM, Paidas M, Harris BH. Prenatal diagnosis and management of gastrointestinal anomalies. Semin Perinatology 1994;18:182–195.
13. Nyberg DA. Intra-abdominal abnormalities. In: Nyberg DA, Mahoney BS, Pretorius DH (eds). Diagnostic Ultrasound of Fetal Anomalies. St Louis: Mosby Year Book, 1990:342–394.
14. Nyberg DA, Mack LA. Abdominal wall defects. In: Nyberg DA, Mahoney BS, Pretorius DH (eds). Diagnostic Ultrasound of Fetal Anomalies. St Louis: Mosby Year Book, 1990:395–432.
15. Nicolaides KH, Snijders RJM, Cheng HH, Gosden C. Fetal gastro-intestinal and abdominal wall defects: associated malformations and chromosomal abnormalites. Fetal Diagn Ther 1992;7:102–115.
16. Paidas MJ, Crombleholme TM, Robertson F. Prenatal diagnosis and management of the fetus with an abdominal wall defect. Semin Parinatology 1994;18:196–214.

17. Nicolaides KH, Cheng HH, Abbas A et al. Fetal renal defects: associated malformations and chromosomal defects. Fetal Diagn Ther 1992;7:1–11.
18. Cendron M, D'Alton ME, Crombleholme TM. Prenatal diagnosis and management of the fetus with hydronephrosis. Semin Perinatology 1994;18:163–181.
19. Patten RM, Mack LA, Wang KY, Cyr DR. The fetal genitourinary tract. In Benacerraf BR (ed). Fetal Ultrasound. Philadelphia: WB Saunders, 1990:115–130.
20. Romero R, Athanassiadis AP, Jeanty P. Fetal skeletal anomalies. In Benacerraf BR (ed). Fetal Ultrasound. Philadelphia, WB Saunders, 1990:75–99.
21. Mahony BS. The extremities. In: Nyberg DA, Mahoney BS, Pretorius DH (eds). Diagnostic Ultrasound of Fetal Anomalies. St Louis: Mosby Year Book 1990, 492–562.

CHAPTER 14

The Breast

Ellen B. Mendelson, MD and Corinne E. Tobin, MD

The development of high resolution transducers well suited to depicting the fine anatomy of the breast has stimulated a re-evaluation of the use of ultrasound (US) in the diagnosis and management of breast disease. Current technical advances have necessitated another look at lesion characterization with sonography. There has also been stimulation of much exciting research in adapting the new tehcnical advances to cost-effective management of benign and malignant breast disease.

Although there are many areas of current research in applying US to breast evaluation, including a prospective study of screening sonography for the detection of occult masses in dense breasts, the currently accepted applications and indications for breast sonography are:

- characterization of nonpalpable and palpable masses as fluid filled or solid where the mammographic diagnosis is uncertain;
- guidance of interventional procedures (cyst aspiration, fine needle or core biopsy, and presurgical localization);
- primary study of palpable masses in young (under age 30), pregnant and lactating patients;
- evaluation of an area of mammographic asymmetric density where a focal abnormality is suspected as the cause;
- confirmation and more complete visualization of a lesion seen in one mammographic projection (e.g. near the chest wall) (1, 2, 3).

These uses for breast sonography are also applicable to the postsurgical patient, after breast conservation and breast augmentation, and to the male breast when a mass is within an area of gy-

cost. When a vascular breast mass is imaged, there is increased confidence in assigning it a higher probability of malignancy (Figure 1) (9). Nevertheless, despite other reports of its promise (10), no convincing confirmation of Doppler-augmentation sonography as the primary mode of distinguishing malignant from benign solid lesions has appeared in the literature (11, 12). Perhaps more important than Doppler capability is the shape and maneuverability of a probe to be used not only as an instrument for diagnosis but also as a guide for the interventional procedures that are becoming increasingly more important.

PERFORMING THE EXAMINATION

Good breast sonography is highly dependent on excellent equipment and technical skills for accuracy of interpretation (11). Improper focal zone and gain settings can cause diagnostic errors. The mammograms and physical findings must also be correlated with sonography.

For the medial breast, the patient is generally studied in the supine position. For evaluating the upper outer quadrant, the woman should be positioned obliquely towards the contralateral side to minimize the thickness of breast tissue to be traversed by the acoustic beam.

Although most often, US is performed to characterize a breast mass, breast sonography is not simply "lumpography". When evaluating masses, the characteristics of the tissue surrounding the mass such as architectural distortion or compression should be noted along with the orientation of the mass with respect to the skin. The mass should be stabilized manually while scanning, fixing it between two fingers if possible. Find the long axis of a mass, if one is present. The entire mass is observed as one moves the transducer slowly from side-to-side. A second projection, perpendicular to the first, should then be sought. The mass should always be measured in its longest dimension. Ideally, three dimensions of the mass might be recorded to enable volumetric follow-up of a carcinoma treated with chemotherapy or of a probably benign mass such as fibroadenoma. The mass should be scanned through in two projections so that a complex component within a lesion and mural excrescences in a cyst are not missed.

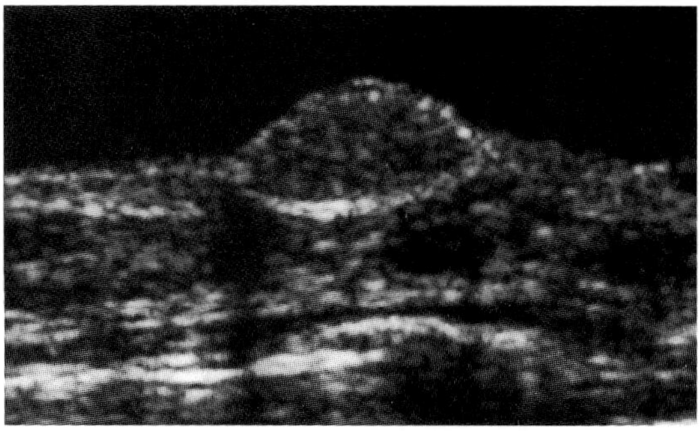

Figure 2 ***Imaging the nipple***
Direct US scanning of the nipple causes posterior acoustic shadowing due to the nipple's fibrous content and crevices. As here, when the transducer is angled at the side of the nipple with its beam toward the retroareolar region, the area behind the nipple can be imaged with minimal refraction shadowing (7.5 MHz transducer with offset pads).

Imaging the nipple-areolar complex requires special technical maneuvers (13, 14). The fibrous elements within the nipple and the abrupt changes in surface contour may cause posterior acoustic shadowing. The transducer should be placed adjacent to the nipple and the US beam angled into the retroareolar area (Figure 2).

Sonographic depiction of multiple lesions may be confusing. The same cysts, for example, can be imaged from more than one location in the breast creating uncertainty regarding the actual number of masses present. An attempt to isolate the mass manually is often rewarding.

To correlate mammographic or palpable findings with sonographic abnormalities, a small radiopaque marker can be placed on the skin over the lesion as it is imaged initially. The area is then reimaged using the correlative technique, either mammography or sonography. To maintain anatomic equivalence, the patient should be upright while being scanned with US as she would be during mammography.

If the lesion is located superficially in the breast or is in the skin or subcutaneous tissues, an offset pad or fluid filled bag or glove should be placed on the skin to diminish artifact in the near field and to place the transducer face at the ideal distance so that the focal zone of the transducer will be at the skin and superficial tis-

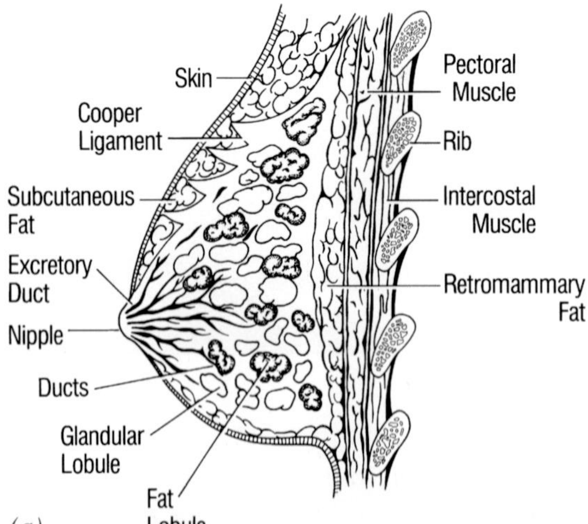

(a)

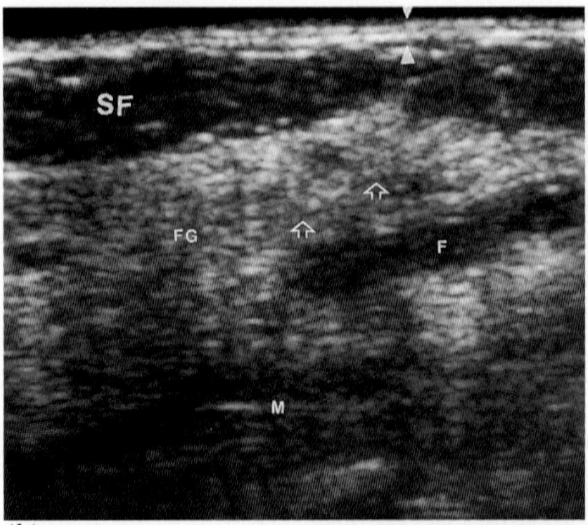

(b)

Figure 3 ***Breast Anatomy***

a. Diagram of normal breast anatomy

b. Sonogram depicting normal breast anatomy with a normal 2 mm skin complex of two echogenic lesions (arrowheads). Beneath the layer of subcutaneous fat (SF) lies dense fibroglandular parenchyma (FG) interspersed with fat lobules. Ducts (open arrows) are seen in the parenchyma. A hypoechoic island in the dense parenchyma is normal hypoechoic breast fat (F) and should not be mistaken for pathology. Turning the transducer orthogonally often helps to elongate a lobule and decrease its mass-like appearance.

c. A tubular anechoic structure beneath the nipple (N) represents a dilated duct.

(c)

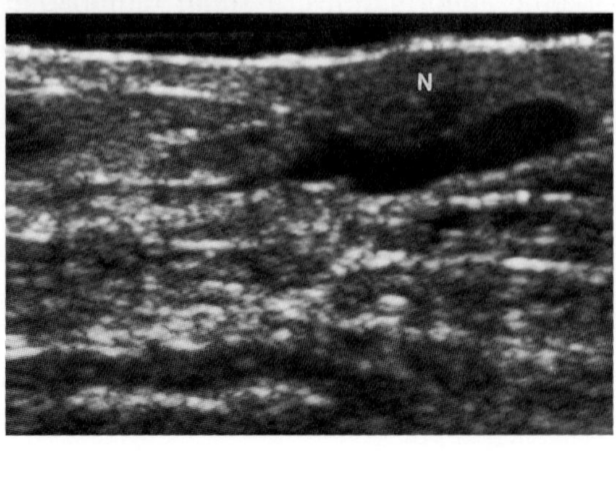

sues, not deeper within the breast (3). Newer probe designs have been successful in reducing near field artifact, minimizing the need for an offset device.

SONOGRAPHIC ANATOMY

Structures of the breast and surrounding tissues – skin, ducts, fat, fibroglandular parenchyma, nipple, blood vessels, retromammary muscle bundles – have recognizable and characteristic sonographic features (Figure 3).

The skin is composed of two thin echogenic lines with a narrow hypoechoic band between them that may represent the dermis. The entire complex measures up to 0.2 cm but can be slightly thicker in the lower breast (3) near the inframammary fold.

Fat lobules, which should not be mistaken for fibroadenomas or other hypoechoic solid masses, are commonly seen subcutaneously. Compared with fat elsewhere in the body, which is generally more echogenic, fat lobules in the breast are hypoechoic relative to the surrounding glandular parenchyma. Fat lobules are well defined by their thin connective tissue envelopes. They often contain a central echogenic focus of connective tissue.

The breast parenchyma is more echogenic than fat and may be interlaced with small, linear, hypoechoic ducts visible as tubular structures that may vary in diameter from 0.1 to 0.5 cm or more. Branching of the ducts can be observed as scanning proceeds from the retroareolar area towards the periphery of the breast. The crevices and fibrous tissue of the nipple, which is of medium level echogenicity, will cause posterior acoustic shadowing that may obscure a column of tissue deep to it (15).

Near the axilla, anechoic or hypoechoic oval or tubular structures often represent axillary vessels. Their elongation and blood flow seen as the transducer is rotated orthogonally will be confirmatory. Color flow imaging, if available, can be used also to identify vascular structures. Other oval masses near the axilla may be lymph nodes. Lymph nodes in the axilla or in the breast are hypoechoic-to-anechoic and may contain echogenic fatty hilar areas. Echogenic foci, in addition to denoting the fatty hilar areas of lymph nodes, may also be seen within fat lobules, fibroadenomas

REFERENCES

1. Jackson VP. Sonography of malignant breast disease. Semin US, CT, MR 1989;10:119–131.
2. Feig SA. The role of ultrasound in a breast imaging center. Semin US, CT, MR 1989;10:90–105.
3. Bassett LW, Kimme-Smith C. Breast sonography: technique, equipment and normal anatomy. Semin US, CT, MR 1989;10:82–89.
4. Mendelson EB. Silicone implants present mammographic challenge. Diagn Imag, September; 1992.
5. Levine RA, Collins TL. Definitive diagnosis of breast implant rupture by ultrasonography. J Plast & Reconst Surg 1991;87:1126.
6. Sickles EA, Filly RA, Callen PW. Breast cancer detection with sonography and mammography: comparisong using state-of-the-art equipment. AJR 1983;140:843–845.
7. Bassett LW, Kimme-Smith C, Southland LK et al. Automated and handheld breast US: effect on patient management. Radiology 1987;165:103–108.
8. Mendelson TB, Tobin CE et al. Marginal analysis of breast masses with high-resolution US. Radiology 1994;193 (P), suppl: p 177.
9. Taylor KKW, Scoutt LM, Quedans-Case C et al. Is there a role for Doppler imaging in breast cancer diagnosis? Radiology 1993;189(P), suppl, p. 154.
10. Schoenberger SG, Sutherland CM, Robinson AE. Breast neoplasms: duplex sonographic imaging as an adjunct in diagnosis. Radiology 1988;168:665–668.
11. Jackson VP. Breast neoplasms: duplex sonographic imaging as an adjunct in diagnosis. Radiology 1989;170:578 (letter).
12. Böhm-Vélez M, Mendelson EB. CT, US, and MRI in evaluating the breast. Semin US, CT, MR 1989;10:171–176.
13. Rubin E, Miller VE, Berland LL et al. Handheld real-time breast sonography. AJR 1985;144:623–627.
14. Hilton SVW, Leopold GR, Olson LK, Wilson SA. Real-time breast sonography: application in 300 consecutive patients. AJR 1986;147:479–486.
15. Harper P. Ultrasound mammography. Baltimore: University Park Press, 1985, pp. 46–47.
16. Dempsey PH. Breast sonography: historical perspective, clinical applications and image interpretation. Ultrasound Quarterly 1988;6:69–90.
17. Stomper RC, VanVoorhis BJ, Raviknar VA, Meyer JR. Mammographic changes associated with postmenopausal hormone replacement therapy: a longitudinal study. Radiology 1990;174:487–490.
18. Sickles EA, Filly CA, Callen PW. Benign breast lesions: ultrasound detection and diagnosis. Radiology 1984;151:467–470.
19. Stavros AT, Parker SH, Dennis MA et al. US of "probably malignant" and "atypical" solid breast nodules. Radiology 1993; 189(P): suppl, p 179.

20. Cole-Beuglet C, Soriano RZ, Kurtz AB et al. Ultrasound analysis of 104 primary breast carcinomas classified according to histopathologic type. Radiology 1983,147:191–196.
21. Logan WW, Hoffman NY. Diabetic fibrous disease. Radiology 1989;172:667–670.
22. Hughes LE, Mansel RE, Webster DJT. Benign disorders and diseases of the breast. London: Balliere Tindall, 1988, pp. 59–73.
23. Kopans DB. Breast imaging. Philadelphia: JB Lippincott, 1989, p. 105.
24. Eklund GW, Busby RC, Miller SH et al. Improved imaging of the augmented breast. AJR 1988;151:469–473.

gree of resoultion required for imaging structures as small as 4 mm is provided. For deeper structures within the neck, a lower frequency 5 MHz transducer may be needed. These real-time imaging probes have mechanical (sector) or electronic (phased or linear) array type tranducers (Figure 1) (1–8). These transducers are either embedded in firm plastic or enclosed within a water bath covered by a flexible membrane. Some favor this latter type of transducer because the membrane is able to conform to the underlying soft tissue components (2).

Occasionally, a stand-off pad in the form of a solid gel block or fluid-filled bag is needed to image very superficially located lesions or in those situations where only a low frequency transducer is available. This interposed pad artificially raises the focal depth of the transducer by increasing the distance from its surface and the target. To accomplish this task, gel is applied between the skin surface, pad, and the probe-pad interface to acoustically couple

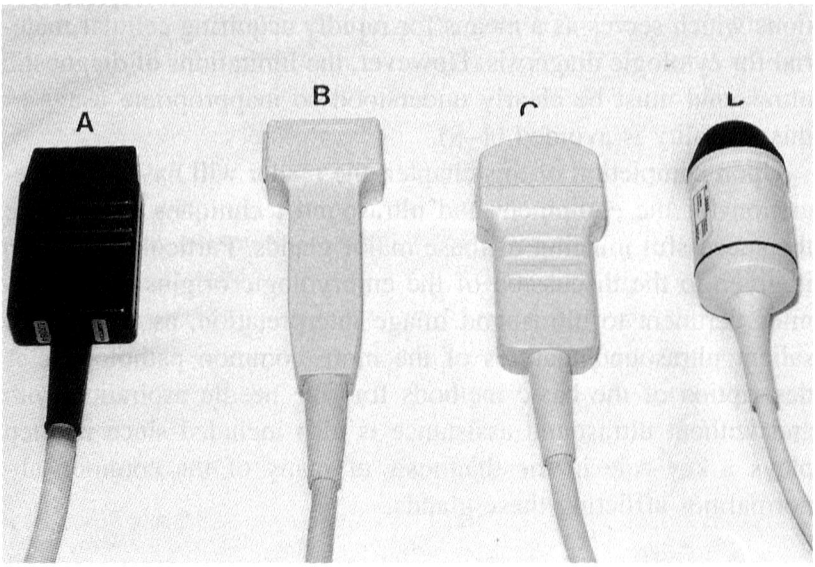

Figure 1 *This figure illustrates the many different types of high frequency small parts probes which produce high resolution images of the head and neck region. From left to right, the first three examples are electronic linear (A and B) and curved (C) array probes. D is a multi-frequency 5, 7.5 and 10.0 MHz mechanical sector probe.*

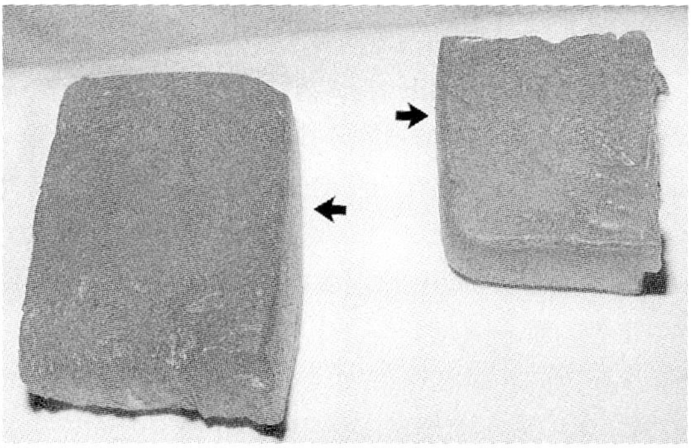

Figure 2 *The two samples of solid gel block stand-off pads (arrows) shown here are used primarily to elevate the focal zone of a lower frequency (5.0 MHz) transducer or to image superficial structures near the skin surface with a higher frequency (7.5 MHz) probe.*

these surfaces so a fairly high quality image results. Frequently, air becomes interposed between these multiple contact points inhibiting sound transmission producing artifacts that degrade the overall image quality and resolution (1–8). In addition, these devices are cumbersome often slipping from the skin surface leading to a loss of acoustical contact (Figure 2).

In general, ultrasound imaging in the cervical region is performed on a supine patient with his neck in extension. Gentle neck extension is maintained by placing a cloth roll or bolster underneath the neck for support. This position also elevates the inferior portion of the thyroid away from the posteromedial aspects of the clavicles and the manubrium. After clothing and personal ornaments are removed from the neck, drapes are placed about the neck and gel is applied to the skin surface so scanning can begin (Figure 3) (1–8).

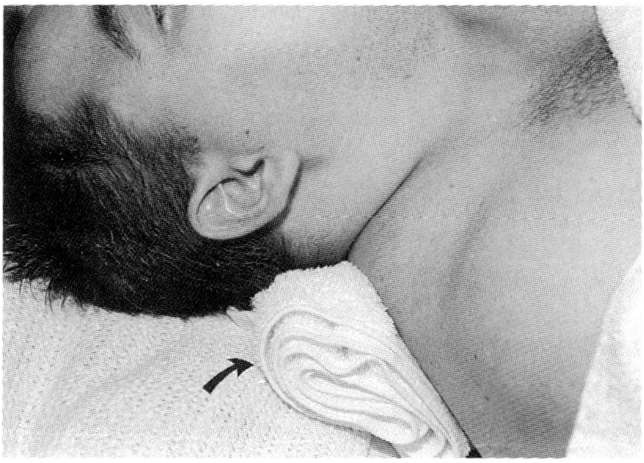

Figure 3 *This photograph shows a patient being prepared for an ultrasound of the neck with his clothing removed, neck extended and supporting neck roll placed (curved arrow).*

Either a physician or sonographer actively scans the patient in both the sagittal and axial planes. In some cases, ultrasound imaging in the coronal or oblique plane is necessary to complete the assessment of these glands especially in the case of the salivary glands. Images representative of both normal and abnormal structures are documented on hard copy or Polaroid film as a permanent record. Each hard copy image has the exact location of the structure in question labeled to avoid confusion. Videotape is an excellent recording option especially in those cases requiring duplex and color Doppler imaging (1–9).

THE THYROID GLAND

The thyroid gland, an important gland of internal secretion, releases two principal hormones, thyroxin and calcitonin. These hormones are essential mediators of body metabolism regulating growth and development. An overabundance or deficiency in the secretion of thyroxin and its associated active components may precipitate a metabolic disturbance such as hyperthyroidism or hypothyroidism (9). In addition, these metabolic aberrations, abnormalities such as congenital anomalies, inflammatory processes and both benign and malignant neoplasms afflict this gland.

Ultrasound offers to the clinician a rapid, non-invasive tool for confirmation and further assessment of many of these latter abnormalities. First, ultrasound rapidly confirms that a mass-like swelling within the region of the thyroid gland actually arise from this gland. Second, findings suspicious for a mass by nuclear medicine imaging are easily verified by ultrasound. Once documented, the number, size, and volume of the mass are accurately measured and then objectively followed. Fourth, ultrasound is capable of assessing the post-surgical soft tissue bed after thyroidectomy for local neoplastic recurrence. Finally, ultrasound assisted fine needle aspiration of a non-palpable mass may be critical to making a nonoperative, definitive diagnosis (1–6, 8, 10).

An appreciation for the limitations in the ability of ultrasound to evaluate the thyroid gland is mandatory so over- and underutilization of this technology are avoided. Ultrasound is frequently requested to make a differentiation between a benign and a malignant mass. For some, this task is accomplished by characterizing the cystic or solid state of the mass. However, this distinction may not always be totally reliable for excluding a malignancy (11, 12). For others, it is desirable to know whether or not multiple solid masses exist. Again, multiplicity is not entirely synonymous with a benign process. In many of these cases, strict ultrasound criteria must be met before a mass is confidently declared to be benign (1–6, 11–18).

Lesion location may also be a limiting factor in ultrasound usage especially in the case of the ectopic, retrosternally positioned thyroid gland. For the ectopically located gland, an alternative imaging modality such as nuclear medicine (NM), computerized tomography (CT), or magnetic resonance imaging (MRI) may be needed (1–6).

Furthermore, some clinicians advocate the opinion that ultrasound has a very limited to nonexistent role in the evaluation of the thyroid and its maladies. Some of their reasoning is based upon the inherent limitations of this technology and the variation in their ultrasonographic experience (19). Contrary to this opinion, ultrasound does supply much useful information when applied intelligently. It is a rapid, efficient and inexpensive adjunct to the physical examination aiding in both the evaluation and therapy of many thyroid ailments (1–6, 11–18).

Embryology and anatomy

Before discussing the anatomic relationships and the ultrasonographic appearance of the thyroid gland, a brief description of thyroid gland embryology is in order. The midline thyroid gland forms from the endodermal tissue arising between the first and second pharyngeal pouches. Developmentally, toward the end of the fourth week, this tissue anlage lengthens and becomes a hollow tubular structure called the thyroglossal duct. This elongation process is a relative phenomenon since it is the forward movement of the growing pharhynx that accounts for it (22). As it advances caudally, the distal portion of the thyroglosssal duct dilates, becomes bilobated and finally rests on the anterior aspect of the trachea. This bilobated portion of the thyroglossal duct is destined to

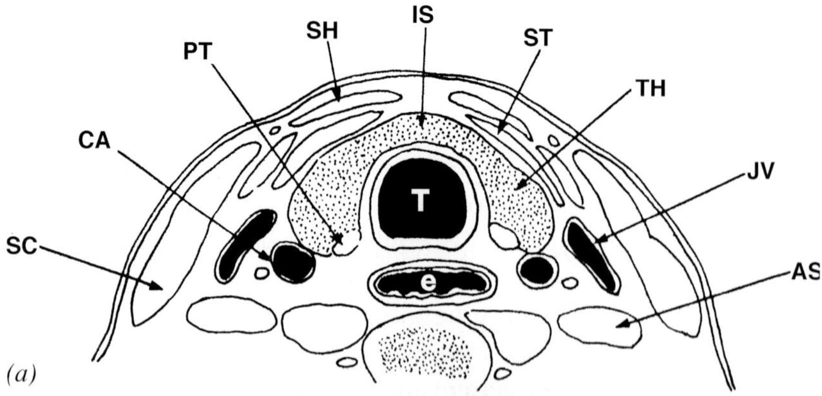

(a)

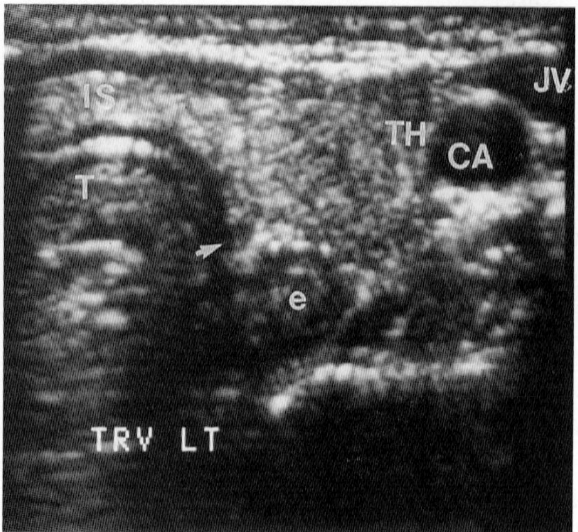

(b)

Figure 4

a. Line drawing done in an axial plane to illustrate the structures of the neck at the level of the thyroid gland commonly imaged by ultrasound. TH = Thyroid gland (left lobe); IS = isthmus portion of thyroid gland; PT = parathyroid gland (right lower gland); CA = right common artery; JV = left internal jugular vein (the small medial structure-vagus nerve); T = trachea; e = esophagus; and neck muscles (SC = sternocleidomastoid; SH = sternohyoid, SH; ST = sternothyroid).

b. A transverse ultrasound image which corresponds to left half of the line illustration. TH = Left lobe of the thyroid gland; IS = isthmus of thyroid gland; arrow = parathyroid gland (lower gland of left pair); T = trachea; e = esophagus (slightly lateral to position in line illustration); JV = left internal jugular vein.

form the crescent shaped right and left lobes of the thyroid. At the base of the tongue, the foramen cecum marks the residual origin of this tissue. Occasionally, a strip of residual thyroid tissue known as the pyramidal lobe, identified in up to 15 % of normal population, lies along the embryologic path of descent (20–23).

Anatomically, the normal thyroid gland consists of two lateral lobes superimposed over the anterolateral surface of the trachea. The right and left lateral lobes are joined at their inferior aspects by a thin slip of thyroid tissue called the isthmus. These lobes are invested by the pretracheal fascia which affixes them to the anterolateral surface of the trachea. The carotid sheath with its carotid artery, internal jugular vein accompanied by the deep cervical chain of lymph nodes and vagus nerve runs along the posterolateral aspect of each lateral lobe. The cervical esophagus is located on the posteromedial aspect of the left lobe of the thyroid gland. Bilaterally, the recurrent laryngeal nerves pass between the trachea and the posterior aspects of the lateral lobes of the gland. Normally, the paired parathyroid glands reside on the posterior surface of the lateral lobes of the thyroid gland except for those cases of parathyroid gland ectopia (Figure 4). The thyroid gland and its adjacent structures are protected by the anterior neck muscles composed of the sternohyoid, posterior belly of the omohyoid, sternothyroid, and the anterior border of the sternocleidomastoid (23, 24) (Figure 5).

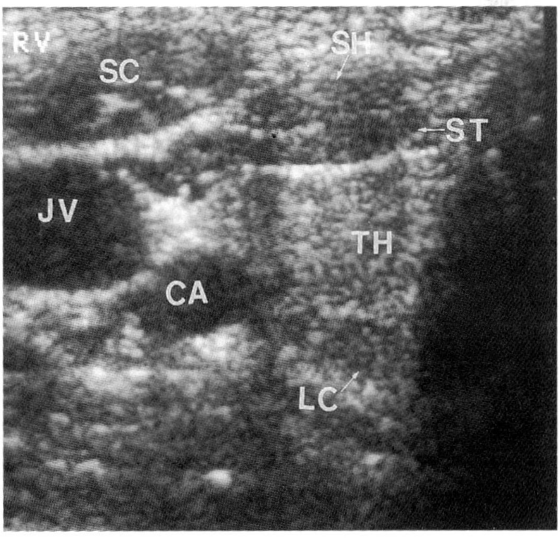

Figure 5 *This transverse ultrasound image over the right lobe of the thyroid gland (TH) shows the cross-sectional appearance of the anterior neck muscles to be hypoechoic (less echogenic). ST = Sternocleidomastoid; SH = sternohyoid; ST = sternothyroid; LC = longus colli; TH = thyroid gland; CA = right common carotid artery; and JV = right internal jugular vein.*

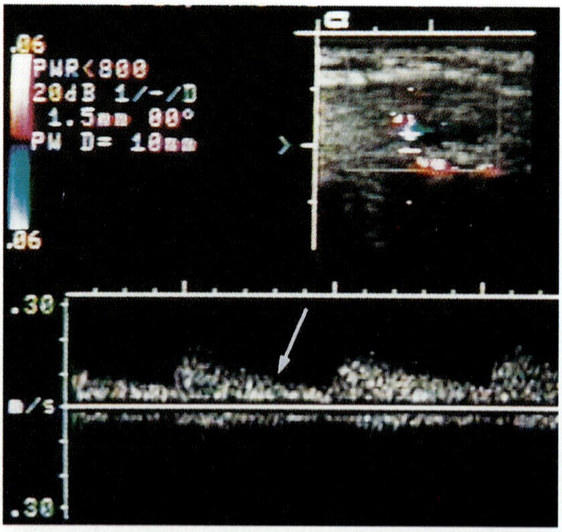

Figure 6 *A color Doppler image in the sagittal plane near the inferior thyroid artery with an arterial waveform from the parenchyma of the gland demonstrating ample diastolic flow (arrow below).*

The arterial supply to the thyroid arises from the superior thyroid artery, a branch of the external carotid artery and the inferior thyroid artery, a branch from the thyrocervical trunk. Venous drainage is accomplished through the superior and middle thyroid veins which drain into the ipsilateral internal jugular vein. The inferior thyroid vein services the inferior portion of the thyroid and drains into the ipsilateral brachiocephalic vein (23, 24).

Indeed, both duplex and color Doppler imaging have demonstrated the increased vascularity of this gland. The shape of the Doppler waveform depends on the arterial segment insonated (25–29). Signals from the thyroid parenchyma will have a high diastolic flow with normal systolic peak frequency shifts being 1.77 KHz ± 1.75 KHz. However, these signals are not always easily acquired (Figure 6) (30).

Ultrasonographically, the echotexture of the anatomically normal thyroid gland is brighter than the hypoechoic appearing neck muscles but less echogenic than the surrounding pretracheal fat and fascia. Internally, the parenchyma has a stipple-like echo pattern which is fairly homogeneous and symmetric throughout. Frequently, very tiny round sonolucent cystic structures are seen scattered about the parenchyma of both thyroid lobes. Less than millimeters in size, these lucencies commonly represent portions of diminutive blood vessels rather than a congenital thyroid cyst (Figure 7) (1, 26). Occasionally, normal thyroid follicles will be identified within the parenchyma as discrete, hy-

Figure 7
a. A photograph of a properly positioned patient having a sagittal image of the right lobe of the thyroid gland acquired.
b. The sagittal ultrasound image of the same right lobe (TH) with a homogeneous, stippled echo echotexture which is not as bright as the surrounding fascia (black arrow). Note the tiny sonolucent structure (white arrow) which represents a portion of a vessel, not a thyroid cyst.

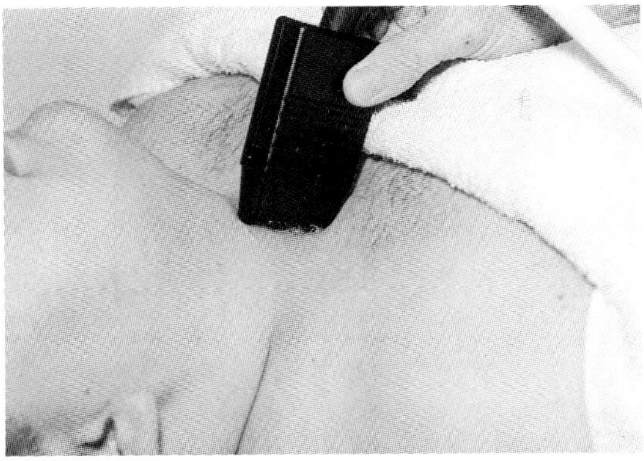

(a)

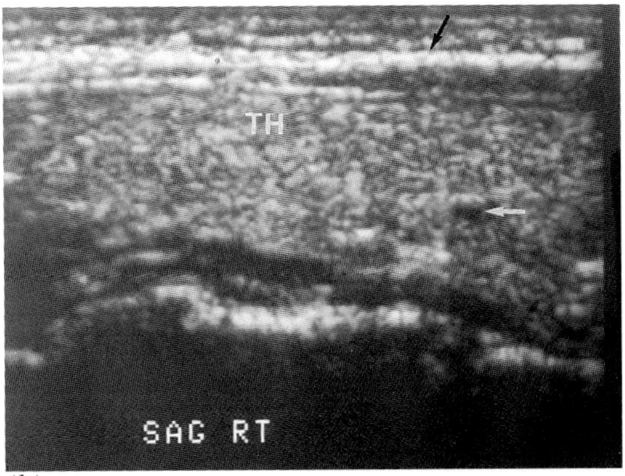

(b)

poechoic masses measuring millimeters in size. The hyperechoic, pretracheal fascia and fat surround the gland while the posterior thyroid cartilage and the trachea appear as hyperechogenic rings with a posterior shadow created by intratracheal air. Remember, the esophagus lies on the left, posteromedially and sonographically, it is a doughnut-like structure possessing an outer hypoechoic ring surrounding an inner echogenic ring. The uninitiated often mistakes the esophagus for a mass but a simple swallow by the patient will reveal its true identity (Figure 8) (1–5).

Thyroid gland anomalies

Developmental anomalies range from a partial or complete absence of thyroid gland to variations in structure and location. When thyroid

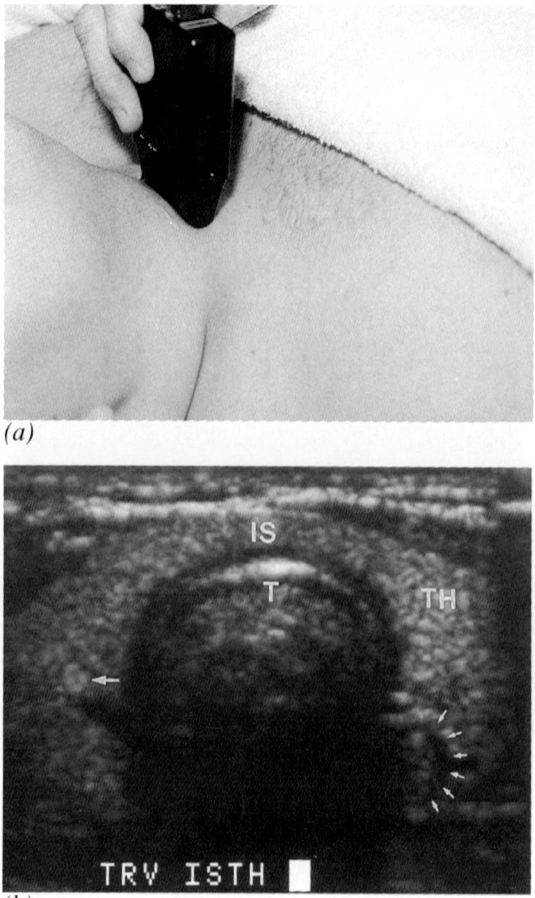

(a)

(b)

Figure 8
a. A photograph of a patient being imaged in the transverse plane with ultrasound image depicted in b.
b. The thyroid gland (TH) has a homogeneous echotexture with the exception of a small colloid nodule (arrow). Isthmus, IS; Trachea (echogenic cartilaginous rings), and multiple arrows = esophagus (hypoechoic-echogenic ring), multiple arrows.

aplasia or complete absence tissue occurs, it usually presents clinically as congenital cretinism, the most common form of congenital hypothyroidism identified within the United States. In suspicious cases, ultrasound rapidly confirms the presence or absence of thyroid tissue without the need for administration of radiopharmaceuticals or ionizing radiation. In partial absence, it is the isthmus portion that is usually absent (5 %). If a lobe is missing, then it is most frequently the left lobe (3). Once ultrasound has determined the presence of the normal echogenic thyroid tissue, then the endocrinologist may focus on the various metabolic causes for this abnormality.

In the case of ectopia, thyroid tissue wanders from its usual pretracheal location in the anterior neck with its final destination being any site along its path of descent from the base of the tongue to the mediastium. Rarely, aberrant thyroid tissue is found in very remote or unusual sites such as the scrotum, vagina, or porta-hepatis (31). If this ectopic tissue remains within the region of the neck, then ultrasound may quickly locate it by looking for the normally echogenic thyroid tissue. However, additional studies such as nuclear medicine imaging, computed tomography or MRI may better evaluate these more distant sites (16, 31, 34).

Another common anomaly, the thyroglossal duct cyst, typically presents as a common neck mass within the pediatric age group but it does escape detection into the adult years. This sac-like, cystic structure represents the remains of the primitive thyroglossal duct. Histologically, the thin wall of the cyst contains either mature thyroid epithelium or metaplastic stratified squamous with or without ciliated columnar epithelium (31). Sonographically, most, if not all, of these masses are purely cystic measuring from 1 to 2 cm. The thin cyst wall is well defined and posteriorly, enhancement through transmission of sound is noted. On occasion, a layer of low level echoes will be identified along the dependent wall of the cyst and now it must be characterized as complex. These low level echoes represent a predominantly cellular component composed of red blood cells after hemorrhage or white blood cells when infected (Figure 9) (1–5, 31–33).

Diffuse thyroid disease

Goiter is a generic term which refers to the diffuse enlargement of the thyroid gland without assigning in an etiology. Environmental, metabolic-hormonal, iatrogenic and inflammatory processes may induce a generalized increase in gland size. The establishment of a diagnosis relies upon clinical, physical and laboratory data along with the appropriate imaging studies (9, 31).

A generalized increase in thyroid gland size is usually the first indication of a diffuse process but enlargement is not specific to any disease process. Furthermore, an accurate assessment for the thyroid gland size is not easily made by the physical examination alone. Compared to palpation, ultrasound more accurately measures the dimensions of the gland providing objective data for the clinician. Measurements are made in three planes: craniocaudad (CC), anteroposterior (AP) and transverse (trans) planes. Both the CC and AP measurements are taken from the sagittal image while the axial image provides the transverse measurement. Both the AP and transverse distances must be measured from the broadest portion of each lateral lobe (Figure 10) (2, 3, 35, 36).

Sizes quoted for the lateral lobes of the adult thyroid gland range from 5.0 to 8.0 cm (CC), 1.0 to 2.5 cm (AP) and 2.0 to 4.0

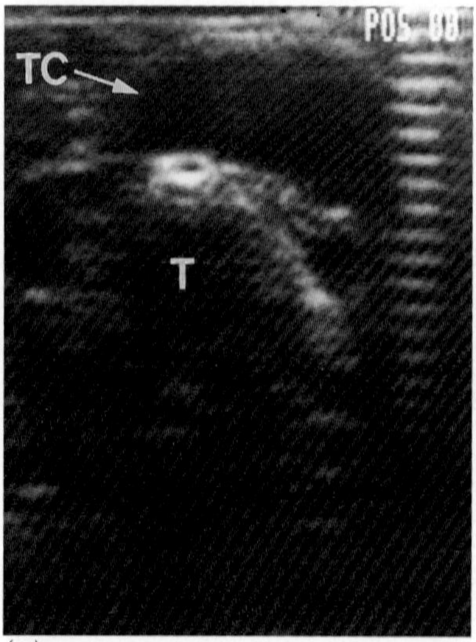

(a)

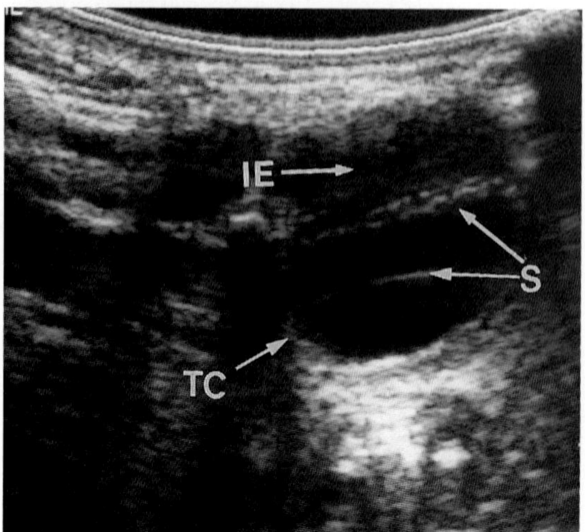

(b)

Figure 9
a. Transverse image of a purely cystic (no internal echoes, well-defined back wall and through transmission of sound) thyroglossal duct cyst (TC) lies anterior to trachea (T).
b. The transverse image revals a thyroglossal duct cyst complicated by infection with low level internal echoes (IE) and septations (S).

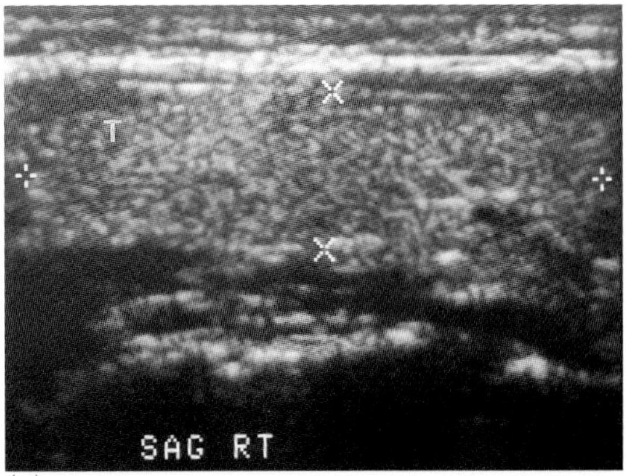

(a)

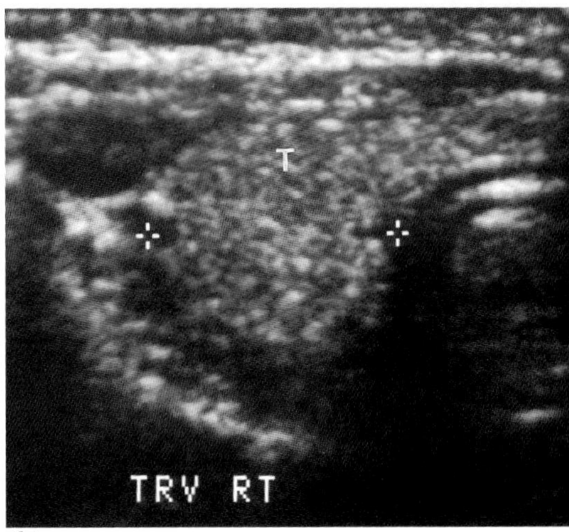

(b)

Figure 10
a. Sagittal ultrasound image demonstrating the proper technique for measuring the cranio-caudad (++) and the anteroposterior (xx) dimension of the thyroid gland (T).
b. The axial image is used to measure the transverse dimension of each lobe. Both lobes should be measured and these same values may be used to generate the volume of the gland.

cm (trans). On the other hand, pediatric (term to 2 years) thyroid lobe sizes range from 2.0 to 3.0 cm (CC), 0.18 to 1.2 cm (AP) and 1.0 to 1.5 cm (trans). Measurements for both the adult and pediatric groups have a dependance on the height, weight, age, and sex of the individual. In fact, some have suggested that thyroid volume determinations may more closely approximate the exact weight and size of the gland (2, 3, 35, 36).

The calculated thyroid volume may be compared to body weight with the final specific values varying among reporting investigators. In one series, the normal adult thyroid volumes were measured with aid of a computer digitizer and listed as 13.4 ± 4.1

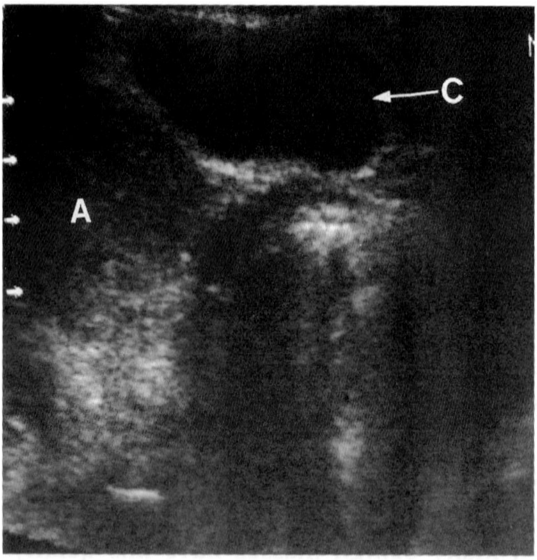

Figure 15 *Transverse ultrasound image of a true, congenital thyroid cyst (C) documented by surgical pathology after its surgical removal with the adjacent adenoma (A).*

through transmission of sound with posterior wall enhancement (Figure 15). With careful scrutiny, most of these "cystic masses" will have a solid component when imaged by ultrasound, therefore they are considered to be sonographically complex. Typically, these are follicular adenomas imaged in various stages of degeneration. Again, the identification of low level internal echoes along the dependent wall suggests the presence of cellular debris or hemorrhage. Internally, septations are imaged as thin or thick linear echo bands and focal soft tissue masses may be encountered along the inner wall. These characteristics are not unique and therefore, a cystic neoplasm must be excluded (1, 2, 5, 14, 15).

Benign, solitary, solid thyroid masses

The most common benign, solitary, solid thyroid mass is the colloid or adenomatous nodule. Basically, this nodule is an enlarged colloid filled follicle. Since it is not a true neoplasm, it lacks a premalignant potential (1). On ultrasound, this hypoechoic nodule is a fairly well defined mass possessing a hypoechoic echotexture with a variable degree of through transmission sound. When hemorrhage or ischemic necrosis occurs, this nodule becomes sonographically complex with a grainy echogenicity (1, 2). Occasionally, coarse foci of calcification are found, however, these more commonly originate from adjacent vascular structures and not from the colloid collections (11, 12). Aspiration of a colloid nodule with a fine needle often yields of bloody specimen and typically, these specimens are classified as unsatisfactory for a cytologic diagnosis (Figure 16) (44).

As a group, thyroid adenomas are the next most common benign thyroid mass frequently found in women. They are outnumbered by the colloid nodule 10 to 1 but unlike the colloid nodule, the follicular adenoma is a true neoplasm. Pathologically, these nodules are subdivided into follicular, papillary, and atypical varieties (1, 31).

Of these adenomas, the follicular type is the most common and, histologically, it may be further subdivided into fetal, colloid, simple embryonal, and Hurthle cell types (31). Most are benign, however, with detailed histologic analysis up to 10 % will show features of capsular invasion (11, 31). Therefore, these lesions often require fine needle aspiration and ultimately surgical excision before malignant invasion is excluded (39–42).

Sonographically, the solitary follicular adenoma is a solid hypoechoic mass with a well defined sonolucent rim measuring approximately 1 to 2 mm in thickness. This rim completely surrounds the mass and is uninterrupted. The ultrasonographic explanation for

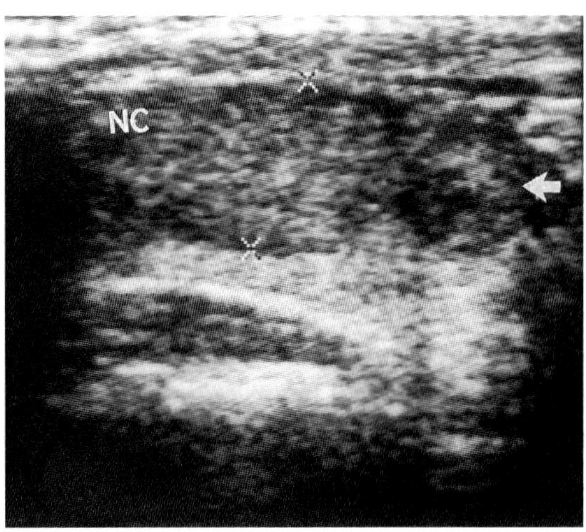

Figure 16 *This sagittal image contains two different types of solid, hypoechoic thyroid masses. The largest of these masses is the more common benign colloid nodule (NC) with an adjacent malignant Hurthle cell tumor (arrow). Sonographically, both have the same appearance which underscores the point that ultrasound is not always able to distinguish a benign mass from a malignant one.*

mens (4). A cytologic distinction between papillary, follicular and Hurthle cell types is not easily made. However, this situation is usually not a problem since the surgically excised specimen provides the answer (39–44).

Both ultrasound and radiopharmaceutical imaging do give valuable diagnostic information prior to biopsy. Ultrasound confirms that the lesion arises from the thyroid and it quantifies its size as well as the number of lesions present. In particular, nuclear medicine imaging provides functional information which may identify a particular lesion in need of a biopsy (1–6, 39).

Before describing the thyroid biopsy technique, a brief discussion of the complications associated with this procedure is needed. The risk for these untoward events following a thyroid biopsy is very low especially in the case of infection or hemorrhage. Although the very vascular thyroid lies in close proximity to the common carotid artery, no fatal hemorrhages have been documented. Hematomas are uncommon and rarely, if ever, cause significant morbidity. Because the trachea sits posterior to the gland, it is occasionally punctured with the biopsy needle. The patient will begin coughing and quiets with speedy removal of the needle, without further sequelae. Some of these mishaps encountered may be avoided with direct visualization of the abnormality with ultrasound during the biopsy (10).

Blind biopsy

To begin the biopsy of any thyroid nodule, the supine patient has his neck extended so access to the thyroid and its nodule is easily obtained. If the nodule is palpable, then ultrasound guidance is unnecessary. Once located, the skin site over the nodule is sterilely prepped and draped. A local anesthetic is injected into the skin and subcutaneous tissues. Afterwards, a fine needle, 25 to 22 gauge, is punctured through the skin into the nodule. In most cases, a 25 gauge intramuscular needle is selected and if an insufficient specimen is obtained, then a larger gauge such as a 23 or 22 gauge is chosen (10).

Next, a 5 to 10 cc syringe is attached to the hub of the needle and approximately 1 to 2 cc of suction are applied by withdrawing on the plunger. Successful acquisition of a cytologic sample results by making several quick up and down motions with the syringe needle unit. If blood wells into the hub of the needle during sampling, then the attempt is immediately completed. Frequently, these bloody samples are unsatisfactory for a definitive cytologic diagnosis (44). Therefore, cell block material is crucial and in most cases a diagnosis is achieved with a minimal amount of this material. For best results, multiple samples are taken with the usual number between 2 and 4. Optimally, a cytotechnologist should be available to determine the adequacy of each sample. If none is on hand, then material should be placed into the proper medium for transport to the lab (Figure 23) (10).

Ultrasound guided biopsy

A nonpalpable lesion, as small as 5 mm may be biopsied using a 7.5 to 10 MHz high frequency ultrasound probe to assist with needle guidance. Prior to the actual puncture, the steps for patient

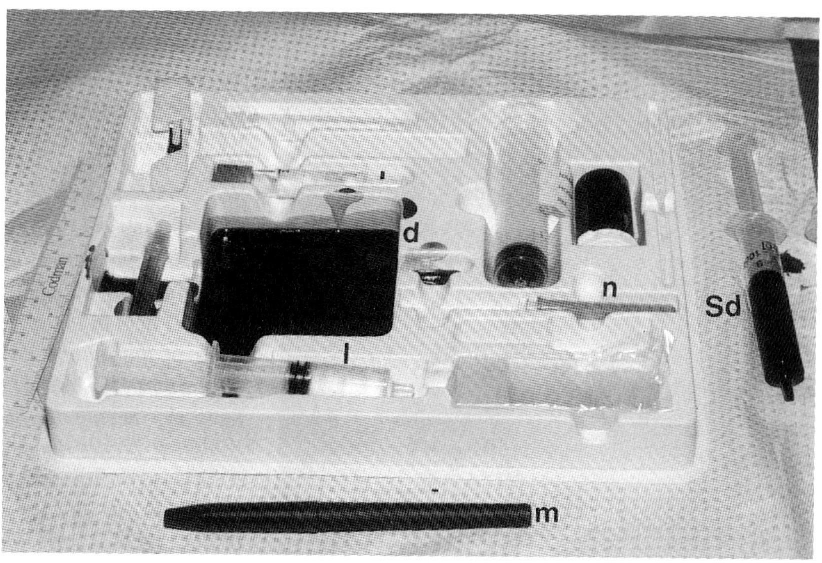

Figure 23 *This photograph of a tray prepared for thyroid biopsy shows the essential items needed which include a local anesthetic, l; 25 gauge needle, n; marking pen, m; topical disinfectant, d and syringe with desinfectant (acoustical coupler), Sd. Remember, this field must remain sterile.*

mally, they lie anterior to the more posterior longus colli muscles and the left sided esophagus. However, the final destination for the upper and lower pair of glands is influenced by their different embryologic origins. The upper pair arises from the fourth branchial pouch and has a more constant location along the dorsal aspect of the upper one-third of the lateral lobes of the thyroid. Because the lower pair of parathyroid glands is derived from the third branchial pouch, it shares a common origin with thymus. Therefore, this pair tends to wander from its usual position along the dorsal surface of the thyroid near the inferior thyroid artery descending into the anterior mediastinum with the thymus (20-24). On occasion, these glands may become invested by the surrounding tissues of the pharynx and esophagus, the carotid artery, and the thyroid fascia. Rarely, they may reside within the parenchyma of the thyroid gland (1, 5, 7).

As in thyroid ultrasound, the successful localization of these glands depends on the availability of high frequency ultrasound probes ranging from 7.5 MHz to 10 MHz with the optimum frequency being 10.0 MHz (1, 5, 7). Lower frequency probes such as a 5 MHz may be necessary when searching for a deeply located ectopic parathyroid gland (1, 2). The supine patient is positioned with his neck extended in a fashion similar to thyroid ultrasound.

Ultrasonographically, success is directly related to the experience of the examiner, the more the better (1, 2, 5, 7, 47). Additional factors ensuring success of the study include the overall size of the parathyroid gland and the presence or absence of disease (45–57). Clearly, sonographic detection improves with enlargment of the diseased gland with reported sensitivities (sens) of 80 to 88 % and specificities (spec) of 92 to 96 % (47).

However, ultrasound is not the only method capable of localizing the parathyroid glands. Nuclear medicine (Thallium 201 chloride / technetium 99m) imaging, computed tomography and magnetic resonance imaging have served as a means of evaluating these glands. Series reports have mentioned sensitivity and specificity values for nuclear imaging (sens 30 to 80 %, spec 49 to 98 %), computed tomography (sens 60-80 %, spec 90-95 %) (53–59) and magnetic resonance imaging (sens 74 %, spec 88 %) (58, 62). While none of these modalities is completely successful, results can be improved when these modalities are combined, especially in the cause of ultrasound and nuclear medicine imaging (56, 59). However, not all authors agree with these statistics and they prefer to forego preoperative localizations in favor of bilateral neck dissections (60, 61).

Of all these modalities, ultrasound provides a rapid, inexpensive method for preoperative localization of parathyroid pathology. Because ultrasound directs the surgeon to the abnormal side, the extent and duration of surgical exploration is decreased. Therefore, surgical morbidity, costs and length of the hospital stay are reduced. In the case of re-operation for failed parathyroid disease, both preoperative and intraoperative ultrasound have improved localizations of retained abnormal parathyroid tissue with better surgical outcome (47–57).

The normal parathyroid glands are rarely imaged with ultrasound even if a high resolution 10 MHz probe is employed (1, 5, 46). When imaged, the normal parathyroid gland usually assumes a pancake-like configuration. The normal echotexture is less echogenic or equivalent to the normal thyroid gland (1, 5, 7, 46–49). The dimensions of the individual, normal parathyroid gland vary with the average adult size being 1.0 × 3.0 × 5.0 mm with the longest dimension up to 12 mm. Since the normal gland has a pancake shape, its thickest point is usually less than 2 mm (0.5–2.0 mm) and its widest is 2 to 5 mm (Figure 25) (1, 5, 7, 47–51).

The clinical presentation common to all abnormalities of the parathyroid glands is one of hyperparathyroidism. The response of these glands to disease is basically limited to enlargement with the extent of enlargement and number of glands affected varying according to the underlying pathology. Differentiation between the hyperplastic, adenomatous and neoplastic glands will depend upon the clinical history and laboratory data along with a recognition of the number and location of the involved parathyroid glands (46).

Typically, the hyperplastically enlarged parathyroid glands arise from a secondary process (secondary hyperparathyroidism) such as chronic renal glomerular insufficiency or vitamin D deficiency. If hyperplasia is the primary event (primary hyperparathyroidism), then the underlying cause usually remains unknown. In this latter situation, most cases have a familial pattern or an association with

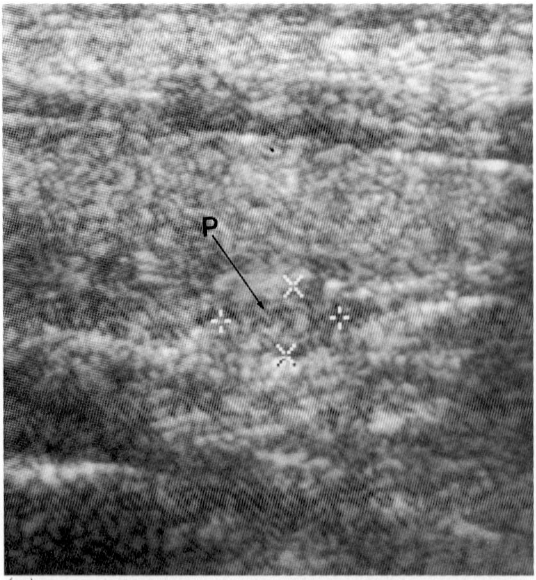

(a)

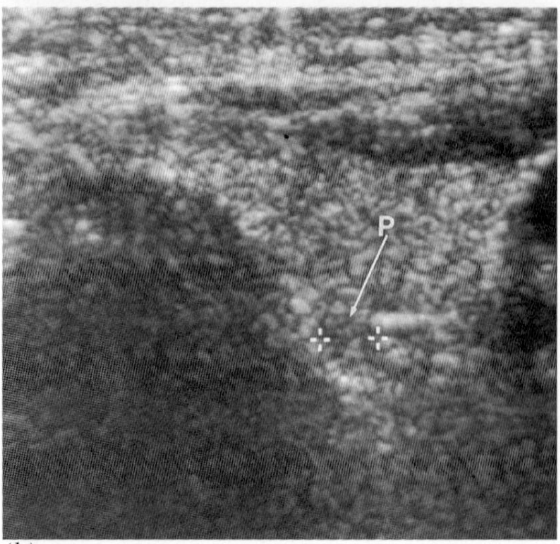

(b)

Figure 25
a. Sagittal image demonstrating one of the normal, pancake-like parathyroid glands (p) with the craniocaudad (++) and anteroposterior (xx) dimensions measured.
b. The transverse appearance of the parathyroid gland (p) is shown with it, marked for a transverse measurement.

multiple endocrinopathies. In either case, hyperparathyroidism leads to an elevation in serum levels of parathyroid hormone and calcium (46).

Sonographically, the hyperplastic parathyroid glands are asymmetrically enlarged with a hypoechoic echotexture. All are hyperplastic to some degree and this latter finding is key to separat-

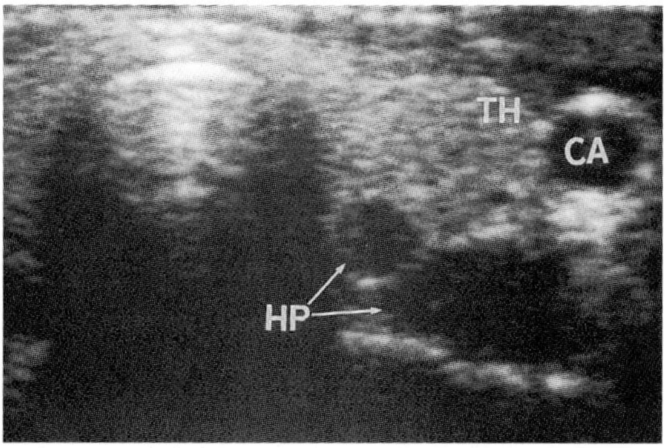

Figure 26 *Transverse image through the left cervical region demonstrating enlarged hyperplastic parathyroid glands (HP) in a patient with chronic renal failure. Ultrasonographically, these enlarged, hypoechoic glands lie behind the normally echogenic thyroid gland (TH) and the centrally anechoic common carotid artery (CA).*

ing the enlarged hyperplastic parathyroid gland from the solitary parathyroid adenoma. However, it is not too uncommon for them to be normal in size and appearance (Figure 26). When surgical removal of these glands is contemplated, a careful search for each gland is required for a successful outcome (1, 2, 5, 7, 47–51).

Parathyroid adenomas are the most common cause of primary hyperparathyroidism responsible for over 80 % of the cases (1, 3, 7). This neoplasm usually arises from the lower pair of glands. Typically a solitary mass, double or multiple adenomas have been reported in 4.5 % of cases (3). Because adenomas commonly originate from the lower pair of glands, ectopia occurs in up to 10 % of cases. Parathyroid adenomas also have a known association with multiple endocrine adenopathies (MEA 1 and MEA II) (1, 3, 9, 31).

On ultrasound, a parathyroid adenoma has an ovoid shape unlike the pancake shaped normal parathyroid gland. Expansion of the effected gland between the surrounding longitudinally arranged tissue fibers produces this configuration (2, 7). Their well-defined, smooth margins often have an almost anechoic appearance. Internally, its echotexture is usually less echogenic than the normal parathyroid gland. Occasionally, a very large adenoma is internally complex with cystic areas secondary to necrosis (Figure 27). The size of an adenoma varies from 6 to 30 mm in its largest dimension with an average measurement of 15 × 10 mm. Likewise, enlargement of the inferior thyroid artery nearest the adenoma has been reported (1, 2, 7, 47–50).

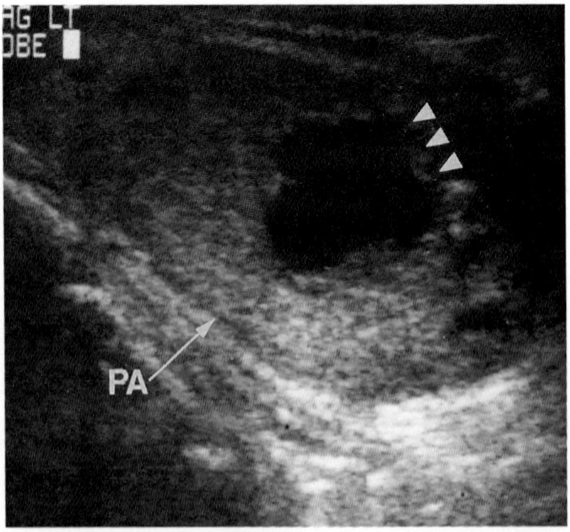

Figure 27 *Left-sided sagittal image reveals a large, well marginated parathyroid adenoma (PA) in a patient with hyperparathyroidism. Internally, the hypoechotexture becomes anechoic in the area of central necrosis (arrowheads).*

Both normal and abnormal structures can mimic a parathyroid adenoma. The normal longus colli muscles and the neurovascular bundles are rarely mistaken for a small adenoma. Confusion is avoided by imaging sagittally, demonstrating the longitudinally oriented longus colli muscles. The small neurovascular bundles are best imaged axially to identify their transverse orientation. Sometimes a posteriorly directed hypoechoic thyroid nodule is difficult to distinguish from an adjacent parathyroid adenoma. In this situation, an echogenic interface between the normal thyroid and the adenoma may aid in making this determination (47). Enlarged cervical lymph nodes may be problematic especially in cases of the ectopic cervical adenoma (Figure 28). In these cases, additional studies such as a nuclear medicine T1 Tc subtraction imaging may yield the desired answer (47, 50, 51). Fine needle aspiration is always an option when the diagnosis remains uncertain (63, 64).

Parathyroid carcinomas are rare with many of these neoplasms being hormonally active with extremely high PTH levels. However, PTH levels may be normal with the hormonally "silent" carcinomas. Fortunately, parathyroid carcinomas are not very aggressive with long term survivals expected. If these neoplasms metastasize, then the usual direction is toward the lungs or liver (46).

The typical sonographic presentation is a large, lobulated, hypoechoic mass. Except for being slightly larger than the usual adenoma, both have similar features which can be confusing for the sonographer (see Figure 27) (1, 5, 7, 65). Frank invasion into the surrounding structures, such as the thyroid gland, is rarely demonstrated and is certainly difficult to discern on ultrasound images (65).

THE SALIVARY GLANDS

Salivary glands may be artificially subdivided into major and minor gland groups. The major salivary glands, including the parotid, the submandibular, and sublingual glands, all have been studied with ultrasound. These glands are responsible for production of the serous and mucus portions of saliva. The primary function of these secretions is aiding and intiating digestion along with facilitating the formation of speech (23, 24).

All salivary glands have a common origin arising from the oral ectoderm. Seen as early as the 6th fetal week, the parotid and submandibular gland are completely developed by the 5th fetal month (20, 21).

The role of ultrasound in the evaluation of the salivary glands is limited to confirming that an area of swelling in the region of a sa-

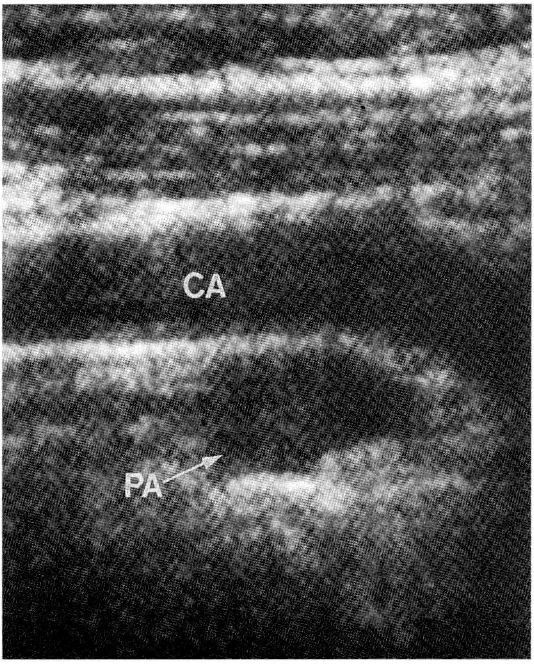

Figure 28 *Sagittal image from a patient with hyperparathyroidism with a hypoechoic parathyroid adenoma (PA) located posterior to the common carotid artery (CA).*

livary gland truly arises from the gland. Of the major glands, the parotid and submandibular glands have received the most ultrasonographic attention. Otherwise, fine detail analysis has been left to imaging with computed tomography and sialography playing a much lesser role (8, 66–70).

The parotid gland

The parotid gland, the largest of the major salivary glands, lies inferior to the external auditory meatus between the sternocleidomastoid muscle, posteriorly, and the ramus of the mandible with its masseter muscle, anteriorly. For the surgeon, the course of the fascial nerve artificially divides this gland into a superficial and deep lobe (23, 24).

The superficial lobe, 80 % of the gland, may be scanned with a high resolution small parts probe with ultrasound frequencies in the 7.5 to 10 MHz range. However, the deep lobe, 20 % of the gland, is less well studied, with ultrasound and computed tomography often needed for a complete study. Initial ultrasound scanning is done in the transverse plane while the sagittal and coronal orientations provide additional planes of information (8, 66–70). The sonographically normal gland has homogeneous hypoechoic appearance compared to fascia but slightly more echogenic than the adjacent muscles (Figure 29).

Parotitis

Clinically, acute parotitis presents as sudden gland swelling, commonly caused by the mumps virus. Ultrasound is usually not necessary for the diagnosis of this problem. On the other hand, if acute sialadenitis is imaged by ultrasound, then one may see the loss of the normal homogeneous glandular echotexture, although this finding is very nonspecific. With the onset of suppuration or abscess formation, ultrasound may aid by characterizing the size and extent of this process (8, 66, 71).

Except for the identification of duct stones and ductal dilatation, the utility of ultrasound in the evaluation of chronic sialadenitis and autoimmune disorders such as Sjogren's syndrome is un-

Figure 29
a. Photograph of an individual having his parotid gland imaged in the transverse plane with a 7.5 MHz probe. The transverse image in b. demonstrates most of homogeneous, less echogenic superficial lobe (S) of the parotid gland (PG). The deep lobe (D) is not as well imaged here. SM = Sternocleidomastoid muscle and MM = masseter muscle.

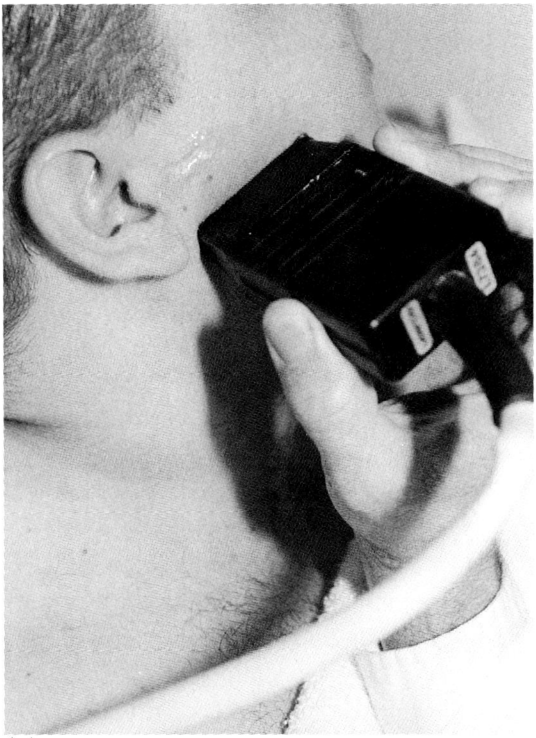

(a)

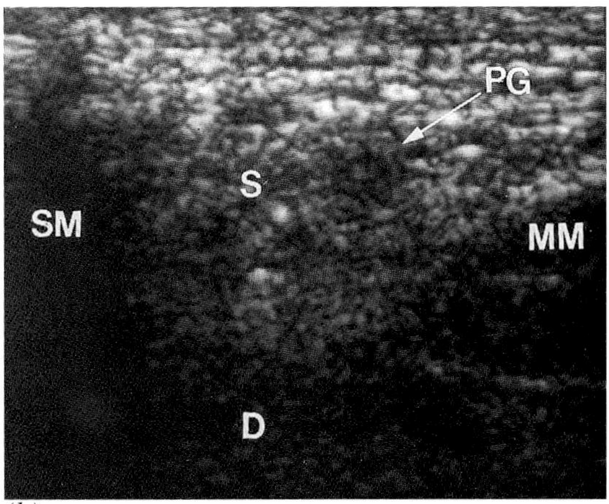

(b)

clear. On ultrasound, cystic areas are scattered throughout the parenchyma of the parotid gland, especially in patients with Sjogren's syndrome. Sialography, on the other hand, better defines the degree and extensiveness of ductal dilatation (71, 72, 73).

Benign and malignant neoplasms

Both benign and malignant parotid neoplasms have been imaged with ultrasound. Neoplasms of the parotid gland account for less than 3 % of all neoplasms with the pleomorphic adenoma, papillary cystadenoma (Warthin's tumor), and carcinoma comprising the major portion of these neoplasms. Clinically, one may encounter a nonspecific mass-like swelling (74). In these cases, ultrasound may be able to differentiate a more superficially located extraparotid mass from a primary neoplasm of the superficial parotid lobe. However, the deep lobe of the parotid gland and deeper pharyngeal lesions are less well evaluated by ultrasound requiring computed tomography for description and staging (66, 67, 68).

Pleomorphic adenomas comprise 60 to 90 % of the benign parotid neoplasms. When encountered, it is frequently a woman past her 5th decade. It is considered to be a benign lesion although it may re-occur after an incomplete excision (74). Ultrasonographically, this neoplasm has a hypoechoic echotexture with a fairly well defined border and somewhat lobulated contour. Recognition of the margins and contour of this lesion is important since it may influence the surgical approach taken (8, 66–68).

The next most common benign parotid neoplasm is the papillary cystadenoma of Warthin's tumor. A neoplasm predominantly found in males after the 6th decade, it usually arises from heterotopic salivary duct epithelium contained within intraparotid lymph nodes (74). These neoplasms tend to have a complex sonographic appearance with low level internal echoes although surely cystic tumors have been described. In the complex varieties, these internal echoes represent septations and mucus components of this neoplasm. Both parotid glands should be studied since, on rare occasions, this neoplasm is known to be present (8, 66, 67, 68).

Malignant parotid neoplasms are rare and certainly less frequent than the benign variety. The type and classification of these neoplasms depends on the predominant histologic pattern present. Of the different carcinomas, mucoepidermoid carcinoma is the most common. Frequently found in females during the 5th decade, these neoplasms metastasize early and local recurrence after surgery may be encountered (74).

The sonographic features of the primary parotid neoplasm are similar to those described for a benign neoplasm. Malignant neoplasms tend to be solid, hypoechoic masses although a more

Figure 30
a. A patient is receiving an ultrasound of the right submandibular gland.
b. The submandibular gland (SG) is normally less echogenic which is similar to the normal parotid gland.

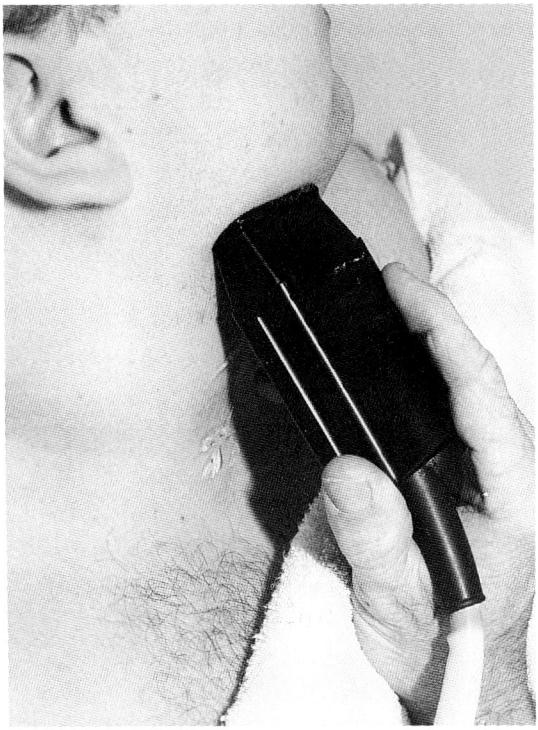

(a)

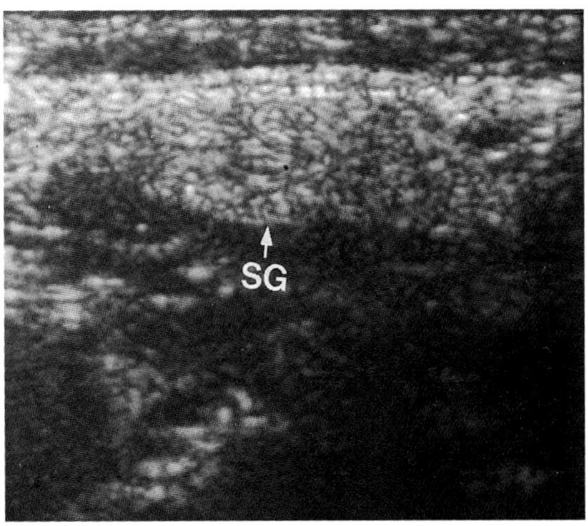

(b)

complex echotexture can be seen. The key to distinguishing between benign and malignant neoplams is made by characterizing the margins and contours of these masses. Commonly, malignant margins are ill-defined and irregular in comparison to the well defined margins of a benign neoplasm (8, 66, 67, 68).

Rarely, a local neoplasm such as a squamous cell carcinoma or lymphoma will metastasize to the parotid gland. Sonographically, their appearance is similar to the primary parotid malignancy. Differentiation between the two entities relies heavily on the historical presence of a known primary lesion (8, 66 67, 68).

The submandibular glands

Submandibular gland sonography is less routinely performed than parotid gland sonography. This gland lies along the inner surface of the mandible in the region of the submandibular fossa (23, 24). It is invested by fascia and surrounded by muscles of the submandibular region. Like the parotid gland, it is artificially divided into a superficial and a deep portion with sonographic appearance similar to the parotid gland (Figure 30) (8).

Inflammatory and autoimmune diseases, benign and malignant neoplasms, and sialolithiasis have all been known to affect the submandibular gland. Of these processes, sialolithiasis is the most common problem accounting for 80 to 90 % of all salivary gland calculi. The role of sonography in the study of sialolithasisis is limited to the identification of the nonradiopaque calculus or the small calculus hidden by superimposed bone of the mandible (8).

Unlike the parotid gland tumors, most submandibular gland neoplasms are malignant. Their sonographic description as a large, indistinct hypoechoic mass is similar to any parotid gland neoplasm. In addition, an ultrasonographic search for enlarged lymph nodes along the deep cervical chain should always be made since neoplastic involvement is common (8).

CERVICAL LYMPH NODES

Lymph nodes of the cervical region are subdivided into regional groups and a major terminal group. Regional cervical lymph node groups are named for their locations, receiving lymphatic drainage from local, as well as remote sites. Regional node groups drain into the important deep terminal group which is intimately associated with the internal jugular vein. These lymph nodes are invested by fascia of the common carotid sheath and follow its course from the skull base to the root of the neck. Reference is occasionally made to two clinically important lymph nodes within this deep group. One is the jugulodigastric node to principally drain the tonsils and tongue, resides behind and below the angle of the mandible. The second important node, called the jugulo-omohyoid node, always receives lymph drainage from the tongue (23, 24).

When cervical lymph nodes become enlarged, they clinically present as neck masses. Both inflammatory and neoplastic processes insight this nonspecific response. Size, number, discreteness, texture, and any adjacent abnormality are important bits of information which are difficult to appreciate by palpation alone. Because of the impreciseness of the physical examination, ultrasound is able to supply much of this desired information to the clinician (8). Small parts, high resolution ultrasound probes with frequency ranges of 7.5 to 10 MHz are a necessity. In general, patients assume a supine position for scanning. Often the neck is placed in extension but the head may be deviated to the side opposite the region of interest (8).

When a neoplastic process is responsible for cervical lymphadenopathy, computed tomography or magnetic resonance imaging are usually assigned the task of staging. These modalities supply a superior topographic map and lead to a better understanding of disease extent. After the initial staging process, ultrasound monitors treatment response more cheaply. Certainly, it is better than the physical examination, especially after head and neck irradiation. Because thickening of the skin after therapy hinders the physical assessment of post-treatment adenopathy, ultrasound has been used to overcome this obstacle. In addition, ultrasound provides rapid and accurate assessement for thrombosis of the internal jugular vein which is often associated with neoplastic disease (8, 74, 75).

Sonographically, normal lymph nodes are less than 5 mm in their longest dimension and may be difficult to image. Oval to kidney bean shape, their parenchymal echogenicity is usually medium to hypoechoic and their hilar fat is echogenic. Abnormally

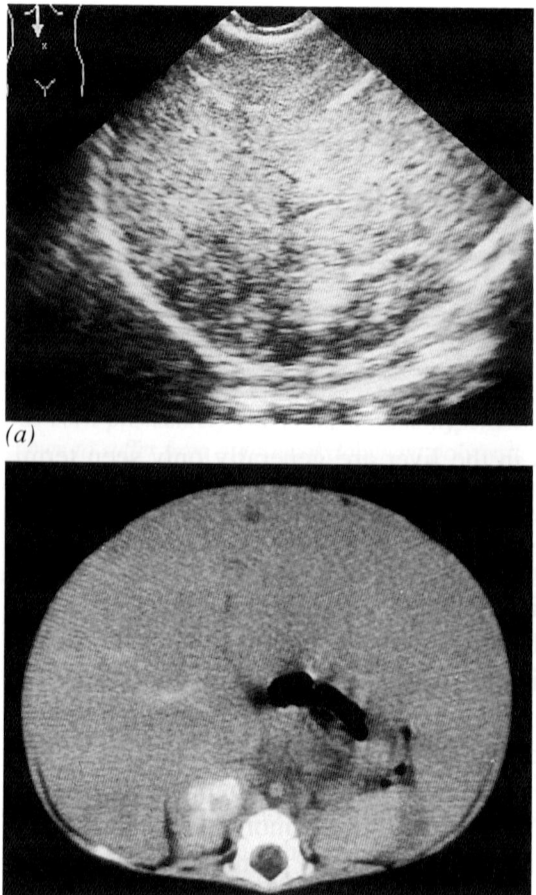

(a)

(b)

Figure 16
a. Neuroblastoma. Longitudinal sonogram of the liver in a neonate who presented with abdominal distention. The liver is markedly enlarged with a heterogenous echotexture. This is classically described as having a "pepper-pot" appearance.There is a small echogenic right adrenal primary neuroblastoma. This form of neuroblastoma has a better prognosis than that occurring in older children.
b. CT on the same child. Notice the small right calcified adrenal tumour and the enlarged liver.

Other adrenal masses

Pheochromocytomas are extremely rare in children. In childhood the tumour differs from that seen in adults, in that they are frequently extra adrenal, multiple and have less malignant potential.

Adrenal carcinomas are also extremely rare in childhood and usually present clinically with evidence of excessive hormonal activity, e.g. Cushing's syndrome and in girls, masculinisation (14).

Hepatic masses

Hepatic masses in childhood are relatively uncommon. Clinically the majority present with what appears to be hepatomegaly, and

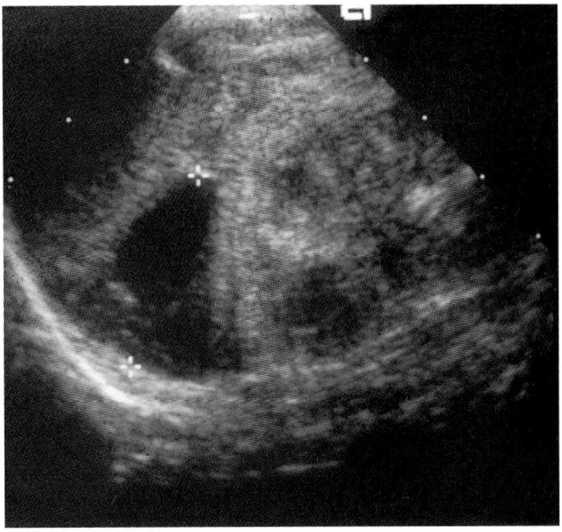

Figure 17 *Longitudinal sonogram of a left adrenal haemorrhage. The adrenal haemorrhage is predominantly cystic (marked with +). This indicates the haemorrhage is not acute as it has had time to start liquefying. The left kidney is enlarged and echogenic and the child had an associated left renal vein thrombosis. Adrenal haemorrhages are more common on the left due to the drainage of the left adrenal vein into the left renal vein.*

on ultrasound examination the sonographer needs to answer a number of questions (16).

- Is the abnormality diffuse hepatomegaly or a focal mass?
- If focal, what lobe/s of the liver are involved?
- Hepatic vascular supply must be carefully examined with particular reference to the size of the hepatic artery and draining veins. Doppler examinations are particularly helpful in differentiating hepatic masses.
- Can the portal vein be identified and what is its relationship to the mass?
- Is the biliary tree normal?

Focal hepatic masses

Hepatoblastomas and hepatocellular carcinoma.

Hepatoblastoma is the third commonest malignancy seen in childhood after a Wilms' tumour and neuroblastoma. The hepatoblastoma is derived from primitive fetal epithelial cells and is more common in young infants and children under 3 years of age. Hepatocellular carcinoma is derived from mature hepatocytes and is more common in children over 3 years of age, often with underlying liver disease. Alpha-fetoprotein levels are elevated in both tumours. Hepatoblastomas are associated with Beckwith-Wiedemann syndrome, hemihypertrophy and polyposis coli.

Hepatocellular carcinoma is associated with tyrosinaemia, biliary atresia, glycogen storage disease and Fanconi's anaemia.

Both occur more commonly in the right lobe of the liver. Calcification may be seen in up to 50 % of masses.

Ultimate prognosis depends on resectability of the lesion.

CT and MRI are performed at diagnosis and before surgery to assess precise extent of the lesion.

Haemangiomas

Haemangiomas are the commonest benign tumours in infancy, and may be solitary or diffuse. Clinically they may present with an abdominal mass, cardiac failure or skin haemangiomas. The cutaneous form is more common in diffuse haemangioendotheliomas. Ultrasound examination of the liver is particularly helpful and this is when Doppler is particularly useful. Depending on the flow within the mass variable Doppler signals may be found but additional information is obtained by carefully examining the hepatic arterial supply and any large draining veins.

The natural history is for these masses to regress in size and intervention would only be indicated if complications were uncontrolable, e.g. cardiac failure, consumptive coagulopathy and haemorrhage.

On ultrasound liver haemangioma presents as a solid heterogenous mass with central calcification or huge hepatomegaly with multiple hypoechoic areas. If doubt remains, a contrast enhanced computed tomogram will demonstrate marked peripheral enhancement of the vessels (17).

Mesenchymal hamartoma

These tumours of the liver are thought to be a congenital anomaly rather than a true tumour and present within the first two years of life. Ultrasound shows a multiloculated cystic mass with cystic spaces of varying sizes and septa. There is a marked male preponderance. Complete excision is usually curative (18).

Adenoma

Adenomas in children are usually associated with glycogen storage disease or are secondary to anabolic steroids for treatment of Fanconi's anaemia.

Infection

Focal infection lesions of the liver are relatively uncommon and may present as areas of mixed echogenicity. They are rarely purely cystic unless associated with an unusual infection, such as hydatid. Of particular importance in children to be aware of, is infection spreading from appendicitis into the portal system and then to the liver. For this reason careful examination should be made of the portal vein for patency and any evidence of collateral channels. Streptococcus mirabilis is an organism implicated in causing a large degree of necrosis (Figure 18). Another cause of a localised inflammatory mass in the liver that should not be forgotten is amoebiasis.

Hepatomegaly

Once hepatomegaly has been found the texture of the liver should be carefully examined. Hepatomegaly with a very echogenic parenchyma in children is seen in Glycogen Storage Disease (GSD), acute fatty infiltration of the liver and long term parenteral nutrition. Virtually, any paediatric malignancy may produce secondary deposits in the liver. The most frequent are those from Wilms' tumour, neuroblastoma, lymphoma or rhabdomyosarcoma. They usually present with hypoechoic nodules. Neuroblastoma stage 45 in the liver has a heterogenous "pepper-pot" appearance.

Other abdominal masses

When an intraabdominal mass is not clearly associated with an intraabdominal organ, it may be more difficult to identify their exact

19. Barr LL, Hayden CK, Jr., Stansberry SD et al. Enteric duplication cysts in children: are their ultrasonograpic wall characteristics diagnostic? Pediatr Radiol 1990;20:326–328.
20. Mason WG, Jr. Urinary tract infections in children: renal ultrasound evaluation. Radiology 1984;153:109–111.
21. Vignault F, Filiatrault D, Brandt ML et al. Acute appendicitis in children: evaluation with US. Pediatr Radiol 1990;176:501–504.
22. Verschelden P, Filiatrault D, Garel L et al. Intussusception in children: reliability of US in diagnosis. A prospective study. Pediatr Radiol 1985;184:741–744.
23. Gomes H, Menanteau B. Gastro-oesophageal reflux: comparative study between sonography and pH monitoring. Pediatr Radiol 1991;21;168–174.
24. Dufour D, Delaet MH, Dassonville M et al. Midgut malrotation, the reliability of sonographic diagnosis. Pediatr Radiol 1992;22:21–23.

CHAPTER 17

The Infant Brain

Henrietta Kotlus Rosenberg, MD, Nancy H.Sherman, MD, †, and Cheryl L. Kirby, MD

Since the advent of high-resolution realtime ultrasonography (US) in the 1980s, this non-invasive, non-ionizing means of imaging the infant brain has become a most important part of our armamentarium (1–9). This chapter will review the technique for performing cranial sonography, normal brain anatomy, and the many applications of this portable, reliable and comparatively cost-effective imaging modality.

TECHNIQUE AND ANATOMY

Routine US of the brain is performed via the anterior fontanelle which remains patent in fullterm infants until approximately nine to eighteen months of age (1, 2). In premature infants and in those with increased intracranial pressure, this sonic window to the brain may remain open for much longer periods of time. Scanning can also be done via the posterior fontanelle in the coronal, sagittal and/or oblique planes (10). In addition, axial images may be obtained via the squamosal suture, anterolateral or posterolateral fontanelles or through other bone windows in patients with closed fontanelles, who have craniotomy or burr hole defects. The choice of transducer is related to the size of the cranial vault and the intracranial content. In order to maximize resolution and allow for maximum depth penetration, the following guidelines are suggested: 3 MHz frequency for

† With great sadness, love and respect, I dedicate this chapter to the memory of my dear friend and collegue, Nancy H. Sherman, MD.
Henrietta Kotlus Rosenberg, MD

the larger older babies, 5 or 7.0 MHz for the average fullterm infant, 7.5 MHz for the premature infant, and 7.5 or 10 MHz for superficial scalp lesions and to assess the internal content of a meningocele or encephalocele. We utilize a sector scanhead for the grey-scale imaging, a phased array or curvilinear probe for the duplex/color Doppler examinations, and sector or linear transducers for superficial structures (with a step-off if necessary).

In order to obtain images that encompass as much of the intracranial contents as possible, it is necessary to scan the brain in a sequential fashion from anterior to posterior in the coronal plane and then from the midline to the far lateral aspects of the cerebral hemispheres in the sagittal plane (Figure 1). The ventricular system and cerebrospinal fluid spaces are used as references for the identification of the cross-sectional anatomy. Additionally, the con-

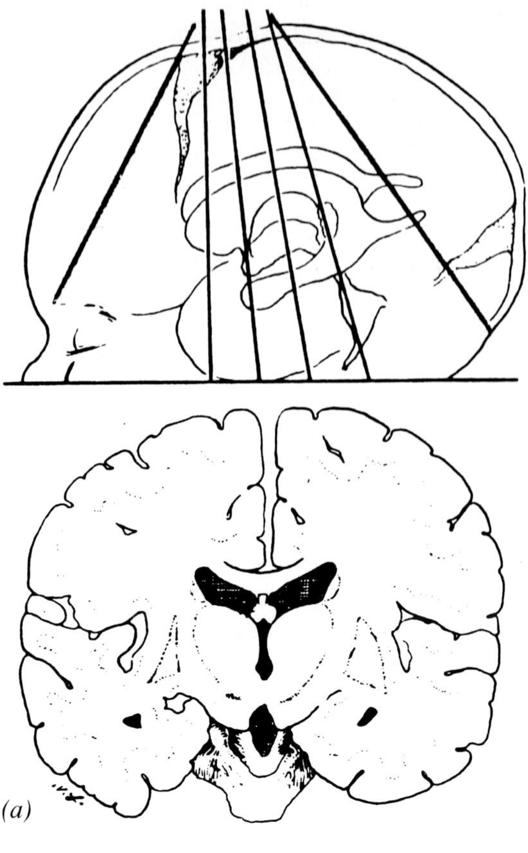

(a)

Figure 1 ***Planes of sonographic sections***
a. Coronal section. The brain is scanned sequentially from anterior to posterior.

vexities of the brain must be imaged as completely as possible with a high frequency probe and by angling the beam as necessary.

A routine protocol for the performance of cranial sonography via the anterior fontanelle is as follows: we survey the entire brain in coronal and sagittal planes and then obtain three sheets of six-on-one hard copy images as well as a brief videotape of bedside examinations when necessary. Image #1 (Figure 2 a) begins with a right parasagittal view of the brain that includes the frontal horns and bodies of the lateral ventricles, as well as the caudothalamic groove, a thin, echogenic band which lies between the slightly more echogenic caudate nucleus anteriorly and the thalamus posteriorly (11). In the premature infant, the highly vascular germinal matrix is found inferolateral to the ependyma lining the floor of the lateral ventricle, anterior and superior to the caudothalamic

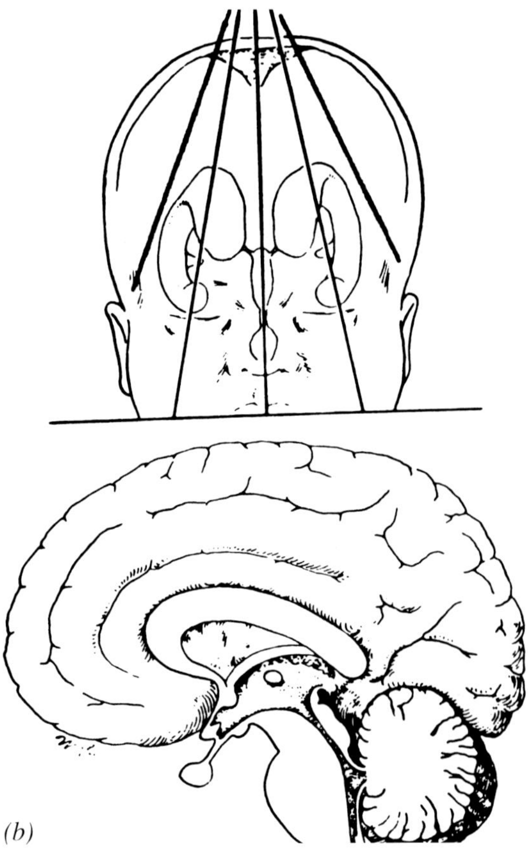

(b)

b. Sagittal section. The brain is scanned in midline (shown here), as well as parasagittal planes.
(Adapted with permission from Slovis et al: Real-time sonography of the brain through the anterior fontanelle. AJR 1981;136:277–286, Figure 1).

roid plexus. The choroid plexus should be a symmetric structure with a smooth, tapered configuration that does not extend into the occipital horn or into the frontal horn anterior to the foramen of Monroe. Clot may become adherent to the choroid plexus, giving it a lumpy, bulbous configuarion. In grade III IVH with ventricular dilatation, the clot is easily detected (Figure 6). With severe hemorrhage, the entire ventricle is filled with blood, forming a cast of the ventricle (1, 25).

As the hemorrhage resolves in both grades II and III IVH, the intraventricular clot gradually decreases in size and echogenicity due to internal liquefaction. The interior of the clot becomes more hypoechoic, surrounded by a densely echogenic clot margin. There is gradual clot retraction away from the ventricular walls. Fragmentation of the clot may occur, resulting in small fragments which move freely within the ventricle. Resorption of clot continues until there is complete clearing. A residual intraventricular septation may persist. Often the ependymal lining of the ventricle becomes brightly echogenic, approximately 7 days after the hemorrhagic event, and usually disappears in about 6 weeks (36).

The ventricular enlargement in grade III IVH is initially due to distention by hemorrhage. As the blood resorbs, ventriculomegaly may resolve spontaneously, persist or progress. Post-hemorrhagic hydrocephalus may result from obstruction of the ventricular sys-

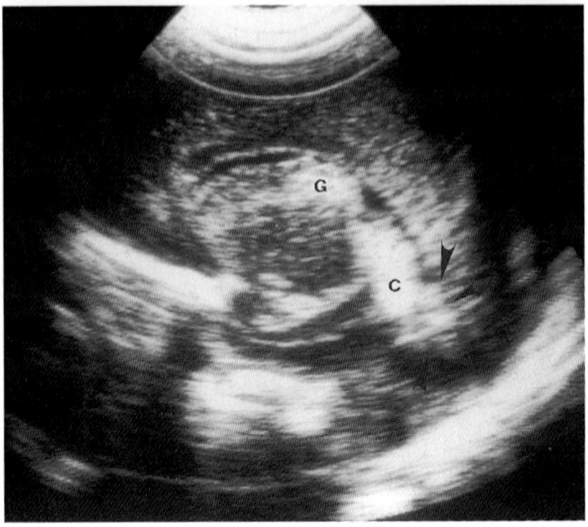

Figure 5
Grade II intraventricular hemorrhage
Sagittal image shows a germinal matrix hemorrhage (G) and an intraventricular hemorrhage within the occipital horn (arrowheads). Note that the lateral ventricle is not dilated. (c = choroid plexus)

tem by clot (usually at the aqueduct). A communicating form of hydrocephalus may develop secondary to arachnoiditis, in which CSF is not resorbed by the arachnoid granulations. An inflammatory ependymitis secondary to the IVH may also result in persistent ventriculomegaly (28). Periodic lumbar puncture or a ventricular shunt may be required to control the hydrocephalus.

Intraparenchymal hemorrhage (IPH) is the most severe grade of ICH in the premature baby. Although IPH was originally believed to be the result of direct extension of IVH into adjacent parenchyma; there is recent work that indicates that it may represent a form of hemorrhagic periventricular infarction (37) (see section on Hypoxic-Ischemic Encephalopathy). As the clot retracts, a porencephalic cyst forms at the site of the originally infarcted hemorrhagic parenchyma, and communicates with the dilated ipsilateral ventricle (Figure 7) (37).

The morbidity and mortality associated with ICH increases with the severity and extent of the hemorrhage. Infants with grades I and II hemorrhage have the same risk for major neurologic damage (12–18 %) as premature infants without hemorrhage (28). There is a markedly increased incidence of major neurologic handicaps in grades III and IV IVH. These include developmental delay, mental retardation, and motor disabilities. A contralateral hemiparesis may result from an IPH (38).

Figure 6
Grade III-A intraventricular hemorrhage
Sagittal sonogram shows an echogenic intraventricular hemorrhage (arrow) within a mildly dilated lateral ventricle.

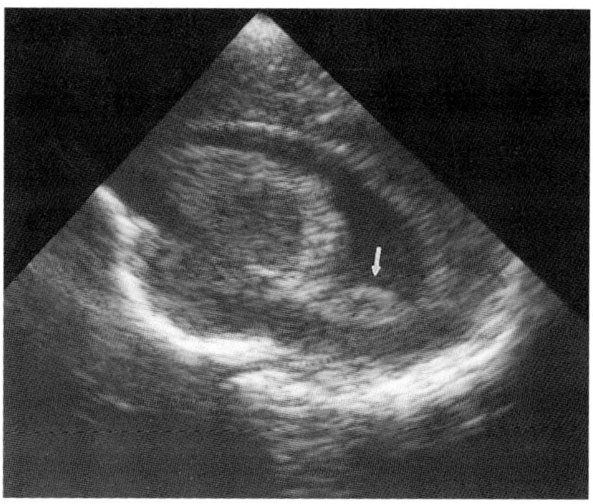

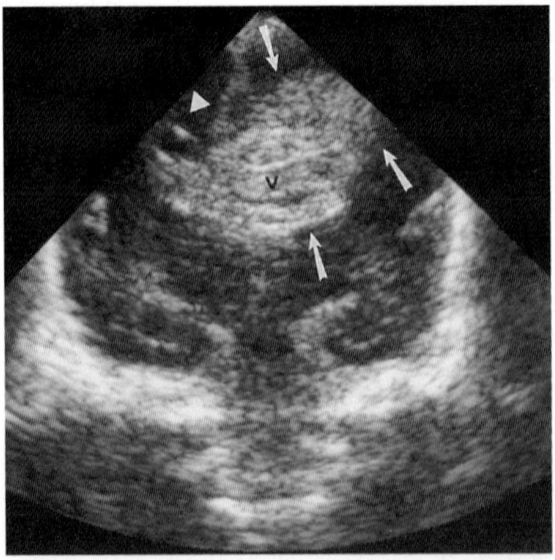

(a)

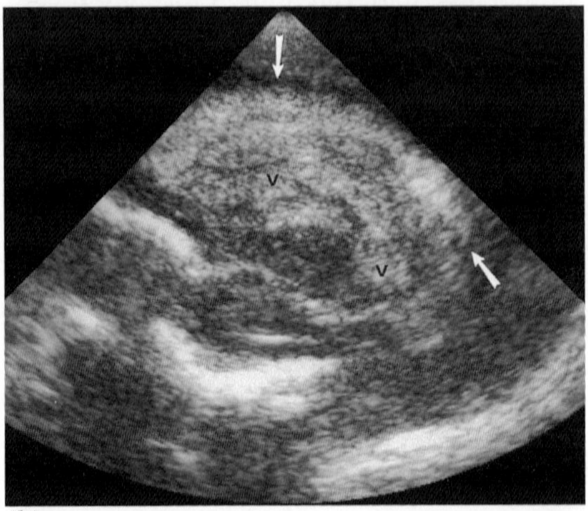

(b)

Figure 7
Intraparenchymal hemorrhage (infarction)
a. Coronal, and
b. left parasagittal sonograms show a large intraparenchymal hemorrhage extending from the frontal to the posterior parietal lobes (arrows). The left lateral ventricle is completely filled with blood (V). Note the mass effect with shift of the interhemispheric fissure to the right on the coronal scan (arrowhead).

Intracranial hemorrhage in the term infant is much less common than in the premature infant. Both GMH and IVH have been reported in term babies. Remnants of the germinal matrix are present at term in the perivascular tissue. Scattered islands of matrix cells may persist in the ventricular wall at term. GMH in the term infant may be clinically asymptomatic. Hayden et al reported that term infants with GMH were usually small for gestational age, vaginally delivered and black (39). IVH in the full-term neonate is thought to arise primarily from the choroid plexus; there is no associated GMH. Etiologic factors associated with ICH in the term

c. Follow-up coronal, and
d. left parasagittal scans show liquefaction of the left intraparenchymal hemorrhagic infarction with a developing porencephalic cyst (P). There is retraction of clot within the frontal lobe and left lateral ventricle and bilateral ventriculomegaly (C = clot)

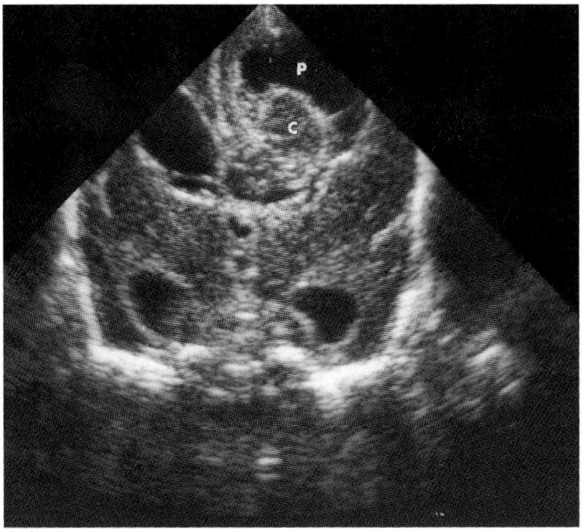

(c)

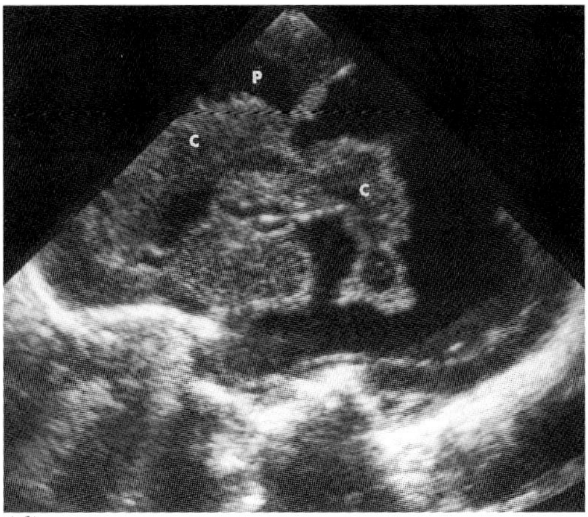

(d)

baby include asphyxia, birth trauma, apnea, seizures and coagulation defects (28).

Other much less common sites of ICH in the neonate are subarachnoid hemorrhage (SAH), intracerebellar hemorrhage, and subdural and epidural hemorrhages (40, 41). Ultrasound is less accurate than CT and MRI in the detection of these types of hemorrhage.

HYPOXIC-ISCHEMIC ENCEPHALOPATHY

Major neurological and developmental deficits in the infant and young child are the result of perinatal hypoxic-ischemic injury to the brain. In the preterm infant, germinal matrix-intraventricular hemorrhage (GMH-IVH) is the most common manifestation of hypoxic brain injury. However, if there is a significant ischemic component to the insult, then infarction may result. Periventricular leukomalacia and periventricular hemorrhagic infarction are the primary manifestations of hypoxic-ischemic encephalopathy (HIE) in the premature infant (42, 43).

Periventricular leukomalacia (PVL) is coagulation necrosis of the deep white matter. This white matter infarction usually occurs at two common sites: the external angle of the frontal horns near the foramen of Monroe, and the level of the optic radiations adjacent to the trigone. The earliest sonographic abnormality in PVL consists of bilateral coarse, globular or broad bands of echodensity in the periventricular white matter (13). This finding usually develops within the first 10 days of life (44, 45, 46). The echodensities may be distributed diffusely in the periventricular white matter or localized along the external angles of the frontal horns and adjacent to the trigone of the lateral ventricles (Figure 8 a, b). PVL is almost always bilateral and symmetrical. Secondary petechial hemorrhages can occur within areas of PVL; this is more common the more premature the infant (43).

The bright periventricular echoes may represent hemorrhagic PVL; US cannot differentiate between the hemorrhagic and non-hemorrhagic forms. Increased periventricular echogenicity is not specific for PVL. This sonographic finding is seen in other types of parenchymal injuries, including white matter gliosis, hemorrhage and cortical infarction which extends into the deep white matter (47). In the evolution of PVL, multiple small cysts develop at the sites of periventricular echodensity (Figure 8 c, d). Cyst formation usually occurs 2–3 weeks after the appearance of the echodensities. The cysts represent areas of necrosis and cavitation. Frequently, the small cavities collapse and disappear on sonography after 1–3 months. White matter gliotic scars develop resulting in decreased cerebral myelin and enlarged ventricles, especially in

Figure 8 ***Periventricular leukomalacia***
a. Sagittal, and
b. coronal scans show bilateral symmetrical triangular bands of echodensity in the white matter adjacent to the frontal horns and trigones (arrowheads)
c. Three weeks later, follow-up sagittal and
d. coronal scans show multiple, small, bilateral cysts in the peritrigonal region (arrows).

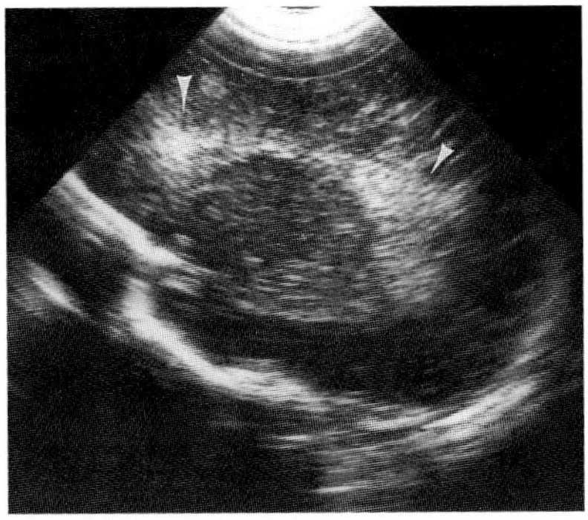

(a)

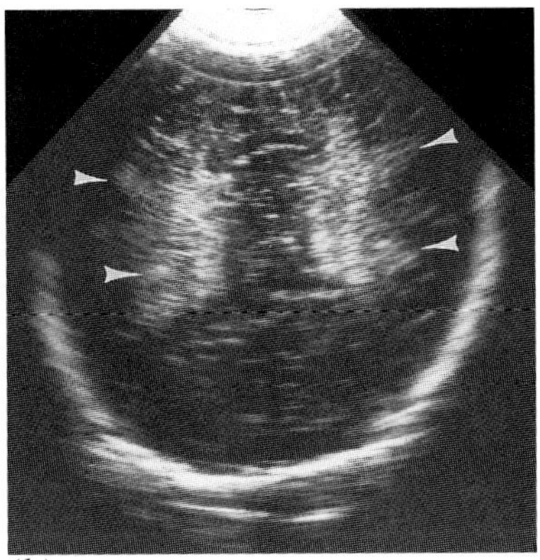

(b)

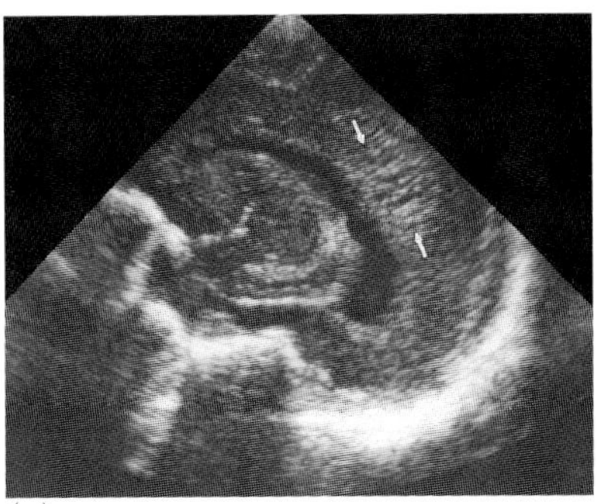

(c)

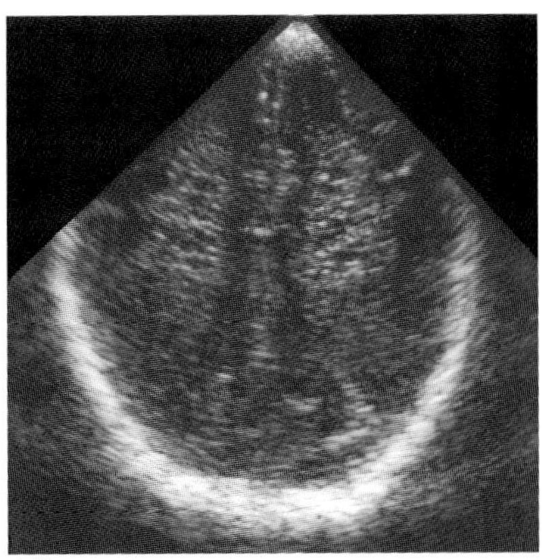

(d)

the region of the trigone and occipital horns. The larger cysts may either resolve or persist and form porencephalic cysts (48).

PVL occurs in approximately 25–40 % of low birth weight preterm neonates. However, only 28 % of lesions are detected in vivo with cranial sonography (43). Although US is more accurate than CT in the detection of periventricular cystic leukomalacia, neither modality is sensitive when compared to neuropathologic series (49, 50).The early detection of PVL is crucial, because PVL is associated with major neurodevelopmental handicaps, in particular cerebral palsy. Spastic diplegia, in which the lower extremities are more affected than the upper extremities, is the most common clinical sequela of PVL. It is the result of necrosis involving the descending fibers from the motor cortex which normally run in the periventricular frontal white matter. With more extensive lesions of PVL, spastic quadriparesis may develop. Severe visual impairment with cortical blindness may result from lesions involving the optic radiations adjacent to the trigone (51, 52, 53). Intellectual deficits are less common but can occur if extensive PVL involves the fibers associated with visual, auditory and somatesthetic functions necessary for learning (Figure 8) (43).

Intraparenchymal hemorrhage (IPH) is a serious sequela of hypoxic-ischemic injury to the brain of the preterm neonate. In most cases, intraparenchymal hemorrhage is associated with germinal matrix and intraventricular hemorrhage. As a result, it was originally thought that intraparenchymal hemorrhage was a direct extension of hemorrhage from the subependymal germinal matrix and/or the ventricle (i.e. grade IV IVH). However, more recent studies have shown that IPH can occur in the absence of IVH; IPH can occur at a site distant from IVH; and IPH can develop 2–10 days after the initial IVH (54, 55). These observations, in conjunction with neuropathologic data, indicate that these intraparenchymal lesions represent areas of hemorrhagic infarction. Volpe uses the term periventricular hemorrhagic infarction (PVHI) to describe this lesion (43).

Periventricular hemorrhagic infarction is an area of hemorrhagic necrosis in the periventricular white matter. It is usually a large, asymmetric lesion that coexists with large IVH in 80 % of the cases. The incidence is highest in very small premature infants. PVHI is most commonly located dorsal and lateral to the external angle

few patients may have significantly impaired cerebral circulation and that this position may aggravate cerebral ischaemia; so if the patient appears to have gone to sleep make sure that he/she is rousable. The patient's chin should be turned a little away from the side being examined so that there is good access, altering the degree of chin rotation may improve visualisation of the bifurcation to some extent during the examination. The examiner sits in the normal position in relation to the patient: that is beside the patient's thorax and scanning "up" towards the neck. Previously it was considered to be advantageous for the examiner to stand above the patient's head and look down towards the patient's feet. This was useful when using continuous wave pencil-type probes as it improved the level of standardisation and reproducibility of the examination but it is not so valuable, or necessary, with modern duplex or colour Doppler equipment.

Technique of examination

The examination begins with a transverse scan of the lower common carotid artery on the right, the transducer is angled inferiorly into the upper mediastinum to visualise the common carotid or innominate artery as far as possible down into the retrosternal region. The transducer is then moved transversely up the neck as far as possible to behind the angle of the mandible. This allows an appreciation of the depth and course of the carotid artery and, importantly, the level and orientation of the bifurcation. Areas of plaques may also be seen and identified for more detailed examination at a later stage.

Colour Doppler is then activated, if available, and the common carotid artery, bifurcation and each branch are surveyed to identify areas of abnormal and normal flow. The transducer is positioned longitudinally and scanning is performed from an antero-lateral approach, although increasingly posterior scan planes may be tried if visualisation is poor, particularly with a high bifurcation. The colour display allows rapid identification of abnormal areas of flow, clearer definition of vessel wall abnormalities – especially hypoechoic plaques and hypoechoic thrombi attached to plaques – and in difficult cases may show the location of the internal and external carotid arteries through a colour signal, even if they cannot be identified on the image. In normal patients representative spectra can be recorded from the CCA 2–3 cm below the bulb, the ICA and the ECA above their origins, ideally 1–2 cm above the bifurcation so that any turbulence has largely settled (Figure 3).

If areas of abnormal flow, or areas of plaques, are identified then careful assessment of these areas must be undertaken using both colour and spectral Doppler in order to assess the severity of the lesion and its likely clinical significance. The criteria used for this assessment will be discussed later in this chapter. Once the right carotid has been examined, the left side is examined in a similar fashion.

After the carotids have been examined attention can be turned to the vertebral arteries. These can usually be identified in the vertebral canal, just lateral to the vertebral bodies and between the transverse processes of the cervical vertebrae. The transducer is aligned longitudinally to show the vertebral bodies, it is then swept laterally until the transverse processes and the gaps between them are seen; the vertebral artery and vein can then be identified within these. Other sites where the vertebral arteries may be identified are in the lower neck as they pass from the subclavian artery towards the cervical spine; or high in the neck behind the mastoid process where they pass around and behind the lateral mass of the atlas.

If colour Doppler is not available then the CCA, bifurcation, ICA and ECA must be examined carefully using spectral Doppler. The sample volume should be set to approximately 2/3 of the total vessel diameter and positioned away from the vessel walls (Figure 3), this will allow a survey of most of the vessel lumen without artefacts from wall motion and the slower peripheral flow confusing the situation. If an abnormal segment of vessel is discovered, the sample volume is reduced to a small size and the relevant segment is interrogated carefully by moving it slowly around the area and listening to the changes in the signal – the human ear is the best spectrum analyser available – so that a picture of the abnormal area is developed in the operator's mind and the optimum position for sample volume placement can be chosen so that the peak systolic velocity can be measured. If the vertebral arteries cannot be located on the image then they may be located by positioning the sample volume in the gap between the transverse processes of the vertebrae and moving the transducer and sample volume by small amounts until the signal is obtained.

ULTRASOUND FINDINGS

A duplex, or colour Doppler examination has two main components: firstly, high resolution imaging, which allows vessels to be located and identified, areas of disease to be imaged and the Doppler sample volume to be positioned in a specific part of a particular vessel. Secondly, Doppler gives information on the blood flow in the vessel. In practice, especially with colour Doppler,

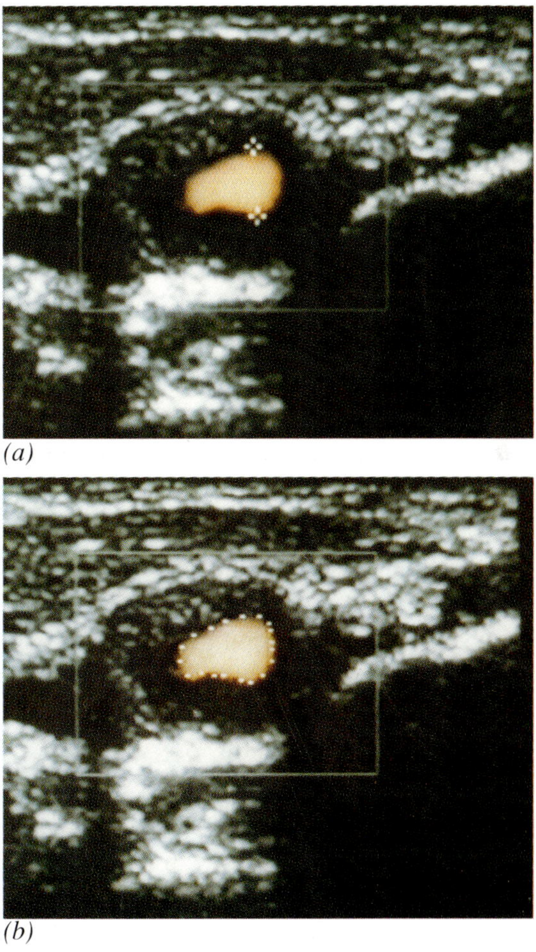

Figure 4 ***Measuring the degree of stenosis***
(a) shows a stenosis of the CCA with the diameter reduction measured by the shortest diameter, resulting in an estimated 56 % diameter stenosis.
(b) shows the same stenosis with the area reduction measured, resulting in an estimated 83 % area stenosis.

these two aspects are assessed simultaneously as the Doppler information is coded in the colour map and displayed together with the imaging information. However, for the purposes of this chapter it is easier to discuss these two components separately, especially in relation to the diagnosis and assessment of atheroma.

High resolution imaging

This provides information on the location and course of the carotids or vertebral arteries, the level of the bifurcation, identification of the carotid branches, areas of disease and their nature, the type and extent of plaque, together with allowing direct measurement of the stenosis and the vessel lumen, if this can be visualised clearly.

Measuring the stenosis

There are two main methods for direct measurement and reporting of the severity of a stenosis: diameter reduction and area reduction (Figure 4). It is important that the sonographer and the recipient of the report of the examination are clearly aware of the method being used, as the numerical values for the same degree of calibre reduction differ significantly: a 50 % diameter reduction is equivalent to a 70 % area reduction. Area reduction measurements are theoretically more precise as they take into account the variations in plaque thickness around the circumference of the vessel but are a little more difficult and time-consuming to perform reliably. Diameter measurements are easier to make but may overestimate, or underestimate overall plaque thickness if they are made at an inappropriate point. It is therefore essential that the vessel is examined transversely, or in several planes if transverse scanning is not feasible, so that the most appropriate diameter reduction is chosen – usually the smallest diameter. As disease becomes more severe it gets increasingly difficult to visualise the stenosis and residual lumen clearly enough to perform an accurate measurement; colour Doppler makes visualisation of the residual lumen easier in some cases but in many cases accurate direct measurement becomes increasingly difficult over 60 % diameter reduction and the assessment of the stenosis must rely on the Doppler wave form changes.

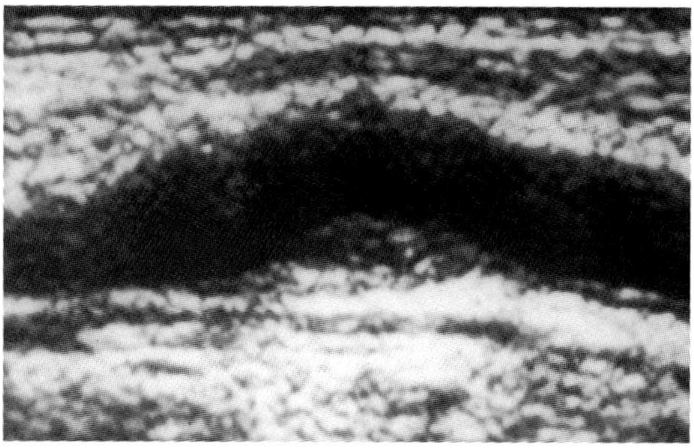

Figure 5
Haemorrhagic plaque
Heterogeneous echoity with areas of anechoity compatible with intra-plaque haemorrhage.

Plaque morphology and characteristics

In many cases of severe disease it is not possible to distinguish plaque details due to the presence of calcification and inadequate visualisation. However, in some cases the plaques can be seen clearly and different types distinguished; in addition, some of the complications of plaque, such as ulceration or thrombus can be diagnosed. Intra-plaque haemorrhage can also be seen as hypoechoic areas within the plaque in a number of cases (18) (Figure 5), although distinction from aggregations of intra-plaque lipid cannot be made with certainty; these heterogeneous plaques are less solid than homogeneous fibrous plaques and are more likely to be associated with symptoms. Steffen and colleagues have categorised plaque appearances into four groups (19); 1/ hypoechoic with a thin rim over the surface (Figure 6); 2/ predominantly hypoechoic but with some more echoic material within it; 3/ predominantly echoic but with some areas of lower echoity within it; 4/ generally

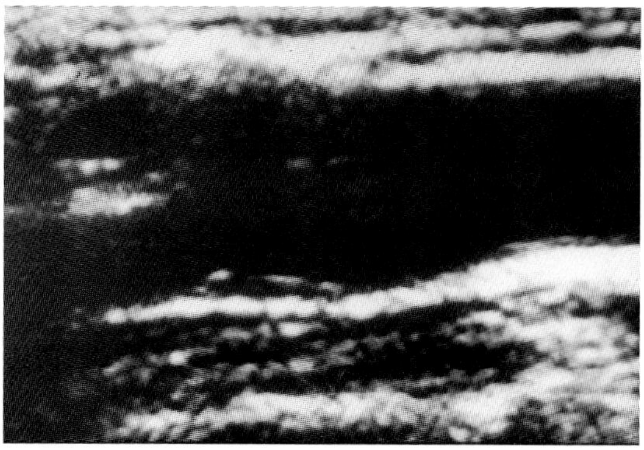

Figure 6
Type 1 plaque
Hypoechoic plaque with a thin echogenic surface.

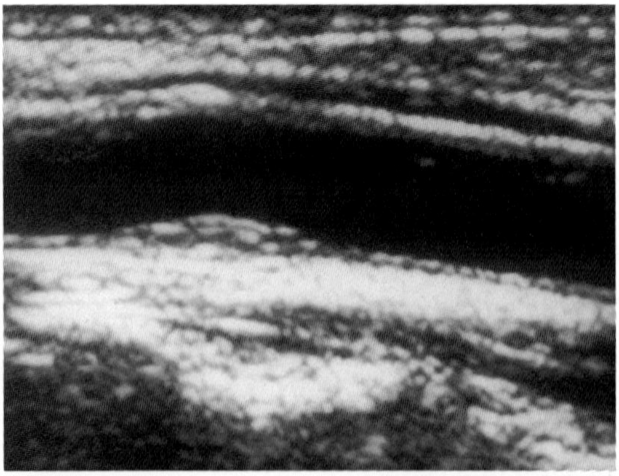

Figure 7
Type 4 plaque
Predominantly hyperechoic plaque with a smooth, intact surface.

echoic (Figure 7). The first two categories have been shown to be associated more frequently with symptoms than the latter two groups and it is suggested that the hypoechoic types correspond to the friable, fragile types of plaque, whereas the more echogenic types are more fibrotic and stable.

In addition, attention should be given to the surface of the plaque as a smooth, intact surface is less likely to be associated with symptoms than an irregular surface which may be associated with uleration and can give rise to small emboli from plaque contents, or small thrombi, even if the plaque is not producing a significant stenosis. Ulceration can be identified in some patients as a defect in the plaque surface, if this can be imaged clearly (Figure 8). However, several pitfalls exist: large ulcers can be missed quite easily, especially in complex plaques with calcification; false positive diagnoses may occur if there are two adjacent plaques and the gap between them is mistaken for an ulcer; surface irregularity can exist

Figure 8
Ulcerated plaque
Circumferential plaque showing a little calcification in its upper (anterior) aspect and a large ulcer crater in the lower (posterior) component.

without ulceration; and complex plaques may have hypoechoic components near the surface which are overlooked and a false impression of irregularity is obtained (1). Care should therefore be taken before making a diagnosis of ulceration.

In many cases, plaque details will not be clearly seen; however, in some cases the plaques will be visualised well enough to allow the operator to comment on whether they are predominantly echogenic with a smooth, well defined surface and therefore likely to be relatively "benign"; or if they are predominantly hypoehcoic with an irregular, possibly ulcerated surface, which would be of greater clinical concern.

Doppler information

The Doppler information is basically very simple. It shows the presence of flowing blood, which way it is flowing, how fast it is flowing, and gives some information on the character of flow – increased diastolic flow, turbulent flow, etc. Colour Doppler represents each of these in the colour map: the presence of a colour signal indicates flow, the colour of the signal indicates the direction of flow, the shade of colour indicates the velocity of the blood and the character of the flow can be indicated, to some extent, by the temporal variation of the colour map; turbulence, or spectral broadening, can be represented in part by variance maps.

Spectral Doppler criteria

Over the years, much work has been done on correlating Doppler findings with degrees of stenosis found on arteriography or at surgery. Moving a small sample volume carefully around the area of disease will allow the operator to build up a mental image of the flow patterns in this area (Figure 9) and, using the audible sound more than the visible spectrum, the point of peak velocity change can be located. Peak systolic velocity, end diastolic velocity and the ratio of peak systolic velocities in the internal and common carotid arteries (IC/CC systolic ratio) are the most useful in routine practice (20). Spectral broadening and filling in of the window under the spectrum are subjective, difficult to quantify and can be af-

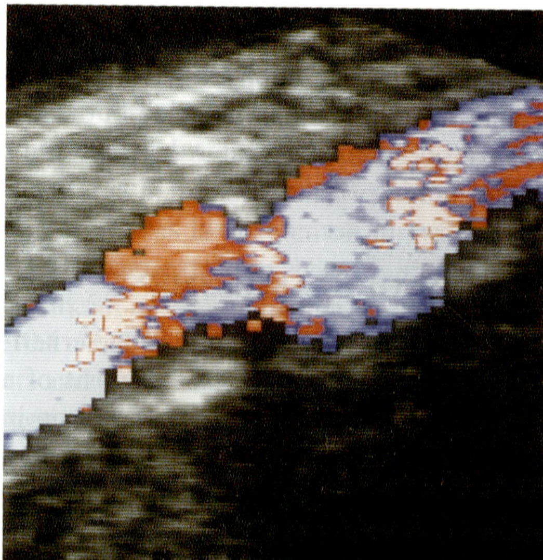

Figure 3 *A longitudinal sonogram of a brachial artery shows turbulence and irregularity, a result of emboli from a mycotic aneurysm more proximal (out of field of view).*

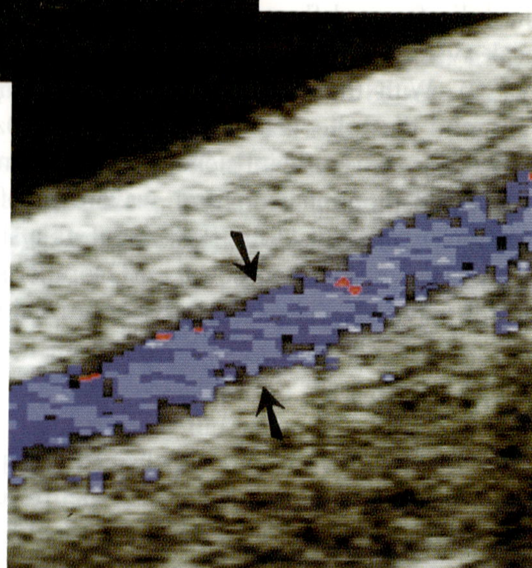

Figure 4 *A longitudinal sonogram shows a greater saphenous vein prior to harvest for a vascular graft (color photographed in black and white).*

ANEURYSMS

Peripheral aneurysms or pseudoaneurysms are followed by ultrasound to determine the size and extent, delineate the presence of mural thrombus and the caliber of the patent channel, as well as determine the relationship of the mass produced to adjacent structures, define associated problems such as dissection or leakage, and detect the presence of adjacent abnormality, such as adenopathy or fluid (26).

Suspected dissection or occlusion are other indications for vascular sonographic studies. Assessment of intraoperative vascular repair is an expanding application (27), as is the evaluation of the results of angioplasty, particularly as a baseline for future developments.

Peripheral aneurysms are not nearly as common as aortic aneurysms, and lower extremity aneurysms far exceed those of the upper extremity (28, 29). Predominantly atherosclerotic and frequently multiple, these aneurysms are usually surgically corrected when the diagnosis is made, because of the inherent risk of thrombosis, distal

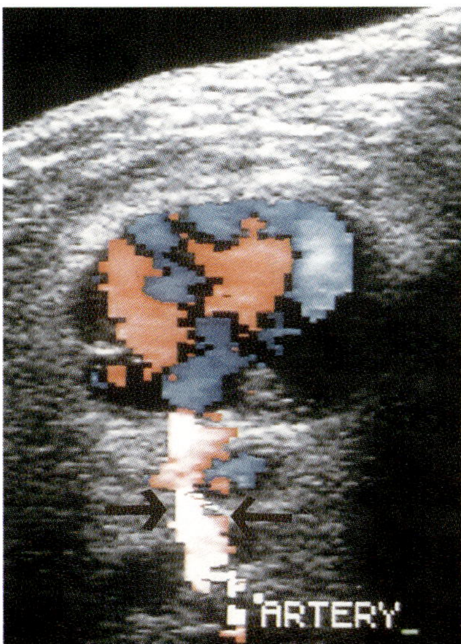

(a)

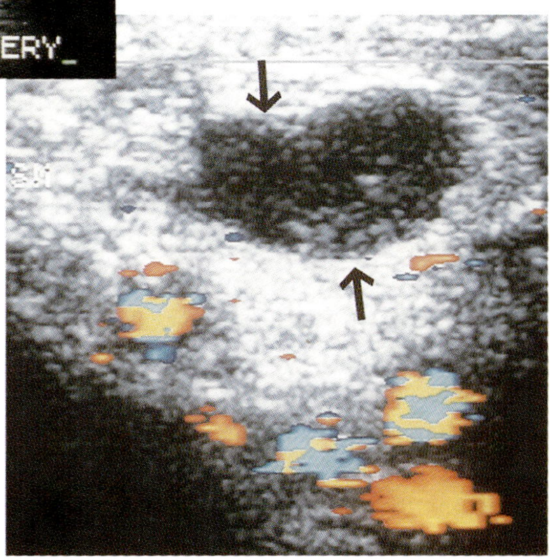

(b)

Figure 5
a. A transverse sonogram shows a false aneurysm of the common femoral artery with a narrow stalk (arrows).
b. Following transducer pressure, the false aneurysm in a. has been converted to a hematoma (arrows).

embolization, and inexorable expansion with the risk of rupture or compression of adjacent veins causing passive congestion.

Popliteal aneurysms are the most common peripheral aneurysms and, in combination with femoral aneurysms, represent the great majority (30). Usually an atherosclerotic disease of elderly males and bilateral in 70 % (30) popliteal aneurysms are frequently associated with symptoms of limb ischemia and may compress adjacent nerves and veins. Thrombosis leads to embolization and limb ischemia. Rupture is infrequent.

Approximately 28 % of those with femoral aneurysms, will have an aortic aneurysm (31), while bilateral popliteal aneurysms, have an association with an aortic aneurysm in nearly two thirds of the cases (32).

Pseudoaneurysms may result from arterial puncture or other trauma and while duplex Doppler is the study of choice to define these lesions, it is not always possible to make a clear distinction between a false and a true aneurysm, since both will have a focal expansion, as well as a turbulent holosystolic arterial waveform (33). Traumatic pseudoaneurysms can be treated successfully in about 70 % simply by isolated compression of the aneurysm, by the ultrasound transducer to eliminate flow while maintaining native vessel flow (Figure 5) (34).

Anastomotic aneurysms occur at the junction between the vascular graft and the host artery (Figure 6). By classification, these are false aneurysms or pulsating communicating hematomas, encapsulated in a fibrous sac, not the expansion of the intima, media and adventitia of the true aneurysm (35). As such, they may rupture, be a source of distal emboli, or thrombose. They originate from a number of different causes, including local infection or communicating hemorrhage, suture failure, or inadequate surgical technique. By color Doppler, a typical pattern of swirling, turbulent flow in a mosaic of colors occurs, connected by a wide neck to the anastomotic site (35).

Upper extremity aneurysms are more likely to be traumatic, rather than atherosclerotic, particularly since needle perforations of the arteries are more common in the arm for access to arterial blood gas determinations. More proximally, the subclavian artery aneurysm is also the exception to an atherosclerotic origin, being primarily related to thoracic outlet disease, usually a result of post-stenotic dilatation from a cervical rib. Mycotic aneurysms, of the peripheral vascular system are rare.

Both axillary artery and radial artery aneurysms are usually related to either blunt or penetrating trauma (36).

HEMATOMA, ADENOPATHY, ARTERIOVENOUS (AV) FISTULA

Hematomas are common following percutaneous transfemoral catheterization (PTC), seen by sonography as adjacent hypoechoic or anechoic fluid collections in the groin. Hematoma and adenopathy must be differentiated from false aneurysm, which communicate with the femoral artery. By color, false aneurysms produce a swirling, turbulent mosaic of color extraneous to the native vessel unless the aneurysms are thrombosed. The spectral waveform of the typical aneurysm is that of holosystolic flow. This pattern is distinctly different from the blood flow of adenopathy, in which case a single hilar vessel branches into an oval hypoechoic, well-circumscribed mass, the node (37). Adenopathy is commonly noted in the inguinal area.

Iatrogenic arterio-venous fistula is a rare complication of percutaneous transfemoral catheterization (38, 39) and rather than the typical triphasic flow of a peripheral vessel produces prominent continuous systolic, diastolic arterial flow, and abnormal venous flow patterns. Another sign of arterio-venous fistula is a bleeding of a mosaic of color beyond the expected vessel boundaries related to turbulent flow (40). Peripheral aneurysms that rupture can form spontaneous A-V fistulae (41).

POPLITEAL DISEASE

Soft tissue tumors of peripheral vessels are rare, although leiomyosarcoma of the popliteal vessels has been reported (42).

Popliteal entrapment is a disease of young men who present with unilateral calf claudication (43). A clinical clue is that the dorsalis pedis pulse disappears with dorsiflexion on the affected side. It is caused by compression of the medial head of the gastrocnemius

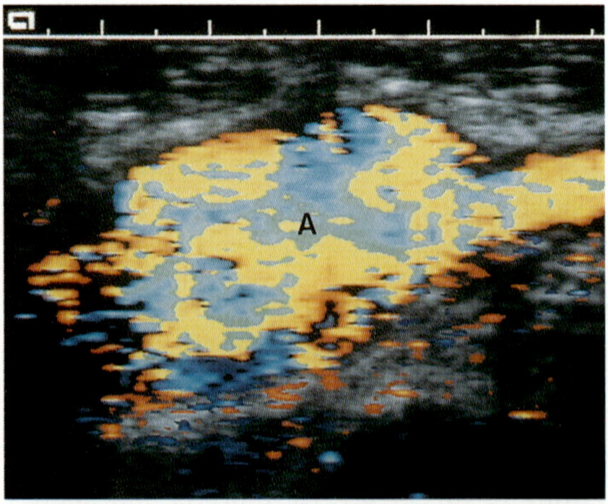

Figure 6 *A longitudinal sonogram shows a distal turbulent anastomotic aneurysm (a) of an aorto-femoral graft.*

which has a tendinuous insertion point on the condyle of the femur more lateral than normal, a condition that leads to stenosis and eventually thrombosis of the popliteal artery from compression. Duplex sonography can be used to define the velocity of flow in the popliteal artery, as well as its morphologic configuration. With color coding, areas of stenosis present with high velocity flow, often white in color, in contradistinction to the normal red flow.

Another disease peculiar to the popliteal artery is adventitial cystic disease. In these cases, the lumen of the vessel is compromised by the gelatinous material laid down in the subadventitia (44) seen by sonography as focal areas of circumferential hypoechoicity (45).

GRAFTS

Infrainguinal bypass grafting is the surgical treatment of choice for incapacitating claudication or limb threatening ischemia in the treatment of peripheral vascular disease of the lower extremity. The procedure has been fine-tuned since the first autologous vein transplant in man was performed by Goyannes in 1906, yet significant problems in maintenance of graft patency remain. Clinical evaluation of the graft cannot define morphological abnormalities nor can such an evaluation assess the character of flow. Rather, physical assessment is limited to the appearance of the wound, the presence of mass effect, the detection of pulsation or its absence.

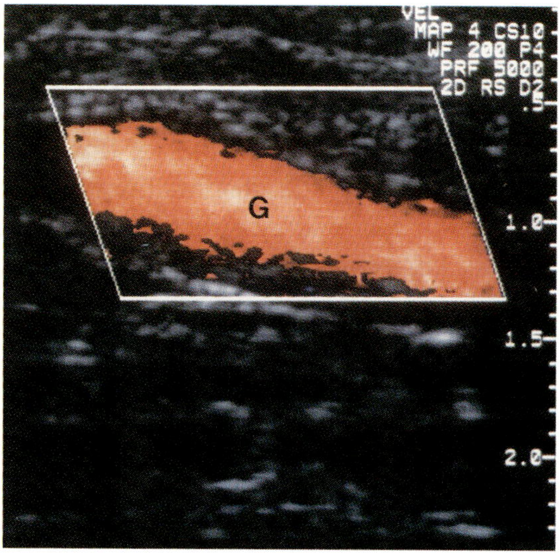

Figure 7 *A longitudinal sonogram of an in situ saphenous graft (G) shows normal flow in the distal calf portion.*

Graft thrombosis and thromboembolic complications are of major importance, as is the specter of graft infection, perioperative hemorrhage that can compromise patency when compressive, anastomotic aneurysms, stenoses, arteriovenous shunts, dissection, and low flow states, all of which are amenable to sonographic detection using duplex and color Doppler.

Peripheral vascular grafts are routinely followed by ultrasound at 1, 3, 6, 9, and 12 months following implantation (Figures 7, 8). When critical stenosis, low flow state, retained venous valve or other abnormality is noted, the next confirmatory step is angiography followed by therapeutic angioplasty when indicated.

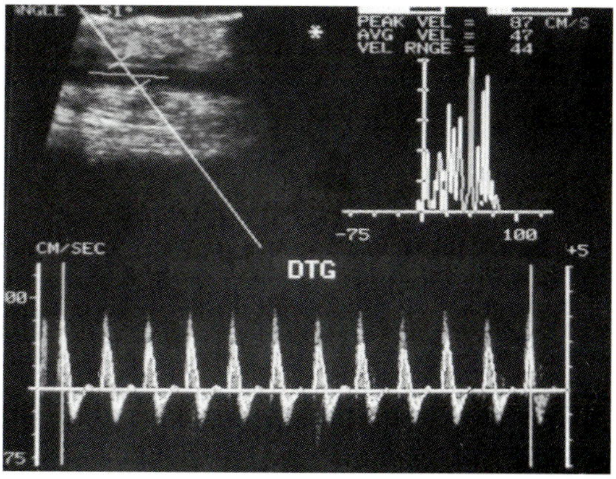

Figure 8 *A longitudinal sonogram of an in situ saphenous graft at the distal thigh shows normal velocity and triphasic flow.*

Lower extremity grafts are superficial. Sonography has excellent near field of view. Grafts have variations in flow. Color and duplex Doppler, using both image and spectral analysis, can be used to evaluate the velocities of flow within the graft and to define the morphologic abnormalities that account for those variations. With sonography, structures can be resolved in two or more planes. Adjacent soft tissues can be assessed. The study is painless, risk free in adults as far as can be determined at this time, time efficient, and has potential to delineate many of the problems inherent in peripheral graft complications. Color Doppler imaging further increases the accuracy of the technique.

Angiography is used to assess the internal lumen of the graft and define in exquisite detail the fine arterial vasculature of the run-off. The procedure is not without risk, not only because of the risk of contrast reactions which occasionally occur, but also for such complications as dissection, false aneurysm, and vascular spasm. The procedure can be uncomfortable, is associated with a significant radiation dose, and is expensive.

Sonography in the study of grafts serves as a noninvasive way to follow the graft to detect low flow (which is an indicator of potential graft failure), irregular cardiac rhythm, focal stenoses (Figure 9), arteriovenous shunting, adjacent fluid (Figure 10) or mass, or confirm occlusion (46–50).

The principal vascular abnormalities that ultrasound is used to detect are: 1/ anastomotic aneurysms (Figure 6); 2/ graft stenosis or native proximal or distal stenosis; 3/ diminished flow from poor runoff or stenosis (Figures 7, 11, 12); 4/ elevated flow such as in focal AV-fistula (Figure 13); 5/ anatomic problems (dissection, venous valve retention) (Figures 14, 15); or 6/ occlusion (Figure 16).

Technique of examination of lower extremity grafts

Grafts are examined by sonography in both transverse and longitudinal planes from the proximal anastomosis at regular intervals down to the distal anastomosis. Included in the study are the proximal and distal native arteries to detect inflow and egress abnormalities.

The longest grafts of the lower extremity extend from the common femoral artery to the dorsalis pedis artery in the foot. With color and duplex scanning, periodic velocity waveforms are taken along the course. Both images and spectral data are recorded at specific regular sites along the graft, e.g., the proximal anastomosis, the mid thigh, the distal thigh, the popliteal fossa, the proximal calf, the mid calf, the distal leg, and the anastomosis at the foot. Without color coded imaging, it is possible to miss a focal area of stenoses because of a failure to sample at the site. With color coding, abnormalities of flow are immediately apparent.

Based on a prospective study of 263 graft examinations over two years using duplex Doppler certain characteristics of the flow are apparent (14). The femoral artery in general has a higher peak systolic velocity than the average PSV of most grafts. The mean peak systolic velocity of the graft tends to diminish over time. Focal fluid collections in the soft tissues adjacent to the graft are common, but usually resolve uneventfully over months. Arteriovenous shunting is associated with a normal peak systolic velocity, a markedly elevated diastole and a large increase in estimated flow. Color images can show the actual branch. Normal peak systolic velocity and elevated diastole flow throughout the length of the graft suggest relative hyperemia in the first weeks post implantation (Figure 17). Stenosis presents gradations of elevation of peak systolic velocity, or with pre-occlusion, low peak systolic velocity with no diastolic flow.

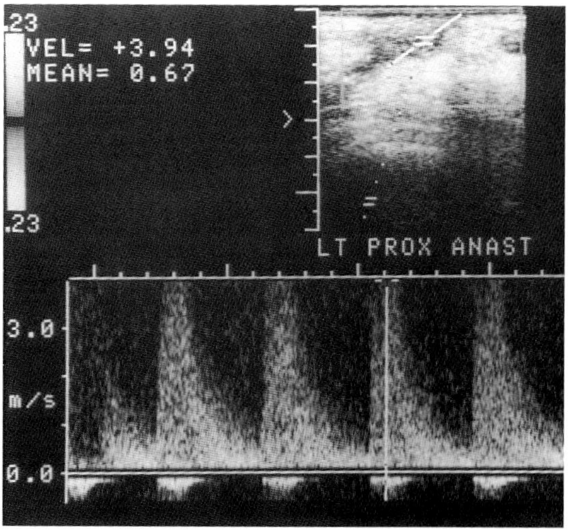

Figure 9 *A longitudinal sonogram of a proximal graft shows a high grade stenosis with a peak systolic velocity of 394 cm/sec and an end diastolic velocity of 67 cm/sec.*

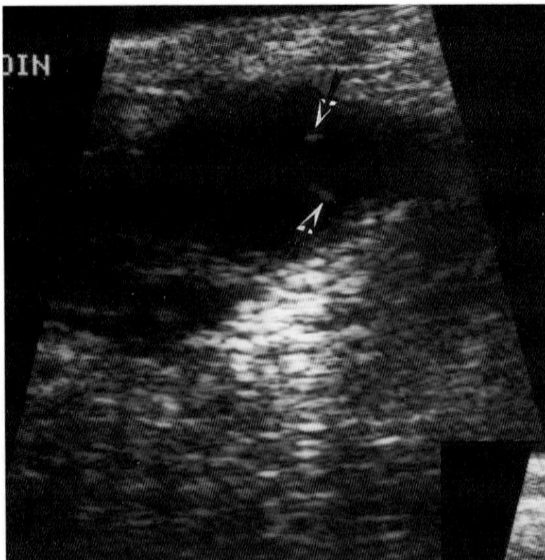

Figure 15 *A longitudinal sonogram demonstrates retained venous valves in the proximal graft anastomosis with the common femoral artery.*

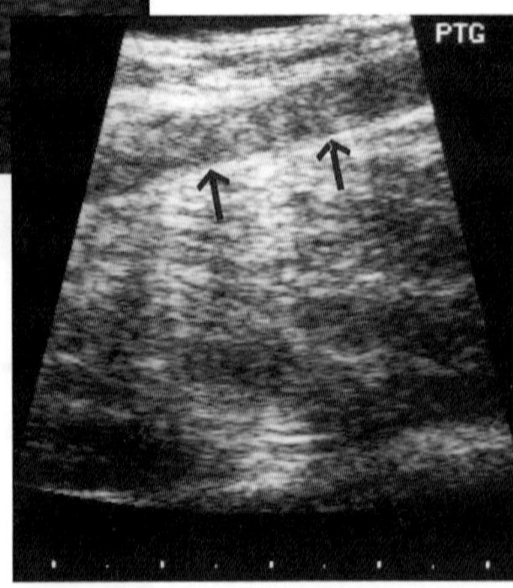

Figure 16 *A longitudinal sonogram of a proximal thigh graft shows complete occlusion (arrows).*

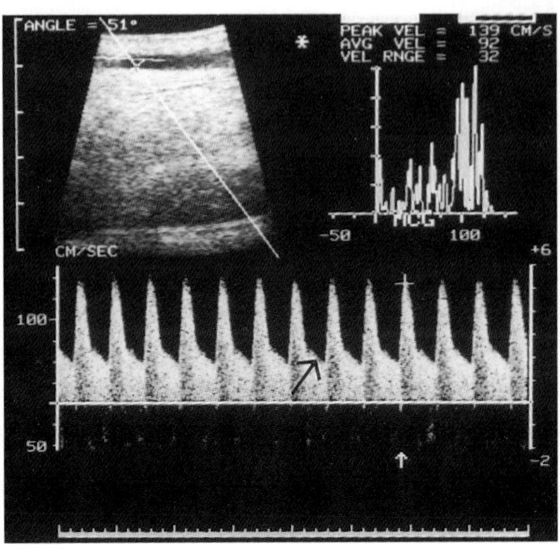

Figure 17 *A longitudinal sonogram of an in situ saphenous graft shows mild elevation of peak systolic velocity but marked elevation of diastolic flow (arrow). If focal, this could be from an AV-fistula. If the marked diastolic elevation is throughout the graft, it could be related to reactive hyperemia following recent graft implantation, and, if so, would be expected to resolve in about 6 weeks.*

Complications of graft therapy

Aneurysms

Unless trauma has disrupted the continuity of the channel, grafts rarely develop aneurysms, except at the anastomosis, the most common site being the femoral anastomosis below the inguinal ligament. The overall incidence of anastomotic aneurysms is low (1–4 %) (51), but these aneurysms are important clinically because of a propensity to expand progressively. These aneurysms can rupture, thrombose, or embolize. Sonography is quite accurate in the diagnosis and is used to differentiate actual aneurysms from adjacent masses, usually fluid collections, such as hematoma.

Adjacent fluid

Adjacent fluid collections are commonly seen following graft implantation occurring in about 30 % of patients during routine follow-up; they tend to disappear without consequence over the first few months, although large collections may take longer to resolve (52). Perigraft fluid may be related to hematoma, seroma, abscess, or even lymphocele (Figure 10) (53).

Low flow

Low flow, below an average peak systole of 40 cm/sec throughout the graft, and absent diastolic flow is an indicator of potential graft failure (54, 55, 56). This may be related to progressive atherosclerosis in the runoff vasculature or intimal hyperplasia which is particularly common distally and reduces the luminal diameter leading to focal stenosis.

Graft stenosis

In postoperative surveillance of bypass grafts for stenosis, color coded sonography has a distinct advantage in that altered flow dynamics can be immediately recognized and these focal areas can then be examined in detail with both image and spectral analysis (Figures 7, 8) (57, 58, 59). Areas of stenosis should be examined at the site of greatest narrowing as well as proximally and distally with docu-

Graft survival

The best results occur in aorto-bifemoral grafts with a 5-year patency rate of 91 % (66). For infrainguinal grafts, in one study the primary patency rate at the first year was about 81 % (50) and 66 % by the fifth year. In that study, if intervention occurred, the secondary cumulative patency rate was 91 % at one year and 80 % at 5 years (50). The greater the number of patent calf arteries and patent pedal arteries, the greater likelihood of a better prognosis for femoropopliteal grafts and femorodistal grafts, particularly if the patient can be convinced to stop smoking (65, 67, 68, 69).

In situ saphenous vein for bypass

In infra-inguinal bypass vascular grafts, the in situ saphenous vein is the frequent choice for the arterial conduit (Figure 3) (70). The vein is autologous, it tapers appropriately, courses in the superficial tissues with easy access and in the case of the greater saphenous, extends the length of the medial leg, allowing revascularization of the arteries of the distal leg and foot. The requirements for harvesting are a non-diseased vessel, at least 2.5 mm in diameter distally, with adequate inflow and egress (71).

Limitations that preclude in situ veins use are a diseased vessel from prior venous thrombosis, a short or narrow vessel, or congenital absence. Once in place, in situ saphenous bypass grafts are subject to problems related to retained venous valves and residual A-V fistulae (71). The former causes stenosis, the latter shunting of flow from arterial graft to vein.

Preoperative mapping of the superficial saphenous veins enables the surgeon to know whether or not these veins are intact and anatomically acceptable, and allows recognitition of anatomic variation in size or location (72–75). Once the vein has been mapped sonographically, the surgeon prepares the site, removes the venous valves with a valvulotome, interrupts the branches to prevent arteriovenous fistulae, and mobilizes the ends for anastomosis to the arteries of choice.

17. Carter SA. Res
and questionab
18. Whelan FF, Ba
comparison wi
ripheral arterial
19. May AG, DeW
sis. Surgery 19
20. Nicholls SC, K
of arterial sten
21. Kohler TR, Ni
dient by Doppl
Vasc Surg 198
22. Moneta GL, Ye
rial occlusive d
duplex mappin
23. Sacks D, Robir
ultrasonograph
24. Leng GC, Why
of duplex ultra
Surg 1993;17:5
25. Pathria MN, Zl
teal fossa and l
26. Liu JB, Merton
iliofemoral reg
27. Sigel B. Opera
Press, 1988, pp
28. Gooding GAW
AJR 1980;134:
29. Gooding GAW.
teries. Sem Ult
30. Evans WE, Ha
EB (ed): Vascu
Saunders, 1989
31. Pappas G, Jane
surgical manag
32. Evans WE,
1976;10:86–91
33. Coughlin BF,
with duplex US
34. Cox GS, Young
pair of postcat
hundred cases.
35. Polak JF, Dona
rounding vascu
ogy 1989;170:

Saphenous vein mapping technique

The saphenous veins are two superficial veins of the leg: the greater and the lesser. The greater, or long saphenous vein, extends from the medial foot anterior to the ankle along the length of the medial leg to empty into the common femoral vein about 3 cm below the inguinal ligament. The lesser saphenous vein begins behind the lateral malleolus of the ankle and empties in the midline posteriorly in the upper calf into the popliteal vein. Both are just under the skin, actually about 1 cm below the skin surface, and are therefore very sensitive to the pressure of the transducer and require a light touch to visualize them. In the lower leg, dependency of the legs accentuates venous filling and therefore venous visualization is enhanced by the effect of gravity.

The superficial veins are marked, with a colored pen and any valves or venous perforators are noted. The veins are mapped and the length of the veins measured so the surgeon knows how much material he/she has to use. The normal saphenous vein suitable for harvesting is 3–4 mm in AP diameter (72, 76). Variations are common. Duplications occur. Irregularities may result from prior venous thrombosis with recanalization.

With intraoperative ultrasound, the saphenous vein can be tracked once again and expeditiously prepared for conversion to arterial conduit (76). If the saphenous veins have been previously harvested, the lateral cephalic vein and the medial basilic vein in the upper extremity may be used, noted sonographically in the superficial soft tissue of the upper arm.

SUBCLAVIAN ARTERY AND VEIN

The normal subclavian artery and vein run parallel to the clavicle along the top of the apex of the lung and by sonography can be traced from the xiphoid, where the bone obscures, to the axilla. The artery is triphasic on spectral analysis (Figure 1). The subclavian artery is associated with an artifact peculiar to its position at the lung apex. A color flow image of the subclavian artery curiously produces in some instances a mirror image artifact of the vessel immediately posterior to the real vessel complete with color and spectral data.

In the sonographic examination of veins of the lower extremity, the patient lies supine initially, rotated slightly toward the side being examined with the leg modestly abducted and externally rotated (15). Some examiners advocate tilting the gurney 25–30° (21) so that the lower extremities are lower than the body (reverse Trendelenburg), others examine the patient without a table tilt. Care is taken to remove any tightly restrictive clothing from the abdomen.

In the supine position, the iliac veins are examined with 3 to 5 MHz transducers while the common femoral, the superficial and deep femoral and the proximal saphenous veins are examined with 5 to 7.5 MHz transducers depending on the venous depth from the surface. The greater saphenous vein, which runs medially from the ankle to empty into the common femoral vein is quite superficial, usually just a centimeter or so beneath the skin surface, so a light touch with the transducer is required to prevent collapsing the vessel which is only a few mm in diameter and very susceptible to collapse from inordinate transducer pressure on the skin.

Thereafter, in lateral or prone position, the popliteal veins are identified. If the calf veins are to be included, the patient may be supine, tilted in reverse Trendelenburg, or sat upright on the side of the bed with the legs over the side to take advantage of gravity, to make the paired calf veins more apparent. Beginning either at the proximal trifurcation from the popliteal vein or distally at the ankle, the posterior tibial, peroneal and anterior tibial veins are traced along the course of the similarly named artery in their entirety.

Not all examiners extend the sonographic examinations to include the calf since many clinicians do not treat calf vein thrombosis with anticoagulants. These veins are small and thrombus there is not considered life threatening until propagation into the popliteal vein and beyond occurs.

An examination of the calf is best obtained with color coded Doppler imaging because visualization is easier, yet the examination in these areas is tedious and time consuming. The anterior tibial veins are best seen with the transducer placed in a longitudinal position along the anterior lower leg lateral to the tibial protuberance. The posterior tibial and peroneal veins are seen with the transducer placed medially on the lower leg. In this position, the peroneal veins are the more posterior.

Non-visualized portions of a particular calf vein engender uncertainty about whether the nonvisualization is technical, a variant, or actual thrombus. However, marked involvement of multiple calf veins with thrombus can be strikingly positive. Overall, accuracy for the diagnosis of DVT in the calf is excellent (98 %), but diminishes to 57 % with technically limited studies which can occur in 40 % (15).

EQUIPMENT

The ideal tool for venous assessment is a linear array transducer, with duplex and color Doppler capability. In the abdomen, visualization of the inferior vena cava and iliac veins may require a sector 3.5 MHz transducer to penetrate appropriately, although a 5 MHz transducer suffices in thin patients. In the leg, the veins are relatively superficial and dependent upon depth from the surface, so 5 to 7.5 MHz transducers are usually sufficient.

A linear array transducer has an oblong shape ideal for tracing the veins along their length in a near field of view. The veins of the leg are examined bilaterally in both transverse and longitudinal planes with compression done in transverse position for better accuracy (21).

Sector transducers have the capability of visualizing peripheral veins, but the near field is shallow, so only small segments can be identified at any one time.

Doppler spectral analysis substantiates the venous signal and defines the response to respiration, augmentation, and Valsalva maneuver.

Color Doppler is complimentary to compression sonography (22) and is the only practical way to examine the calf veins expeditiously (8). Anatomic variations are easier to identify with color. If the venous system is totally occluded, no color in the lumen is noted, but color Doppler is particularly well suited to defining partial thrombus and venous collateralization.

PATHOLOGY

The clinical diagnosis of DVT is inaccurate. The process may be silent and unsuspected, or present initially with pulmonary embolus (PE), or develop with focal localized signs and symptoms in the calf.

The major risks for the development of DVT are significant trauma (23), coagulopathy, prolonged surgery (especially surgery of the lower extremities and surgical procedures for cancer), extended periods of bed rest, marked obesity, pregnancy, and prior thromboembolism. External compression can also be a factor.

Pregnancy tends to be associated with ilio-femoral thrombosis, particularly on the left (24). Ovarian vein thrombosis is another peripheral complication of pregnancy (25).

Those at high risk for deep venous thrombosis include patients with acute hip fractures. Often elderly, immobilized, with local swelling and edema, these patients develop pulmonary emboli as the major complication (26).

Orthopedic procedures of the hip and lower extremity evoke susceptibility to deep venous thrombosis (26, 27).

Because of the propensity to develop DVT after surgery, ultrasound has gained acceptance as a surveillance tool in the perioperative period (28).

A young person having minor surgery has a negligible risk of either deep venous thrombosis (DVT) or pulmonary embolism (PE). For a middle-aged person with a more complicated surgical procedure the risk of DVT increases (10–40 %), but PE is still unlikely (0.1-0.4 %) (29). An elderly person who undergoes prolonged surgery has a 40–70 % risk of DVT and a significant chance, 1–5 % of developing pulmonary embolus. It is in this latter group that ultrasound can be particularly effective in distinguishing normal from abnormal veins. Also, the technique lends itself not only to portable bedside examinations, but also to repeated examinations in follow-up of regression or extension after therapy has begun.

DIAGNOSIS OF DEEP VENOUS THROMBOSIS

Loss of venous compression following transducer pressure is the hallmark of peripheral deep venous thrombosis (Figures 3, 5).

The advantages of color in the diagnosis of DVT is the capability to see small veins, and recognize collaterals and to see the visual effects of gravity, augmentation, compression and Valsalva (22).

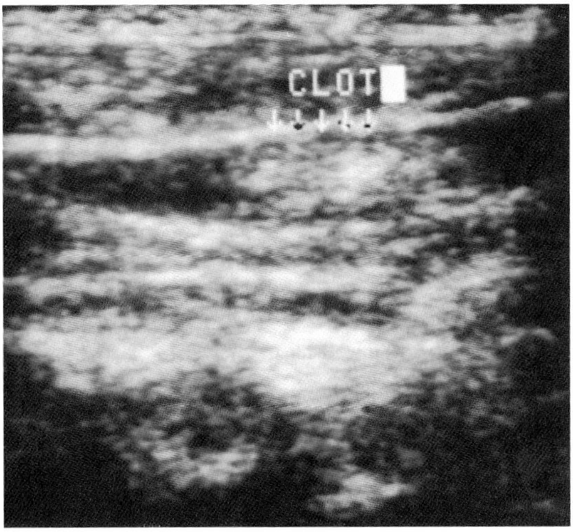

Figure 5 *A longitudinal sonogram of the superficial vein demonstrates an echogenic thrombus that fails to be compressed by the transducer indicating the presence of deep venous thrombosis (arrows).*

The accuracy of diagnoses of deep venous thrombosis using color coding is approximately 99 % above the kncc. In those technically adequate below the knee (60 %), the accuracy of color sonography was, in one study, 81 % below the knee (15).

Proximal venous obstruction whether from intrinsic thrombus or external compression causes distal loss of venous phasicity (Figure 6).

Iliac vein occlusion or compression has an indirect effect on the more distal veins. Respiratory phasicity is lost distally and the response to a Valsalva maneuver is damped in the distal external iliac and common femoral veins.

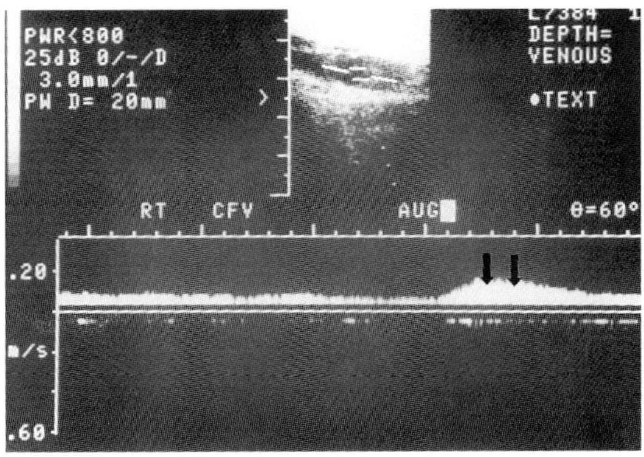

Figure 6 *A longitudinal sonogram of the right common femoral vein shows an abnormal loss of phasic flow on spectral analysis and a dampened augmentation response (arrows) consistent with deep venous thrombosis. Lack of phasicity suggests proximal venous disease and depressed augmentation suggests disease distally.*

The thrombotic process is hypothesized to develop at the site of the venous valve cusp and extend from there. Thrombus may be completely occlusive or partial. Complete venous occlusion is characterized by a spectrum of findings sonographically (30, 31). The vein loses its venous Doppler signal. It fails to respond to any respiratory maneuvers or to augmentation. Although actual luminal thrombus may or may not be seen, the hallmark of occlusion is a failure of the vein to compress after transducer pressure is applied to it (32). With color Doppler no color is evident in the venous lumen, although significant venous collateralization may be evident.

The deep veins of the lower leg have an adjacent artery that should be documented as present. This will prevent mistaking a patent collateral vein which does not have an artery adjacent to it, for an occluded deep vein.

The thrombosed vein may or may not be enlarged. Focal enlargement of the affected vein suggests an acute process (33). The thrombosis may be focal, e.g. at the junction of the greater saphenous vein and the common femoral vein or at the adductor canal, or be diffuse, involving a significant portion of the ilio-femoral system, either unilaterally or bilaterally.

The response to a Valsalva maneuver is an adjunctive measure of venous dynamics. The normal expansion of the common femoral vein in response to a Valsalva maneuver is related to the sudden increase in intra-abdominal pressure which effectively results in cessation of venous inflow into the abdomen. This is graphically depicted with color Doppler imaging; at rest, the normal common femoral vein is blue. With a Valsalva maneuver, the same vein rapidly enlarges but no flow is present within it, and therefore, no color in the vein is appreciated. When the patient releases the Valsalva, a natural augmentation phenomenon ensues and the common femoral vein is noted with high velocity white venous flow and the color spills over the edges of the actual lumen briefly, before returning to the original blue color confined to the true venous lumen. The Valsalva maneuver holds the most value when a baseline normal response has been established before the diagnosis of DVT is suspected, e.g. a normal Valsalva response before surgery which becomes markedly abnormal, i.e. non-reactive, thereafter. It is affected by the patient's ability to understand the in-

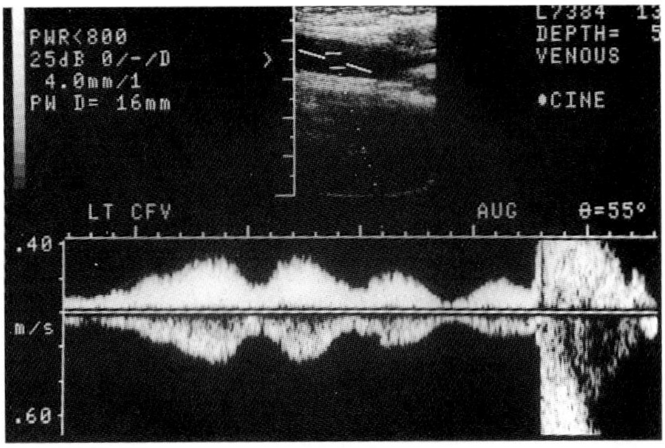

Figure 7 *A longitudinal sonogram of the left common femoral vein shows a patent vein, but on spectral analysis the waveform is pulsatile, a finding consistent with congestive heart failure or other causes of elevated right heart pressure. A normal augmentation response is shown on the right.*

structions and willingness to perform the maneuver, which can be painful after pelvic surgery. When the patient can cooperate and adequately perform a Valsalva maneuver in the study of the common femoral vein, a normal response to compression yet an abnormal Valsalva suggests the possibility of either significant ascites or a pelvic mass compressing the iliac system; such as a lymphocele or hematoma, or iliac thrombus.

In general, compression of the peripheral veins is a simple, uncomplicated maneuver. However, in large obese patients some compressive effects in the soft tissues are already operative and veins can be difficult to see without augmentation or positional changes to take advantage of gravitational dependency.

Patients with congestive failure have an increased venous capitatance (Figure 7) (34, 35). The veins are full. The typical atrial contractions noted in the normal proximal IVC are transmitted down to the leg, noted by a zigzag configuration of the venous spectral analysis (35). With elevated right atrial pressure, the peripheral veins are larger than normal and not as freely compressible as normal, offering some resistance.

PARTIAL DEEP VENOUS THROMBOSIS

Partial deep venous thrombosis produces some flow within the affected vein either along the side or within the thrombus, best seen with color Doppler (Figure 8). The vein is partially compressible. A Doppler signal can be obtained from the portion of the vein that has some

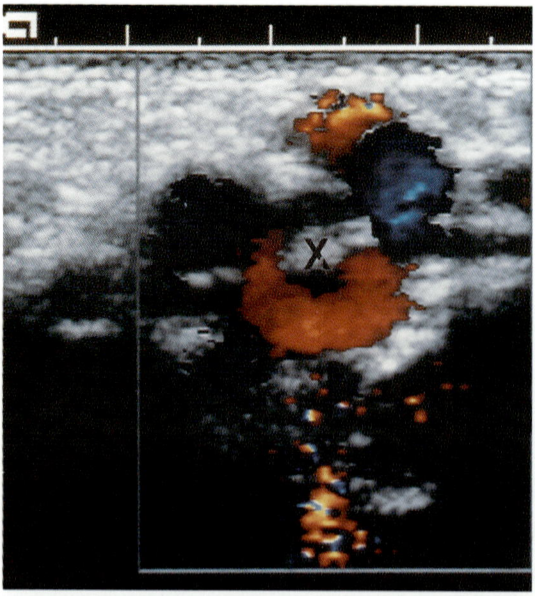

Figure 8 *A transverse sonogram of the right common femoral vein in color shows evidence of partial deep venous thrombus with hyperechoic thrombus (X).*

flow but it is weak. The augmentation response, normally immediate, is damped. The response to Valsalva is present but markedly diminished to less than a 50 % increase in A-P diameter compared to that at rest. Respiratory phasicity is absent. The veins may be irregular.

COMPLETE OCCLUSION

Occluded veins are not compressible with transducer pressure (Figure 9). Occlusive deep venous thrombosis can be focal or diffuse. A common site for focal occlusions is at the confluence of the superficial greater saphenous vein into the deep common femoral vein. Focal expansion of the vein suggests acute disease.

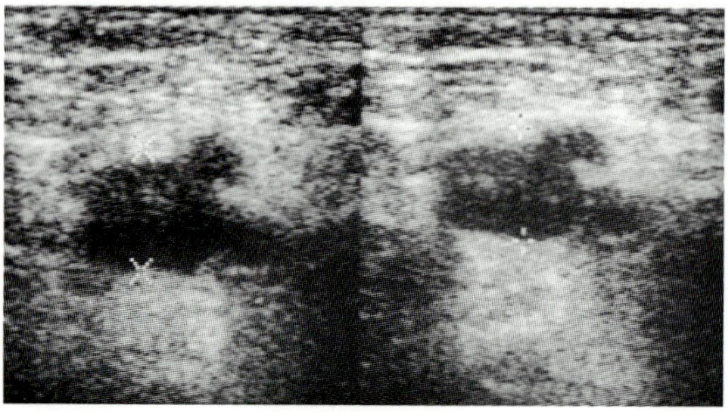

Figure 9 *A transverse sonogram shows a left superficial femoral vein, on the left at rest which is shown to be, on the right, noncompressible consistent with deep venous thrombosis.*

Figure 10 *A longitudinal view of the superficial femoral artery demonstrates in color a patent artery and an occluded superficial femoral vein. There are low level echoes within the vein, as well as a bright echogenic focus in the center which in some views casts a shadow consistent with calcification. This finding denotes chronic deep venous thrombosis. Of interest is the bright leaflets of the more proximal valve which open and close normally. The focal occlusion does not extend to this more proximal valve (arrows).*

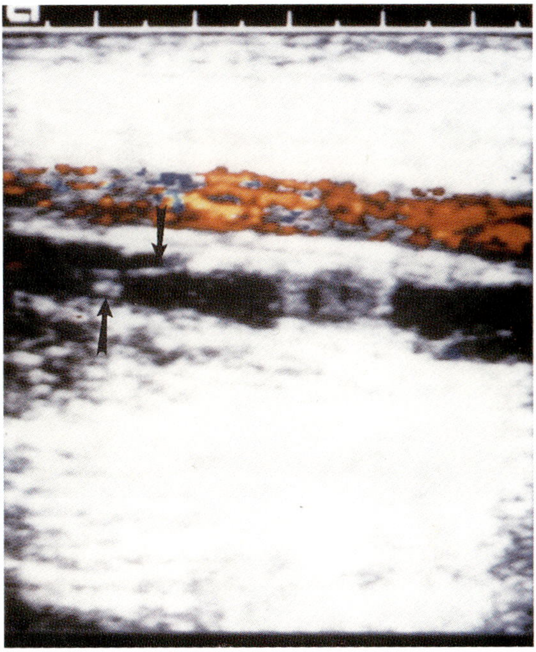

Veins with chronic changes of deep venous thrombosis can be irregular with heterogeneous, often hyperechoic, intraluminal material (Figure 10). The lumen may be patent, partially occluded, or occluded. Valves are incompetent.

Chronic occlusion may cause the affected vein to blend with the soft tissues and not be detected by sonography. This occurrence is usually associated with collateral flow which veins are distinguished

Figure 11 *A longitudinal sonogram in color demonstrates multiple collateral veins from an occlusion of the superficial femoral vein. On the right side of the image the superior red tube is the superficial femoral artery. The serpiginous vessels are the collateral vessels.*

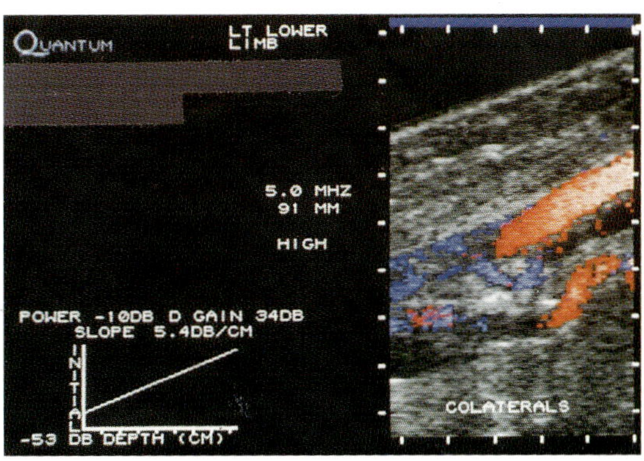

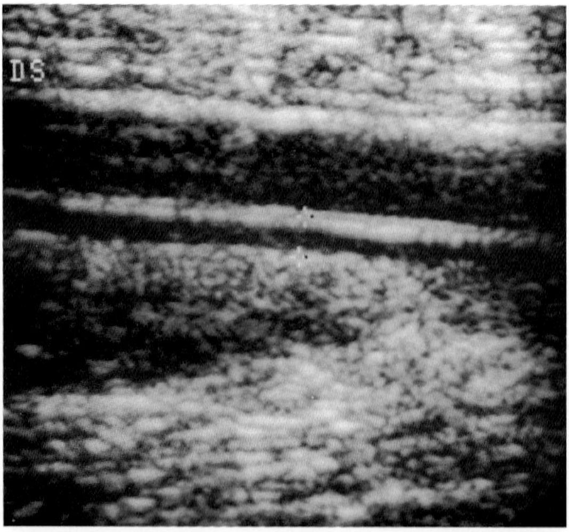

Figure 12 *A longitudinal sonogram of the right superficial femoral vein shows marked diminution in size (++) consistent with chronic venous disease.*

from the deep veins by lack of an adjacent artery (Figure 11). Collateral flow may have a normal response to compression and augmentation. Calcifications in the vein wall also indicate chronic disease as does narrowing and thickening of the wall (Figure 12).

Most fatal pulmonary emboli arise from the ilio-femoral system (36). Propagation of thrombus in the leg occurs before embolization. Fatal pulmonary embolization most likely occurs only after propagation of clot in the popliteal vein and beyond.

Since the ilio-femoral system is well seen by sonography some advocate, especially if color coded imaging is not available, that the examination routinely stop at the popliteal vein with repeated follow-up examinations for those thought to be a high risk (2). However, if the patient has pain in the calf, the area specifically should be examined to eliminate the possibility of Baker's cyst, hematoma or soft tissue tumor.

Undoubtedly, small silent pulmonary emboli arise in the calf (37). Minor calf thrombi are not considered dangerous unless they ascend. The calf veins are small. Propagation of thrombus to larger more proximal veins in calf DVT occurs in only 22 % (38).

Put in perspective, many clinicians do not treat calf DVT unless there is involvement of the femoral popliteal system (39). There is no doubt that including the calf veins adds significantly to the time of the examination. Each calf has 3 pairs of deep calf veins that must be visualized from the ankle to the trifurcation at the popliteal vein to be able with certainty to conclude that the calf veins are normal (40).

TREATMENT

Treatment of deep venous thrombosis is directed toward preventing pulmonary embolism. A prompt, positive diagnosis generates immediate treatment with heparin followed by a maintenance oral dose of warfarin (Coumadin) for 6 weeks to 3 months, to maintain a prothrombin time of 1.5 to 2 times normal or an INR (international normalized ratio) of 2 to 3 (1). Vigorous, prompt treatment is thought to reduce venous insufficiency.

Filters placed in the IVC serve as a barrier to the propagation of thrombus to the lungs. The venous site of percutaneous insertion of the filter is affected by new thrombus in a few instances (14 %) (41, 42) most of which resolve without long range complications.

NATURAL HISTORY

Ultrasound can be used to follow the natural history of DVT after the initial diagnosis is made (43, 44) although it may not be as reliable in patients who develop post thrombotic changes from prior DVT (9). Since acute deep venous thrombosis cannot always be distinguished from chronic DVT, and because recurrence and recrudescence do occur, a baseline sonogram of the peripheral veins may be helpful following the patient's completed therapeutic regimen. Some cases of venous thrombosis resolve completely with therapy. In others, extension of the involvement under therapy occurs (1, 45). Valvular incompetence tends to develop as a complication in about 2/3 of those with DVT (46). Ultrasound has the potential to define the natural history of clot propagation and holds promise to define a response to therapy with different drug regimens.

Compressing a local thrombus that appears to be only partially attached to the wall is associated with risk of pulmonary embolism; one case report documents such a case. Of 15 patients with free floating clots noted by duplex scanning, 20 % suffered pulmonary emboli (47).

nicians. Iliofemoral DVT, in particular, is apt to cause varicose veins. Venous valvular reflux can be segmentally evaluated quantitatively by duplex Doppler (50) by applying distal limb compression and then abruptly releasing it (51). Sonography is used to assess the level of incompetence (52).

In normal patients, a retrograde bolus of flow greater than 30 cm/sec is required to initiate venous valve closure in the leg (53). This can be achieved with a Valsalva maneuver at the common femoral vein but not reliably more distally. Normal flow in the femoral vein is reversed by a Valsalva maneuver; because of a pressure differential, the reversed velocity in the femoral vein rises to greater than 30 cm/sec, which in turn triggers the abrupt closure of the venous valve cusps with cessation of reflux (53). More distally, a Valsalva maneuver has less effect on the venous system and the venous valves may fail to close so that reflux can be demonstrated normally.

Since manual limb compression alone is usually insufficient to test for venous valve competence (50), a pneumatic cuff around the upright limb, inflated to at least 80 mm Hg, then released, transiently creates a reversed venous bolus at the thigh, calf, and ankle. At each level of the leg examined, the duplex transducer is put in position distal to the cuff to note the duration of reflux which occurs at deflation of the cuff. In normal patients, this is less than 0.5 sec, indicating intact valves (50, 54).

Varicosities are treated medically with elastic support or in intractable symptomatic cases with surgical removal or sclerotic therapy. Ultrasound can be used to monitor the injection of sclerosing agents intravenously.

Patients with superficial venous incompetence can be treated with surgery by ligation and stripping or as an alternative, plication of the sapheno-femoral junction. Initial studies suggest duplex sonography can be used to define the level of venous incompetence initially and quantify it and can be used, after surgical plication and reduction of the venous lumen, to indicate improvement in the hemodynamics of venous valve function (55).

The natural history of DVT is over time to either resolve completely or organize with recanalization and collateralization with resultant decreased venous resistance. Over time, just as venous obstruction tends to subside, valve incompetence tends to increase.

RESULTS OF SONOGRAPHIC VENOGRAPHY

Ultrasound for deep venous thrombosis is highly sensitive and specific, ranging from 93–99 %, respectively (2, 6, 11, 12, 14, 56, 57, 58).

PITFALLS IN VENOUS SONOGRAPHY

Absence of phasicity or decreased response to Valsalva in the common femoral vein in the presence of normal compression suggests either more proximal clot in the iliac veins or significant compression of them by pelvic mass or hematoma (58).

Occasionally, a vein may be duplicated with one branch occluded, the other normal, a finding which can lead to a false negative designation for deep venous thrombosis (59, 60, 61). Variation in size and location of peripheral veins can be sources of potential error in assessment.

Visualization and compression of the superficial femoral vein at the adductor canal can be difficult (5, 6, 7, 33, 62). External compression of veins by soft tissue masses and soft tissue edema can also be a factor (63) in their lack of visualization. Failure to recognize partial compression of a thrombosed vein also leads to false negative assessment.

Relying on visualization of thrombus rather than compression is another source of error since thrombus is often anechoic (58). Visualization of thrombus *per se* is not a particularly sensitive way to make the diagnosis of venous thrombosis (45). Remember that the duplex Doppler technique was developed when it was appreciated that carotid occlusion or aortic occlusion could appear as normal vessels with B-mode alone.

UPPER EXTREMITY

The upper extremity venous evaluation is focused upon the subclavian (SV), axillary and brachial deep veins and the basilic and cephalic superficial veins and uses both imaging and spectral analysis in the diagnostic assessment, which should be bilateral. The subclavian vein is examined with the transducer below the clavicle aimed toward the head using a 5 to 7.5 MHz linear array transducer. Because of the inability to compress the subclavian

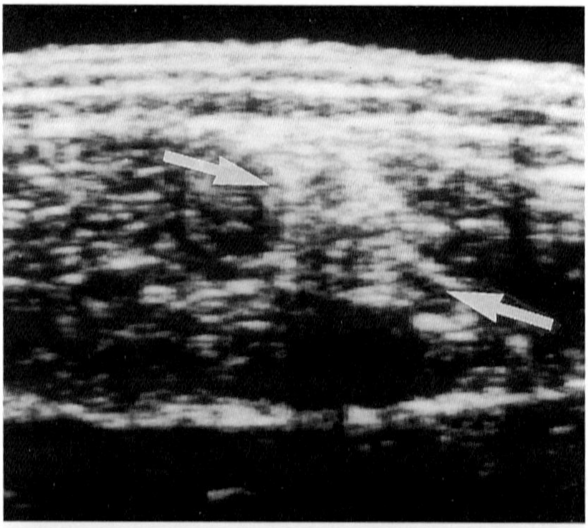

Figure 4 *Intramuscular fibrous scar resulting from a neglected partial rupture of the rectus femoris muscle. Transverse scan of the thigh shows an echogenic, stellate area in the rectus femoris muscle (arrows).*

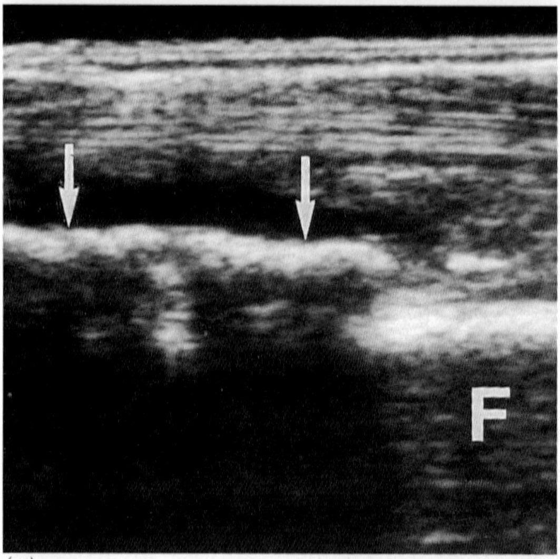

(a)

Figure 5 *Posttraumatic myositis ossificans in the vastus intermedius muscle.*
a. Longitudinal scan shows a brightly echogenic linear interface (arrows) with acoustic shadowing obscuring the femur shaft (F).
b. Low-kilovoltage lateral radiograph confirms the heterotopic ossification.
F = femur.

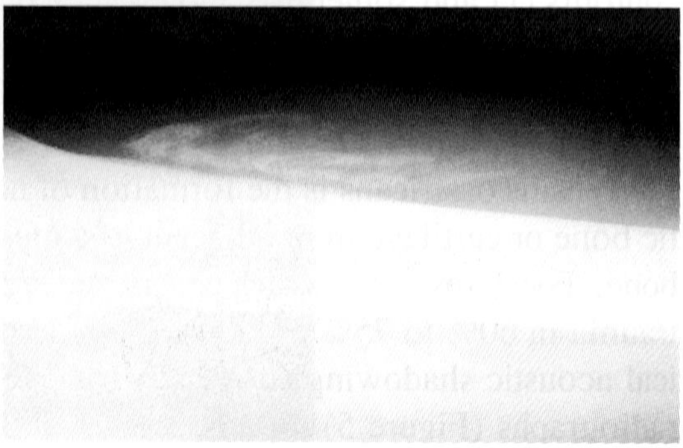

(b)

Muscle hernias bulge through a weakened or ruptured aponeurosis. Real-time sonography during contraction of the involved muscle readily demonstrates that the palpable lump is made of normal muscle tissue.

Infection

Pyomyositis and other muscle abscesses are rare in nontropical countries. These lesions appear as hypoechoic collections, which may contain echogenic debris and occasionally gas bubbles that cause shadowing, or as complex masses. Diagnostic aspiration and drainage can be performed with ultrasound guidance (12). Special attention should be paid to the examination of the adjacent bones for osteomyelitis.

Tumors

Among benign tumors of the muscles, lipomas and hemangiomas are the most common. The presence of areas of increased echogenicity suggests a fatty tumor (Figure 6), although lipomas can also

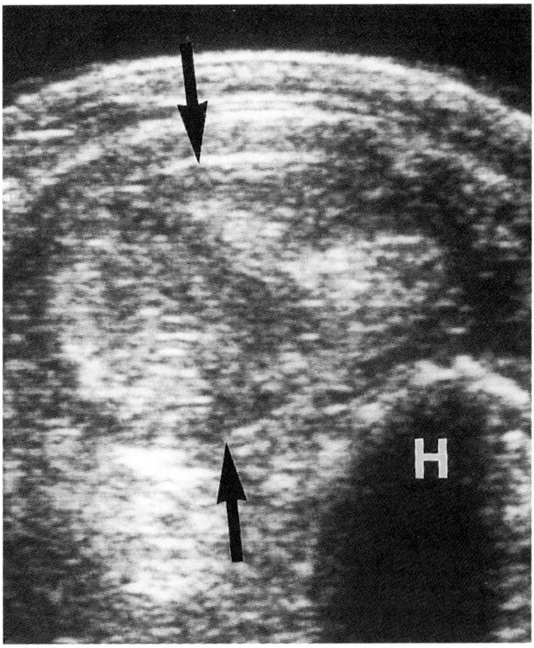

Figure 6 *Transverse scan of the posterior aspect of the arm shows a well-defined, echogenic lipoma (arrows) in the triceps brachii muscle. H = humerus.*

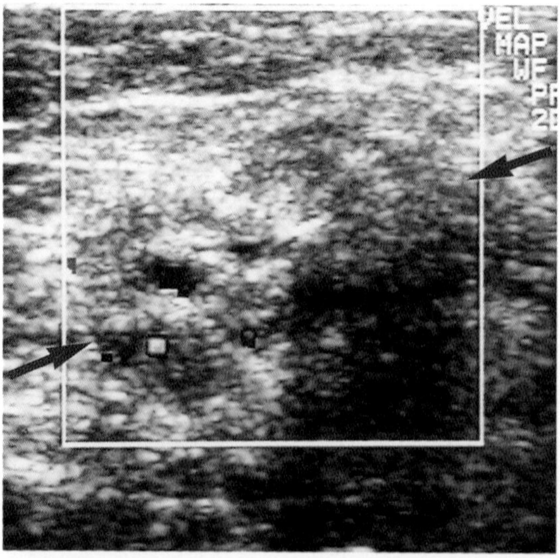

Figure 7 *Hemangioma of the thigh. Transverse scan shows a poorly defined nonhomogeneous, hypoechoic mass (arrows). Note the absence of color Doppler signals.*

be hypoechoic or isoechoic (13, 14). Intramuscular hemangiomas also have a variable echogenicity ranging from markedly hypoechoic to hyperechoic and may be well or very poorly defined (Figure 7) (15). Sonography can demonstrate typical calcified thrombi. Angiolipomas are hyperechoic, because of their fat content, and show an infiltrating pattern. MRI usually shows the extent of intramuscular hemangiomas better than sonography does.

Other less common benign intramuscular tumors include desmoid tumors (fibromatosis), which are often associated with marked shadowing, and intramuscular myxomas, which are markedly hypoechoic and may even appear cystic (16).

Except for well-differentiated liposarcomas, which are often echogenic, malignant tumors, whether primary or metastatic, usually appear as hypoechoic masses (Figure 8).

Soft-tissue sarcomas derive from various anatomic soft-tissue components, including muscles. As a rule, soft-tissue sarcomas are relatively well circumscribed, and calcifications and areas of necrosis can be seen. Sonography is the best technique for guiding percutaneous needle biopsy (Figure 9). Color Doppler imaging demonstrates increased, chaotic vascularity in the majority of soft-tissue sarcomas and metastases to soft tissues from various primary tumors.

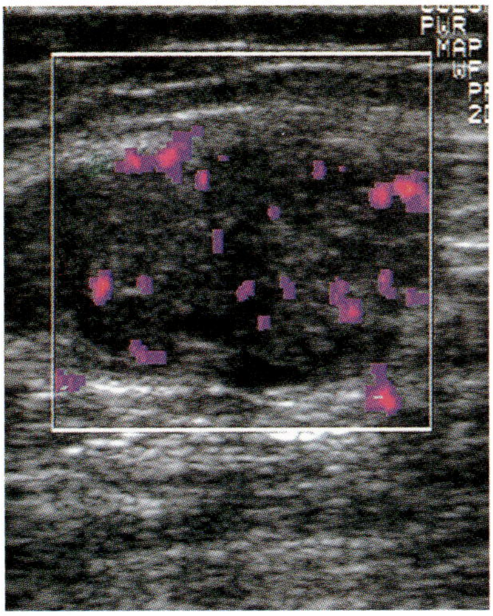

Figure 8 *Metastatic melanoma in the quadriceps muscle. Longitudinal power Doppler scan shows a hypoechoic mass with intense internal hypervascularity.*

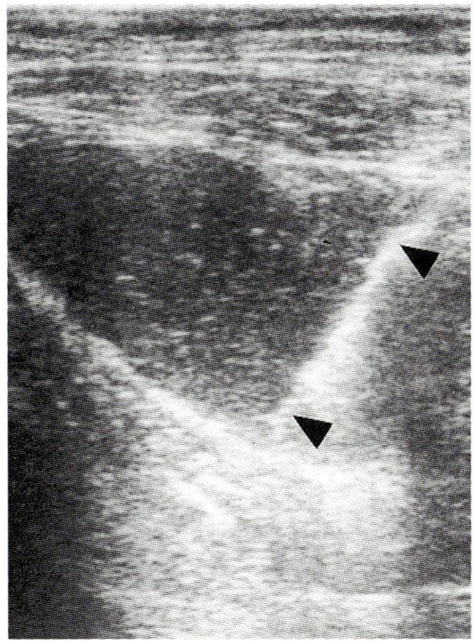

Figure 9 *Ultrasound-guided large-core needle biopsy of recurrent liposarcoma in the thigh. Scan obtained after the automatic spring-loaded biopsy device has been fired into the hypoechoic mass shows the bright cutting needle (arrowheads) inserted obliquely from the right side of the scan.*

Muscular dystrophies

In patients with muscular dystrophies, there is a marked increase in echogenicity of the affected muscles resulting from replacement of muscle fibers by fat and connective tissue. However, CT and MRI are more effective than sonography in imaging these conditions because they provide more objective and reproducible mapping of the lesions. Hopes that sonography would permit screening of carriers of hereditary myopathies have not been realized.

TENDONS

Normal ultrasound anatomy

All tendons are echogenic, with a fibrillar echotexture well seen on longitudinal sonograms (Figure 10) (3–9). On transverse sec-

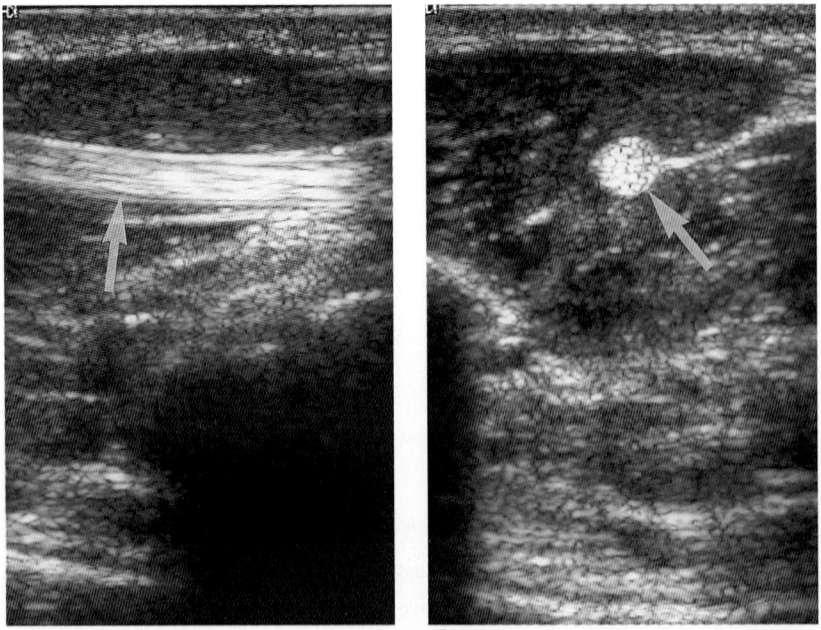

(a) (b)

Figure 10 *Normal tendon of flexor pollicis longus muscle.*
a. Longitudinal scan of the thenar area shows the fibrillar texture of the echogenic 3-mm-thick tendon (arrow).
b. Transverse scan shows the bright tendon (arrow) surrounded by hypoechoic muscle.

tions, most tendons are round to oval. Exceptions include the meniscus-shaped patellar tendon and the flat, convex rotator cuff. Tendons are less clearly visualized when they are surrounded by echogenic fat instead of hypoechoic muscles. A false hypoechogenicity of the tendon may result from the slightest obliquity of the beam in relation to the tendon axis (Figure 11) (17). This is more likely to occur when non-linear-array transducers are used or when the tendon is curved (e.g. rotator cuff, flexor tendons in the fingers). This artifact also occurs on transverse scans.

When high-frequency transducers are used, the synovial sheath is barely visible as a subtle hypoechoic underlining of the tendon; however, the ulnar bursa in the carpal tunnel is particularly prominent when the wrist is flexed. Major synovial bursae (e.g., the deep infrapatellar and the deep calcaneal bursae) appear as hypoechoic, flattened structures adjacent to the tendons, thinner than 2 to 3 mm

(3, 5). Intratendinous sesamoid bones are identified by their acoustic shadowing. During active or passive mobilization of a tendon, real-time sonography demonstrates the gliding of the tendon.

Tendons of the extremities that can be examined with sonography include the rotator cuff (18–25) and the tendon of the long head of the biceps brachii muscle in the shoulder (26, 27); the lower tendons of the biceps and triceps brachii muscles and the common tendons of the flexor (epitrochlear) and extensor (epicondylic) muscles of the forearm at the elbow (5, 28); the flexor and extensor tendons of the fingers at the wrist and in the hand (4); the quadriceps and patellar tendons at the knee (29); and the Achilles tendon and other major tendons of the ankle (30–32).

Pathologic conditions

Disorders of tendons are generally due to trauma or inflammation and are most often associated with athletic or occupational activities.

Trauma

In complete tears, the two tendon fragments are separated by a gap of variable length and echogenicity, which corresponds to the hematoma subsequently colonized by granulomatous tissue (Figure 12) (33). A bone avulsion may accompany a complete detachment of a tendon. In that case, the bone fragment appears as a bright echogenic focus with an acoustic shadow (6).

A recent partial rupture appears as a focal hypoechoic defect in the body of the tendon or at its attachment (3).

Rotator cuff tears

Because of its convex shape, which causes artifacts, the rotator cuff is difficult to examine sonographically (19). The unequivocal diagnostic criterion for a complete tear is the nonvisualization of the avulsed rotator cuff retracted under the acromion process (25). Focal thinning and discontinuity are two other criteria used in the diagnosis of rotator cuff tears. Although described initially as a major diagnostic criterion, the presence of foci of increased echogenicity in the cuff is the least reliable sign of rotator cuff tear (21,

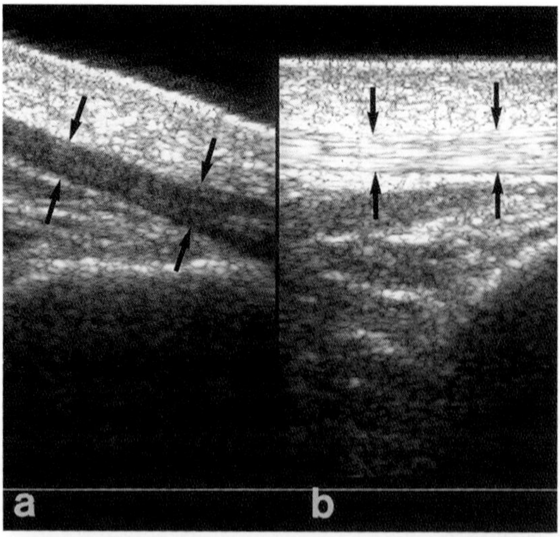

Figure 11 *False hypoechogenicity of normal patellar tendon.*
a. Longitudinal scan obtained with the ultrasound beam oblique to the fibers shows the falsely hypoechoic tendon (arrows).
b. Longitudinal scan obtained with the beam strictly perpendicular to the tendon's axis displays the tendon's normal echogenicity (arrows).

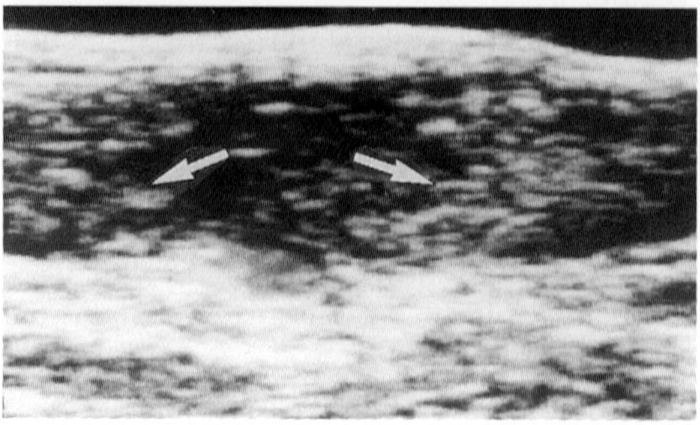

Figure 12 *Complete rupture of the Achilles tendon. Longitudinal scan shows the two frayed tendon fragments (arrows) separated by an organized hematoma.*

25). After early enthusiastic reports claimed that sonography's accuracy was close or even superior to that of arthrography, subsequent studies have indicated a sensitivity of about 60% or less in the diagnosis of rotator cuff tears (21–23). It appears that sonography is accurate in the diagnosis of normal rotator cuff and complete tears but is less reliable in the diagnosis of partial tears.

In complete ruptures of the biceps tendon, sonography can demonstrate an empty bicipital groove, the differential diagnosis being a dislocated tendon (27).

Patellar tendon tears

Partial tears of the patellar tendon are usually detachments of the tendon at the apex of the patella, resulting in a small, well-de-

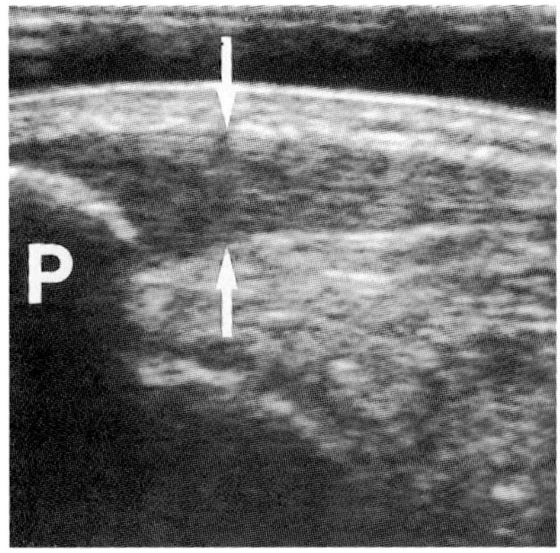

Figure 13 *Acute patellar tendinitis. Longitudinal scan shows the thickened, hypoechoic tendon (arrows). P = patella.*

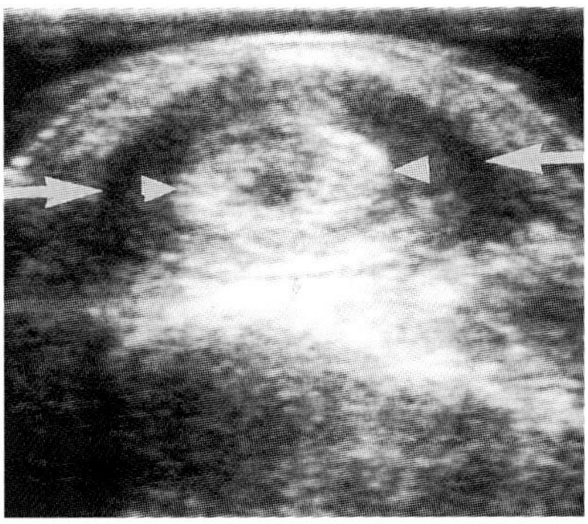

Figure 14 *Chronic tenosynovitis of the anterior tibialis tendon. Transverse scan of the anterior aspect of the ankle shows marked, hypoechoic thickening of the sheath (arrows) around an enlarged nonhomogeneous tendon (arrowheads).*

fined, hypoechoic hematoma whose midline location is best demonstrated on transverse scans (29).

Achilles tendon tears

Most Achilles tendon ruptures occur in the midportion of the tendon, about 2 to 3 cm from the calcaneal attachment. In complete tears, the gap between the torn fragments is variable, and the hematoma may extend along the tendon over a long distance (Figure 12). The tendon fragments show jagged margins, resembling a frayed rope (30–32).

Inflammation

Inflammatory conditions involving tendons include tendinitis, tenosynovitis, and bursitis. In all these conditions, sonography can be used for monitoring the effect of treatment, as well as for diagnosis.

Tendinitis

In acute tendinitis, the tendon is swollen, its echogenicity is decreased, and its contours are often blurred (Figure 13) (33). Minute calcifications can be demonstrated sonographically in chronic tendinitis.

Tenosynovitis

In acute traumatic or infectious tenosynovitis, the synovial sheath is filled with fluid (34, 35). The presence of internal echoes suggests the presence of pus (36). Although significant amounts of fluid can also be found in chronic tenosynovitis, that condition is most often associated with a marked, hypoechoic thickening of the synovium, with little or no fluid (Figure 14). A typical example is rheumatoid tenosynovitis, in which the proliferating pannus appears as a markedly hypoechoic peritendinous sheath (37).

Bursitis

Inflammation of an adjacent bursa can be isolated or, more frequently, associated with tendinitis. Subdeltoid, olecranal, patellar, and calcaneal bursae are most frequently involved. Sonograms show a swollen, rounded, fluid-filled bursa with ill-defined margins. In chronic bursitis, the bursa may exhibit a complex appearance, while calcifications give rise to hypoechoic foci with shadowing.

Miscellaneous

For several months or years after surgery, tendons may remain significantly enlarged on sonograms, with ill-defined contours, nonhomogeneous echotexture, calcifications, and echogenic suture material.

Ganglion cysts occur mainly in the hand and wrist. They are oval and sonolucent and are typically adjacent to the tendons in the palm and fingers (6, 8, 38, 39).

The rare benign tumors that may develop from or in tendons or their sheaths include giant cell tumors (the localized form of pigmented villonodular synovitis) and osteochondromas.

JOINTS

Normal ultrasound anatomy

In adults, the subchondral bone appears on sonograms as an echogenic, smooth, regular line with the overlying articular cartilage appearing as a thin anechoic layer (40). Except in the hip, the articular capsule is rarely identified on sonograms. The menisci of the knee are markedly echogenic with a homogeneous echo pattern (41) and a typical triangular shape on longitudinal cross sections.

Pathologic conditions

Joint effusions

Sonography readily demonstrates intra-articular fluid collections. Septic effusions may contain debris, but there is no clear-cut relationship between the echogenicity of the fluid and the presence or absence of infection. Sonography is ideal for guiding aspiration of small effusions, e.g. in the hips of children.

Synovial proliferations

In proliferative diseases of the synovium, such as pigmented villonodular synovitis or rheumatoid arthritis, high-frequency sonography shows the hypoechoic thickened synovium (Figure 15) (9, 42).

Synovial cysts

Synovial cysts develop from joint spaces or adjacent bursae. Popliteal cysts (Baker's cysts) are due to an abnormal distension of the gastrocnemius-semimembranosus bursa. They are frequently associated with rheumatoid arthritis. Popliteal cysts typically appear as fluid-filled collections, often wrapping around the origin of the gastrocnemius medialis muscle (Figure 16). Inflamed cysts may contain echogenic fibrinous debris, and in patients with rheumatoid arthritis, the cysts may be filled with pannus and mimic solid masses. Sonography can diagnose a ruptured cyst by showing fluid dissecting into the calf.

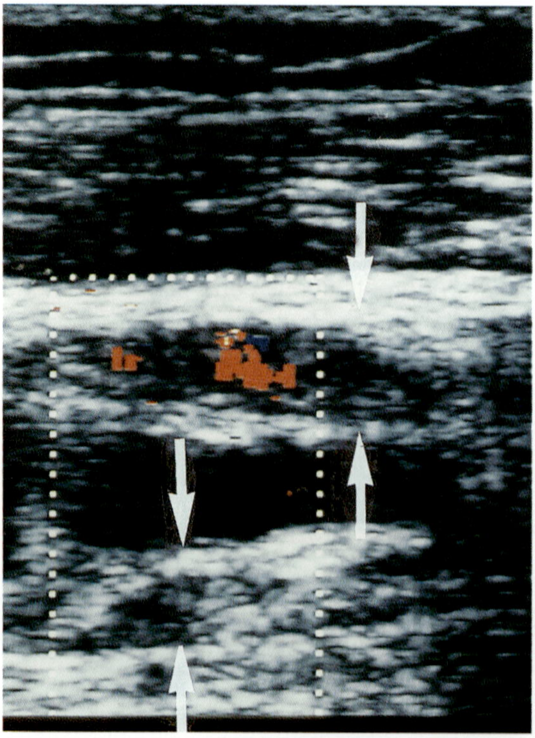

Figure 15 *Pigmented villonodular synovitis of the knee. Longitudinal scan above the patella shows the hypoechoic thickening of the synovium (arrows). Color Doppler shows increased vascularity.*

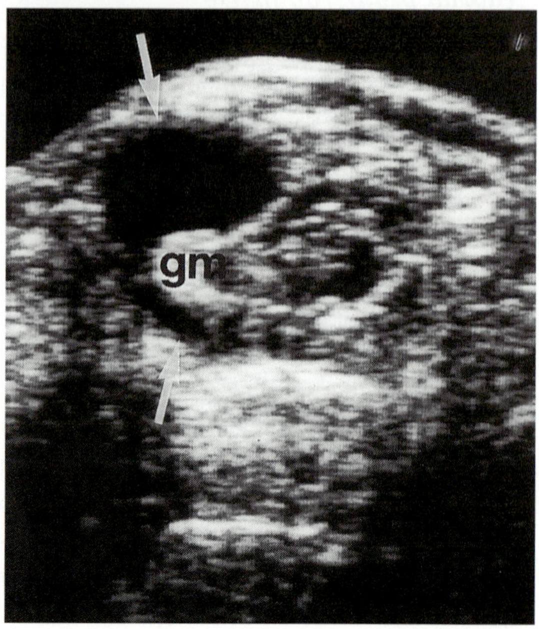

Figure 16 *Baker's cyst. Transverse scan of the popliteal fossa shows the cyst (arrows) surrounding the origin of the gastrocnemius medialis muscle (gm).*

Congenital dislocation/dysplasia of the hip

In neonates, sonography has become the technique of choice with which to examine the hips. Harcke has recently proposed a four-step (four-view) examination technique comprising a coronal view with the hip in neutral position, a coronal view with the hip flexed, a transverse view with the hip flexed, and a transverse view with the hip in neutral position. The goal of the study is to assess the position of the femoral head at rest in neutral and flexed positions (normal, subluxated, dislocated), the relative stability of the hip with motion and stress (normal, lax, dislocatable, reducible, not reducible), and the anatomic development of the hip components (43).

In older children, hip sonography is performed to detect joint effusions.

Miscellaneous

Except for the diagnosis of meniscal cysts (44), sonography has not proved to be a reliable modality for evaluating meniscal disorders, which are best diagnosed using MRI.

PERIPHERAL NERVES

Normal ultrasound anatomy

The trunks of large peripheral nerves can be clearly delineated in specific locations of the extremities using sonography (45). They appear as echogenic tubular structures with a fibrillar texture, similar to that of tendons on longitudinal scans (Figure 17). Their cross section on transverse scans is oval to round, with internal punctate echoes.

Pathologic conditions

Nerve sheath tumors

Benign nerve sheath tumors (neurofibromas and schwannomas) are readily visualized as well-defined, round-to-oval, hypoechoic masses (Figure 18) (45, 46). Marked distal sound enhancement, well-defined margins, and the presence of minute cystic areas are

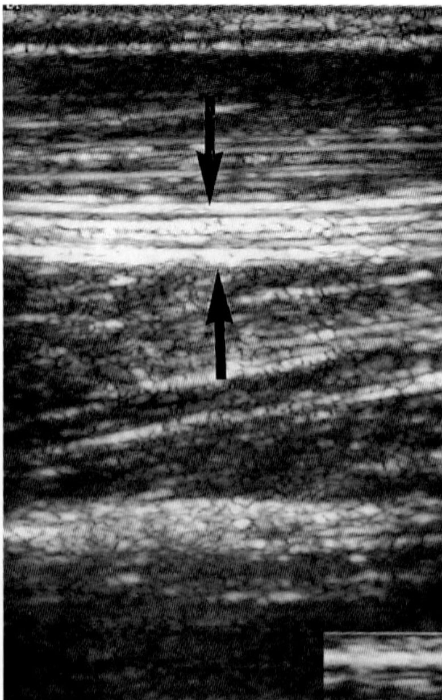

Figure 17 *Normal median nerve in the forearm. Longitudinal scan shows the markedly echogenic median nerve (arrows).*

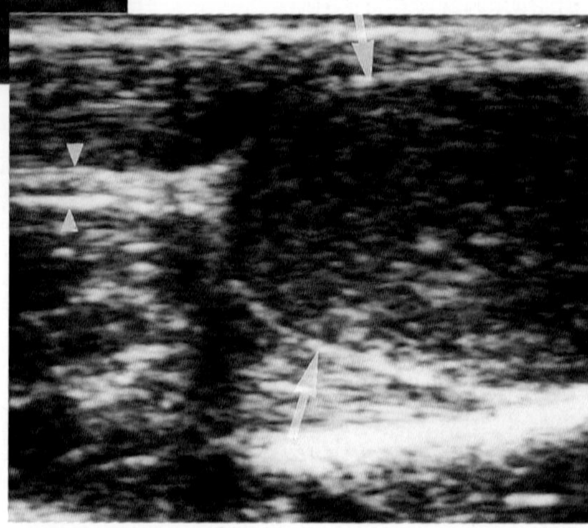

Figure 18 *Benign schwannoma of the median nerve. Longitudinal scan of the anterior aspect of the forearm shows a well-defined hypoechoic mass (arrows) with some sound-through transmission. Arrowheads point to the normal nerve.*

thought to be suggestive of schwannomas. Sonography can depict the junction between the normal nerve and the tumor, thus establishing the diagnosis of nerve sheath tumor (Figure 18).

Miscellaneous

Traumatic neuromas may develop after a direct injury to the nerve. They appear sonographically as ill-defined hypoechoic masses (45).

Morton's neuromas result from the compression of a branch of the interdigital plantar nerve on the head of a metatarsal bone. They appear as well-defined hypoechoic masses on sonograms (47).

SUBCUTANEOUS TISSUES

Normal ultrasound anatomy

Highly detailed images of the subcutaneous tissues can be obtained with conventional 7.5 or 10 MHz transducers. The subcutaneous fat is hypoechoic and contains thin linear echoes representing strands of connective tissue.

Pathologic conditions

Tumors

The most frequent benign tumors in subcutaneous tissues are lipomas and angiomas. Their sonographic appearance is like that of the intramuscular lipomas and angiomas described above.

Numerous other benign tumors in the subcutaneous tissues can be studied with sonography; the vast majority of them appear as hypoechoic masses, so a reliable diagnosis of their nature cannot be made based on the sonographic appearance alone (48, 49).

High-frequency sonography has proved to be as accurate as MRI in the detection of recurrent soft-tissue sarcomas (50). Color Doppler imaging usually demonstrates a chaotic hypervascularity within the malignant mass (Figure 19). Sonography can also demonstrate minute, nonpalpable metastases in the subcutaneous tissues (Figure 20) (51). Whenever such a lesion has been detected, an ultrasound-guided fine-needle aspiration biopsy can be performed, within minutes.

Inflammation

A common problem in evaluating inflamed subcutaneous tissues is differentiating clinically between cellulitis and abscess. Sonography is useful in this situation. In cellulitis, sonograms show a

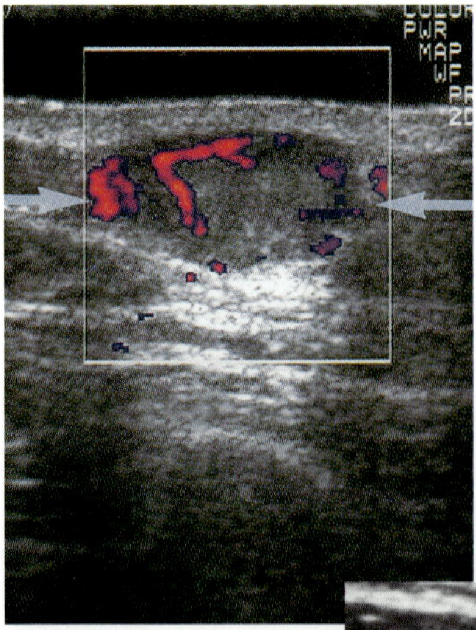

Figure 19 *Metastatic leiomyosarcoma in the subcutaneous tissues of the abdominal wall (arrows). Power Doppler scan shows the intense, disorganized vascularity of the mass.*

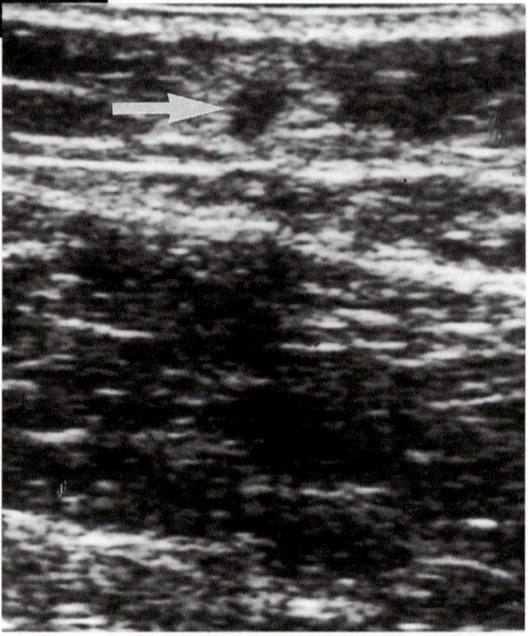

Figure 20 *Nonpalpable metastatic melanoma (arrow) in the subcutaneous fat of the thigh.*

diffuse increase in the echogenicity of the subcutaneous fat, which often becomes indistinguishable from the skin. Color Doppler examination identifies increased blood flow (Figure 21). In contrast, abscesses appear sonographically as fluid-filled collections, often with internal echoes or a complex appearance, irregular walls, and increased vascularity at the periphery of the lesions on color Doppler scans. If an abscess is small or not easily defined by pal-

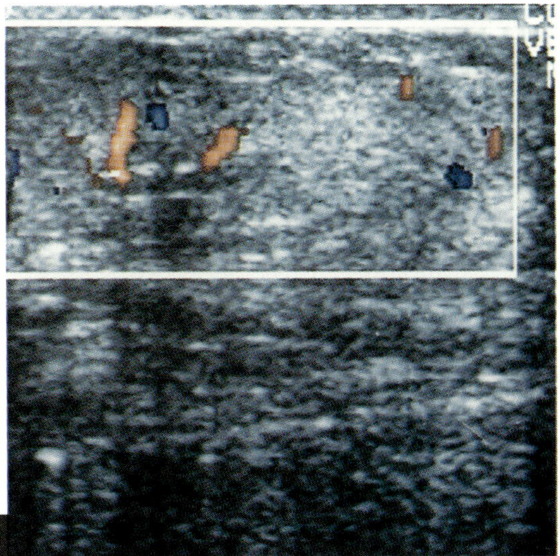

Figure 21 *Cellulitis. Color Doppler scan shows increased echogenicity of the subcutaneous fat with increased vascularity. There is no fluid collection.*

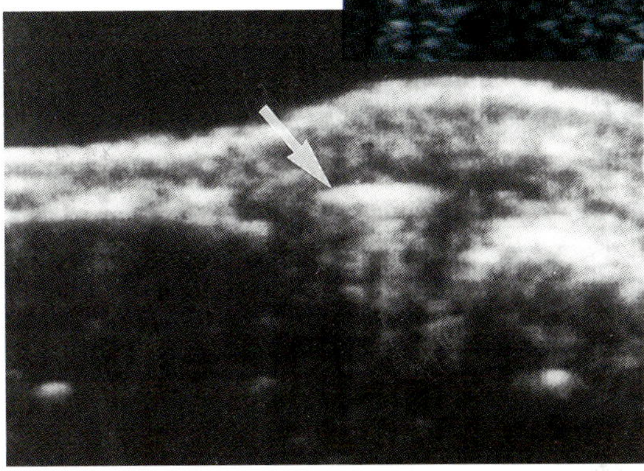

Figure 22 *Metallic foreign body in the hand. Scan shows a bright interface (arrow) followed by a comet-tail artifact.*

pation, sonography can be used to guide a confirmatory fine-needle aspiration and subsequent percutaneous drainage.

Fat necrosis can develop following trauma; it is also seen in patients with systemic diseases such as scleroderma or lupus erythematosus. On sonograms, the involved fat has a dirty appearance with an ill-defined focal area of increased echogenicity.

Foreign bodies

Post-traumatic retained foreign bodies are common in the subcutaneous tissues of the distal extremities. Sonography has proved to be an accurate imaging modality for visualizing foreign bodies in the subcutaneous tissues, including low-density, radiotransparent materials such as wooden splinters. Foreign bodies appear as brightly echogenic foci associated with acoustic shadowing, reverberation echoes, both, or neither, depending on their nature (Figure 22) (52–54). When present, inflammatory changes in the surrounding tissues give rise to an ill-defined hypoechoic area (52). Sonography is instrumental in the preoperative or intraoperative localization of foreign bodies (55, 56).

BONES

Normal ultrasound anatomy

Bones are strong reflectors that interrupt the propagation of the sound beam and cause shadowing. However, because of the strong reflectivity at the proximal surface, the shape of the superficial aspect of a bone can be appreciated in part on sonograms (Figure 23).

Bone lesions that involve the bone surface can be visualized on sonograms.

Pathologic conditions

Trauma

In neonates and children, sonography can diagnose fractures and dislocations involving nonossified epiphyses (57, 58). In the adult, fractures with displacement appear as a typical step-like deformity

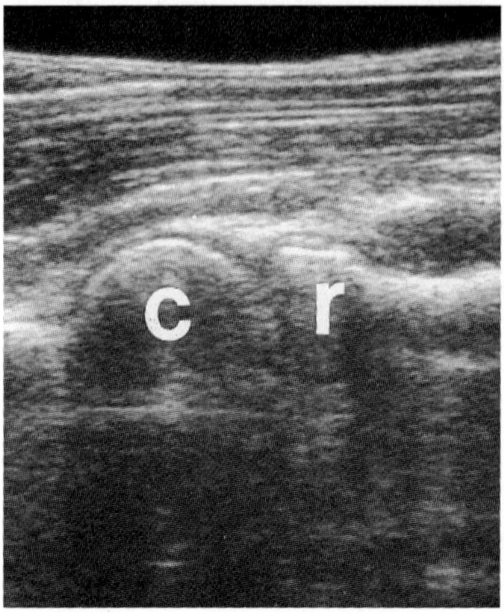

Figure 23 *Normal elbow. Longitudinal scan of the anterior aspect of the elbow silhouettes the capitellum (c) and the radial head (r).*

of the cortex (Figure 24). Sonography has been helpful in detecting such fractures in areas not easily evaluated with conventional radiographs, such as the shoulder or the ribs (59, 60). Bone formation at the fracture site can be seen many weeks before it appears on radiographs, and sonography has been used successfully to monitor bone production at the distraction site in Ilizarov limb-lengthening procedures (61).

Through the specific reverberation artifacts associated with metallic bodies, sonography can identify bone fixation devices and localize them in three dimensions (6).

Osteomyelitis

In the proper clinical setting, the sonographic demonstration of a fluid collection abutting the bone is a reliable sign of osteomye-

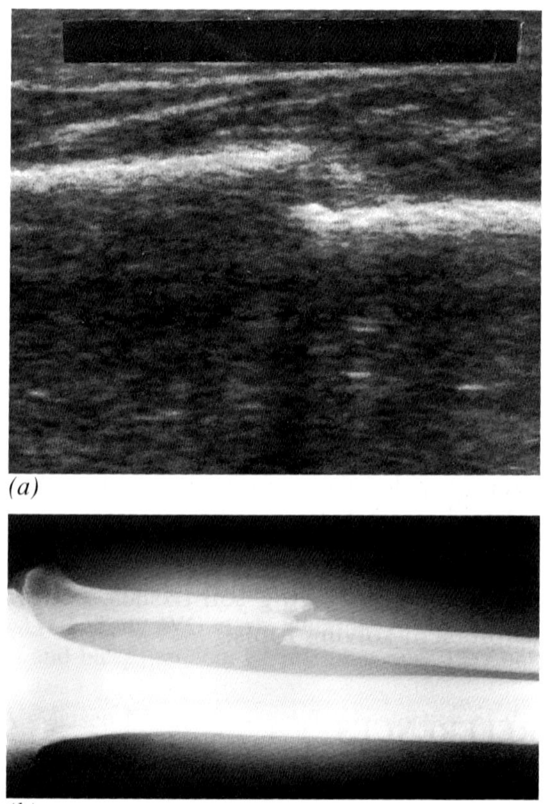

(a)

(b)

Figure 24 *Bone fracture in a soccer player examined after a direct contusion to the leg to rule out a hematoma in the soft tissues.*
a. Longitudinal scan shows the step-like deformity of the shaft of the fibula, which is pathognomonic of a fracture.
b. Radiograph confirms the fracture.

this needle. We use the 2.0 mm needle in such cases and today this is almost the only indication for using such a large diameter needle.

Contraindications

For 1.2 mm (18 G) needle biopsies we apply the same rules as for FNAB but for 2.0 mm needle biopsies a coagulation or bleeding disorder is an absolute contraindication.

The biopsy procedure

Pre-biopsy procedures are the same for coarse needle biopsies as for FNAB. The lesion is localised with the ”sterilised” transducer with mounted needle guide unit. As in FNAB the closed route to the lesion is usually preferable even if the needle passes through another organ like the liver or an intestinal loop.

Local anaesthesia is applied to the puncture site and a small skin incision is made with a knife. A skin incision is needed as a relatively steep bevel angulation is necessary to obtain a good specimen.

During puncture, with the needle tip echo at the edge of the lesion the trigger is depressed and the needle is forced into the lesion automatically. The whole biopsy event from ”skin to skin” is a very fast procedure, a mere two to three seconds and this may be a further reason for the low complication rate with this technique.

When the needle has been withdrawn it is opened and the tissue core is expelled into a suitable medium.

To summarise, automatic cutting biopsy using an automatic biopsy device is a very fast technique with few sampling errors. Further, it achieves large amounts of material with tissue architecture preserved. This makes it a very competitive technique which is capable of replacing FNAB in most instances.

NEPHROPYELOSTOMY

Ultrasonically-guided nephropyelostomy has been performed for many years (17, 18, 19) and is a well accepted technique for drainage of the obstructed urinary tract. Today, nephrostomy is not limited to drainage of obstructed kidneys. It is also used therapeut-

Figure 13 a-d *Nephropyelostomy by the one-step technique. Usually an 8F pig-tail catheter is used (a-b). The catheter on the trochar is introduced into the dilated renal pelvis by direct puncture (c-d).*

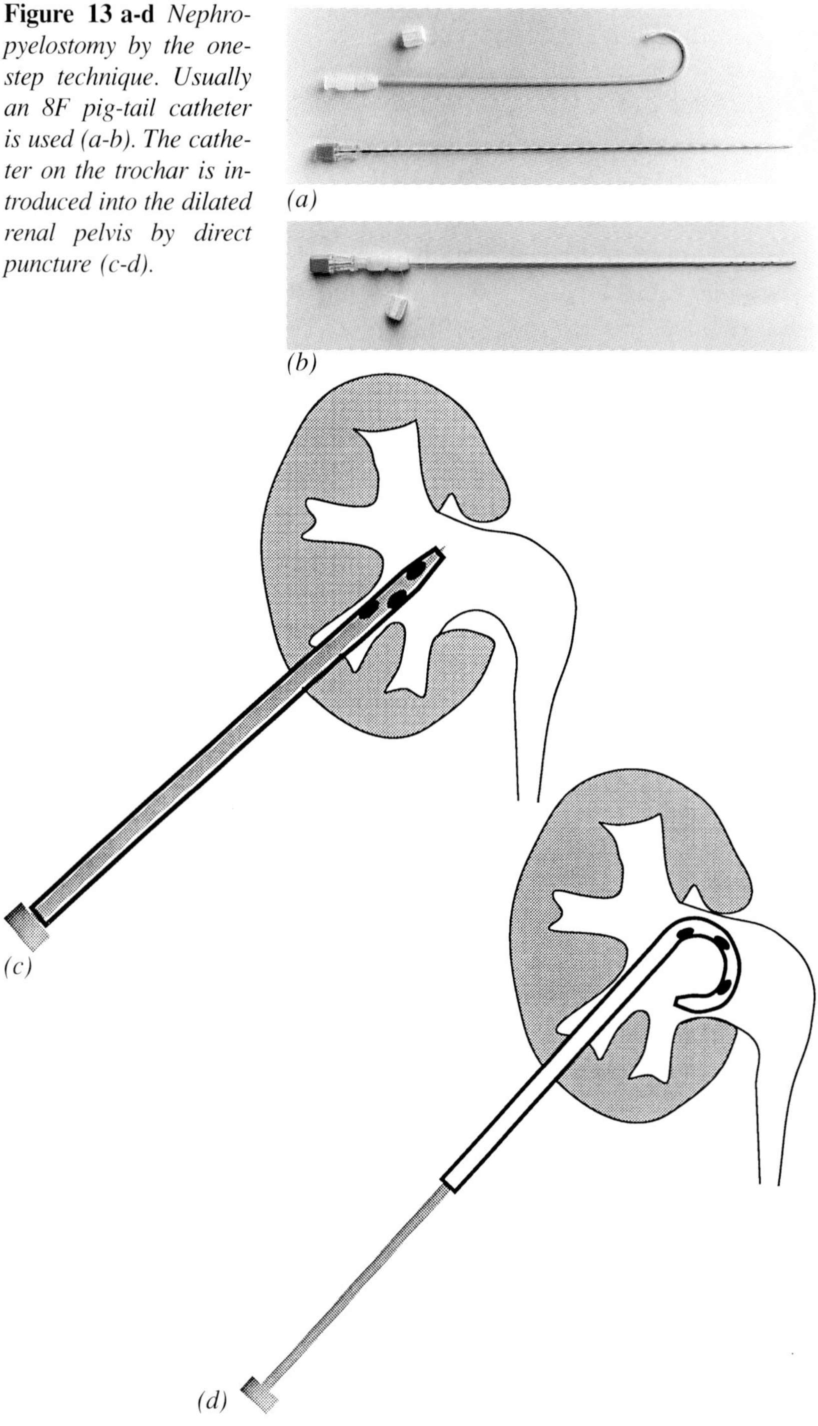

(a) (b) (c) (d)

ically in the removal of stones from the renal pelvis or ureter and in stent insertion (20).

There are two main techniques and which one is used depends on the length of time the urinary tract is to be drained and on the degree of dilatation.

For short term drainage, less than 1–2 weeks, and when the dilatation is marked, a one-step procedure is often chosen. With this technique a pig-tail catheter on a trochar is introduced into the dilated renal pelvis by a direct puncture (Figure 13 a-d). It can be performed without fluoroscopy and is thus a very quick and simple technique. The pig-tail catheters are, however, usually not well suited for long term drainage.

For long term drainage, a Seldinger technique performed under ultrasound guidance in combination with fluoroscopy is often preferred, especially if the dilatation is moderate or negligible. Initial ultrasound guided puncture of a calyx with a fine needle (20 G) is performed and a guide wire is introduced into the pelvis. Over this, a 10 F dilator is introduced to create a channel for a softer catheter to be positioned in the renal pelvis. We prefer a loop catheter for permanent drainage although it is also possible to use Foley catheters (Figure 14).

The best nephropyelostomy track is achieved if the puncture is performed in the posterior axillary line and directed towards a posteriorly directed calyx. This route minimises the risk of colon perforation and bleeding. To avoid pleural penetration, a puncture

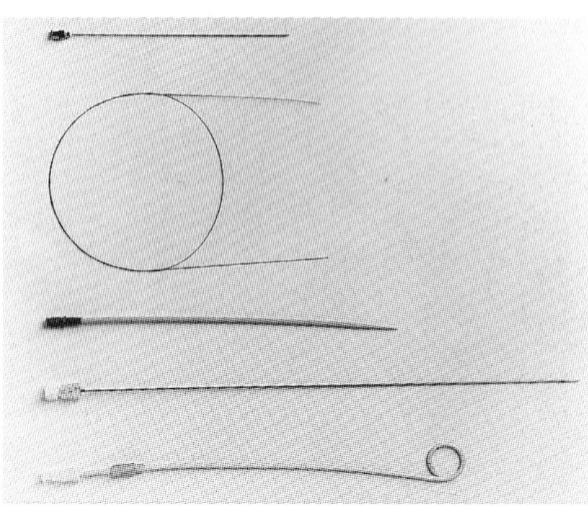

Figure 14 *Material used for nephropyelostomy using the Seldinger technique. From top to bottom; fine needle 1.2 mm (20 G), guidewire 0.46 mm, dilator 10 F, pig-tail catheter with a trocar.*

below the ribs towards a lower calyx should be attempted, but an intercostal approach is sometimes necessary if an upper calyx is to be reached especially if the catheter to be placed there is intended to allow removal of ureteric stones.

FLUID COLLECTIONS: ABSCESSES, ASCITES, PLEURAL EFFUSIONS, PERICARDIAL EFFUSIONS

In principle, all fluid collections can be drained. The same basic technique as described above can be used for drainage of dilated kidney collecting systems.

Abscesses

Percutaneous puncture and drainage is the method of choice for abscess therapy in the abdomen and retroperitoneum. The drainage procedure is usually preceded by a fine needle diagnostic puncture.

Usually the one-step technique can be used for drainage (21). Even if the fluid is pus the diameter of a 6–10 F catheter is usually adequte for drainage (Figure 15). The shortest route from the skin surface to the fluid collection is generally selected.

An infected gallbladder, containing pus, can be drained either with the one-step technique or with the Seldinger technique (22). Particularly patients at high surgical risk are selected for the ultrasonically-guided percutaneous technique instead of surgery. Pre-

Figure 15 *With the one-step technique, an 8 F catheter is placed inside a liver abscess.*

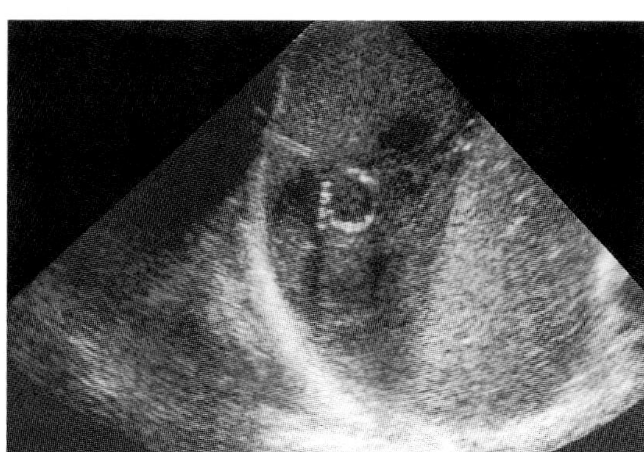

viously it was recommended that a transhepatic route should be used to avoid leakage of pus and bile but it is now claimed that a direct transperitoneal route can be safely used (23).

Pericardial effusions may be punctured using a 0.9 mm needle through the chest wall but if catheter drainage is needed a substernal route is most commonly chosen. It is important to perform the puncture with the patient on a table where catheter position can be checked with fluoroscopy.

CYST THERAPY

Benign renal cysts are very common in adults over 50 years. The majority of them cause no problems and can safely be left untreated. A few may cause pain or may lead to renal obstruction and should therefore be treated.

In Scandinavia, renal cysts have traditionally been treated by injection of bismuth. However, bismuth has now been abandoned in favour of alcohol, as the sclerosing agent (24).

The cyst is punctured under ultrasound control. The one-step technqiue can be used to position a thin catheter, e.g 4 French, inside the cyst. Half of the cyst fluid is then withdrawn and replaced with 95 % ethanol which is left for 10–15 minutes. The cyst is then emptied and the catheter removed after being flushed with saline.

A 95 % success rate is achieved with this technique (24).

TUMOUR THERAPY

Practically all tumours detectable with ultrasound can be punctured. This means that therapeutic agents can be deposited within a tumour with the aid of ultrasonic guidance. The most common such agent today is ethanol.

Liver tumours

Hepatocellular carcinomas predominantly occur in chronically diseased livers and are thus more common in Asian countries than in the West. Surgery is the most common form of therapy but is not suitable in many patients, because of high operation risk. As an alternative, injection of ethanol has been used by a number of authors. Shiina et al (25) reported their experience of ultrasonically-guided ethanol treatment on 146 patients suffering from hepatocellular cancer. They injected, as many others have done since, ethanol to a total volume (V) where $V = 4/3(r+0,5)^3$ ml, in small doses of 2–8 ml, on several occasions, usually 2–3 times per week (r=radius of the tumour). To these 146 patients with 242 lesions, 1048 treatments were given. Post-treatment histopathological examination, angiography and serum levels of alfa-fetoprotein showed that the technique was valuable and that the long-term survival of the patients increased. Minor complications occurred. The best results were achieved if the tumour diameter was less than 3 cm.

Good results have also been achieved by Livraghi et al (26) who treated 20 patients with hepatocellular carcinoma and 10 with hepatic metastases by injection of ethanol under general anaesthesia in a single session. The largest tumour had a diameter of 10 cm and the maximum volume of ethanol used was 165 ml.

Other ultrasonically-guided techniques for treatment of primary and secondary liver tumours include cryosurgery (27) and interstitial laser photocoagulation (28). Both of these techniques have yielded promising results.

Liver hydatid cysts

Sixteen cysts in 14 patients were treated with injection of ethanol by Georgio et al (29). They used a two-session technique, initially injecting ethanol after aspiration of the cyst contents and after three days repeating the procedure without aspiration. No anaphylactic reactions occurred and the results were good.

Parathyroid adenomas

Giangrande et al (30), among others, reported good results after injecting alcohol into parathyroid adenomas in the treatment of secondary hyperparathyroidism. Ethanol was injected into enlarged parathyroid glands under ultrasonic guidance in 50 uraemic patients, all of whom were hyporesponsive to calcium supplements and active metabolites of vitamin D.

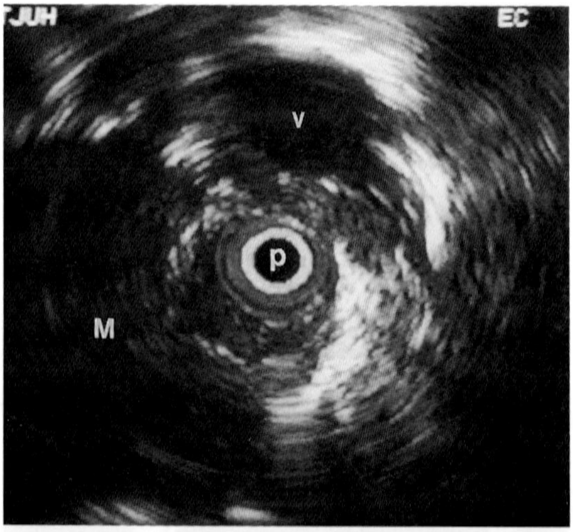

Figure 21 *Endoluminal ultrasound image obtained from the periphery of the lung demonstrates an eccentric mass (M). Note an adjacent blood vessel (V). P = probe*

suggesting normal nodal architecture. Abnormal lymph nodes are usually larger than 1 cm in diameter. Blood vessels are imaged as either anechoic tubular or oval structures and their position relative to the bronchus, tumor or lymph nodes can be delineated (Figure 21). With this information it is possible to avoid puncturing blood vessels by choosing a site for transbronchial biopsy away from these vital structures (41).

These preliminary results suggest that this new bronchoscopic ultrasound procedure will improve the capability to transbronchoscopically localize central and peripheral masses.

POTENTIAL DEVELOPMENTS

Three-dimensional (3-D) analysis and display of imaging data have been employed to evaluate many parts of the human anatomy. Endoluminal ultrasound, in particular, lends itself to 3-D reconstruction. Most attempts at 3-D imaging using catheter-based transducers have been in intravascular ultrasound (42, 43). Reliable and consistent reconstructions which correlated well with angiography have been obtained. Three-dimensional intravascular imaging allows for evaluation of vascular pathology in multiple planes. These advantages also apply to endoluminal 3-D ultrasound images (Figure 22). By providing more details of the longitudinal distribution of lesions, it should be possible to enhance diagnostic capabilities in a variety of nonvascular luminal abnormalities.

While the current catheter-based probes are designed for one-time use, ultimately, separate single use catheters will be coupled with a reusable transducer assembly to avoid catheter contamination while, at the same time, keep costs at a reasonable level.

High resolution endoluminal sonography is a promising new ultrasound imaging approach for the investigation of a variety of vascular and nonvascular lumina throughout the body. The major advantages of this technique are increased resolution and the ability to image mural and submural structures. Its current major limitation is lack of penetration of the ultrasound beam limiting its ability to detect structures beyond two centimetres. Future development of Doppler and 3-D capabilities should significantly improve the diagnostic capabilities of endoluminal ultrasound imaging.

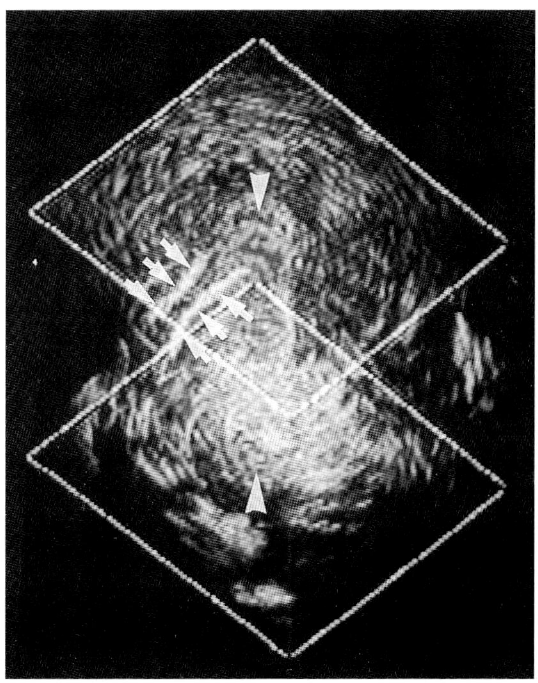

Figure 22 *Preliminary 3D reconstruction image from 2D endoluminal ultrasound shows the relationship of the ureter (arrowheads) to a crossing blood vessel (arrows). A linear interpolation was made of approximately 60 endoluminal 2D images and produced by moving the catheter by hand.*

REFERENCES

1. Wild JJ, Reid JM. Diagnostic use of ultrasound. Br J Phys Med 1956;19:248–257.
2. Bom N, ten Hoff H, Lancee CT et al. Early and recent intraluminal ultrasound devices. Int J Card Imaging 1989;4:79–88.
3. Omoto R. Intracardiac scanning of the heart with the aid of ultrasonic intravenous probe. Jap Heart J 1989;8:569–581.
4. Ebina T, Oka S, Tanaka M et al. The diagnostic application of ultrasound to the disease in mediastinal organs. Ultrasono-tomography for the heart and great vessels. Sci Rep Res Inst Tohoku Univ 1965;12:199–212.
5. von Micsky LI. Ultrasonic tomography in obstetrics and gynecology. In: Grossman CC, Holmes JH, Joyner C et al (eds). Diagnostic Ultrasound. New York: Plenum, 1966:348–368.
6. Bom N, Lancee CT, van Egmond FC. An ultrasonic intracardiac scanner. Ultrasonics 1972;10:72–76.
7. Hisanaga K. Hisanaga A, Nagata K, Yoshida S. A new transesophageal real-time two-dimensional echocardiographic system using a flexible tube and its clinical application. Proc Jap Soc Ultrasonics Med 1977;32:43–44.
8. DiMagno EP, Regan PT, Wilson DA et al. Ultrasonic endoscope. Lancet 1980;March:629–631.
9. Souquet J, Hanrath P, Zitelli A et al. Transesophageal phased array for imaging the heart. IEEE Trans Biomed Engin 1982;BME-29:707–712.
10. Natori H, Tamaki S, Izumi S et al. Clinical application of ultrasound endoscope using linear array transducer for transesophageal ultrasonography of the diseases of the mediastinum. In: Lerski A, Morley P (eds): Ultrasound '82. Oxford: Pergamon Press; 1983:339–343.
11. Fukuda M, Hirata K. Saito K et al. On the diagnostic use of echoendoscope in abdominal disease. I. Diagnostic experience with a new type of echoendoscope on gastric diseases. Proc Jap J Med Ultrasound 1980;37:409–410.
12. Murata Y, Suzuki S, Hashimoto H. Endoscopic ultrasonography of the upper gastrointestinal tract. Surg Endosc 1988;2:180–183.
13. Holm HH, Northeved AA. A transurethral ultrasonic scanner. J Urol 1974;111:238–248.
14. Bom N, Slager CJ, van Egmond FC et al. Intraarterial ultrasonic imaging for recanalization by spark erosion. Microsensors and catheter-based imaging technology. SPIE 1988;904:107–109.
15. Ellis R. Crowley RJ, Eyllon MM. Ultrasonic imaging catheter. Microsensors and catheter-based imaging technology. SPIE 1988;904:127–130.
16. Gussenhoven EJ, Essed CE, Lancee CT et al. Arterial wall characteristics determined by intravascular ultrasound imaging: an in vitro study. J Am Coll Cardiol 1989;14:947–952.

17. Dake MD. Intravascular ultrasound. Curr Opin Radiol 1991; 3:181–187.
18. Goldberg BB, Liu JB, Merton DA et al. Endoluminal US: experiments with non-vascular uses in animals. Radiology 1990;175:39–43.
19. Strup S, Rivas DA, Liu JB et al. Endoluminal ultrasonographic and histologic evaluation of periurethral collagen injection. Proc Fifty-second Annual Meeting of Mid-Atlantic Section of the American Urologic Association, Philadelphia, PA, Sept 21–25, 1994; pp 68–69.
20. Chancellor MB, Karusick S, Erhard MJ et al. Placement of a wire mesh prosthesis in the external urinary sphincter of men with spinal cord injuries. Radiology 1993;187:551–555.
21. Chancellor MB, Liu JB, Rivas DA et al. Intraoperative endoluminal ultrasound evaluation of urethral diverticula. J Urol 1995;153:72–75.
22. Goldberg BB, Bagley D, Liu JB et al. Endoluminal sonography of the urinary tract: preliminary observations. AJR 1991;156:99–103.
23. Liu JB, Bagley DH, Goldberg BB. Endoluminal sonography of the urinary tract. In: Thrall JH (ed): Current Practice of Radiology. St Louis: Mosby, 1993.
24. Bagley DH, Liu JB, Goldberg BB. Use of endoluminal ultrasound of ureter. Sem Urol 1992;3:194–198.
25. Grasso M, Bagley DH, Liu JB et al. Using endoluminal US to treat a variety of upper tract disorders. Contemporary Urology 1994;6:24–32.
26. Goldberg BB, Liu JB, Kuhlman K et al. Endoluminal gynecologic ultrasound: preliminary results. J Ultrasound Med 1991;10:583–590.
27. Malignant tumors of the uterus. In: Mattingly RF, Thompson JD (eds): Te Linde's Operative Gynecology. Philadelphia: JB Lippincott, 1985:845.
28. Fayez JA, Mutie G, Schneider PJ. The diagnostic value of hysterosalpingography and hysteroscopy in infertility investigation. Am J Obstet Gynecol 1987;156:558.
29. Lehtovirta P, Cacciatore B, Wahlstrom T, Ylostalo P. Ultrasonic assessment of endometrial cancer invasion. J Clin Ultrasound 1987;5:519–524.
30. Ragavendra N, McMahon JT, Perrella R et al. Endoluminal catheter-assisted transcervical US of the human embryo. Radiology 1991;181:779–783.
31. Liu JB, Miller LS, Goldberg BB et al. Transnasal US of the esophagus: preliminary morphologic and function studies. Radiology 1992;184:721–727.
32. Liu JB, Miller LS, Feld RI et al. Gastric and esophageal varices: 20 MHz transnasal endoluminal US. Radiology 1993;187:363–366.
33. Miller L, Liu JB, Klenn PJ et al. Endoluminal ultrasonography of the distal esophagus in systemic sclerosis. Gastroenterology 1993;105:31–39.
34. Alexander AA, Miller LS, Liu JB et al. High frequency endoluminal sonography of the anal sphincter complex. J Ultrasound Med 1994;13:281–284.

35. Shapiro MJ, Bonn J, Sullivan KL et al. Endoluminal biliary ultrasound: initial clinical experience. J Vasc & Intervent Radiol 1991;2:11–12.
36. Engstrom CF, Wiechel KL. Endoluminal ultrasound of the bile ducts. Surg Endosc 1990;4:187–190.
37. vanSonnenberg E, D'Agostino HB, Sanchez RL et al. Percutaneous intraluminal US in the gallbladder and bile ducts. Radiology 1992;182:693–696.
38. Shure D, Fedullo PF. Transbronchial needle aspiration of peripheral masses. Am Rev Respir Dis 1983;128:1090–1092.
39. Shure D. Fiberoptic bronchoscopy: diagnostic applications. Clin Chest Med 1987;8:1–12.
40. Hurter TH, Hanrath P. Endobronchial sonography in the diagnosis of pulmonary and mediastinal tumors. Dtsch Med Wochenschr 1990;115:1899–1905.
41. Goldberg BB, Steiner RM, Liu JB et al. US-assisted bronchoscopy with use of miniature transducer-containing catheters. Radiology 1994;190:233–237.
42. Burrell CJ, Kitney RI, Rothman MT. Intravascular ultrasound imaging and three-dimensional modelling of arteries. Echocardiography 1990;7:475–484.
43. Klein HM, Gunther RW, Verlande M et al. 3D-surface reconstruction of intravascular ultrasound images using personal computer hardware and a motorized catheter control. Cardiovasc Intervent Radiol 1992;15:97–101.

CHAPTER 24

Contrast Agents and 3D Ultrasound

Flemming Forsberg, PhD and Barry B. Goldberg, MD

Extensive efforts are currently under way to develop efficacious ultrasound contrast agents. Such agents hold forth the promise of a variety of improvements to the diagnostic capabilities of current ultrasound scanners. The enhancement of Doppler signals from small and/or deep lying vessels have been investigated, as well as increases in the difference in echogenicity between normal and adjcacent abnormal (e.g., tumor) tissue in organs such as the liver and spleen (1, 2). The former is achieved with vascular ultrasound contrast agents, while the latter requires organ- or tumor-specific agents. The many different types of ultrasound contrast agents will be reviewed in the following along with an introduction to the associated artifacts and the possibility of contrast-specific imaging.

In other imaging modalities, such as computed tomography (CT), magnetic resonance imaging (MRI), and single photon emission computed tomography (SPECT), three dimensional (3D) data displays are well established and increasingly used in the diagnostic decision making; not so in ultrasound. Due to the real-time (or at least near real-time) requirements of ultrasound imaging the time available for acquisition and processing of a 3D volume of data is very limited. Consequently, while many experimental prototype systems for 3D imaging have been described, it is only recently, with the improvements in computer processing powers, that preliminary reports on the clinical use of 3D ultrasound scanning have appeared (3). The developments in the field of 3D ultrasound imaging will also be described in this chapter.

ULTRASOUND CONTRAST AGENTS

Physics

Conventional ultrasound imaging relies on differences in backscattering (i.e., echogenicity) to distinguish between different types of tissue. Hence, the most important mechanism for contrast effects is to increase the energy of the backscattered signal. The majority of contrast agents achieve this by introducing microbubbles of air into the bloodstream.

Because the acoustic properties of air are so different from those of blood, microbubble based ultrasound contrast agents can enhance Doppler signals by up to 25 dB. The enhancement typically lasts 3–8 minutes, indicating that the contrast media recirculates through the heart, as well as the pulmonary and systemic capillary circulations. Hence, the microbubbles used must range from 1 to 10 μm in diameter. Moreover, in order for the agent to survive the presssure changes in the heart encapsulated microbubbles (i.e., with an outer shell) have to be employed.

Further increases in the backscattered energy are possible with gas-based contrast agents. Free air microbubbles can act as harmonic oscillators within a liquid. This means that they will resonate at a specific frequency (the fundamental frequency), which can produce enhancement of the echo-signals by an additional three orders of magnitude. A rough estimate of the resonance frequency, f_r in kHz, can be calculated as $f_r = 6500/d$; where d is the bubble diameter in μm (4). Bubble sizes of 1 to 10 μm thus produce resonance frequencies ranging from 650 kHz to 6.5 MHz. However, due to the need for stabilized (i.e. encapsulated) bubbles, which dampens the oscillations, the resonance frequencies are somewhat higher in practice. This is only an advantage, since it brings the fundamental frequency of bubbles 3–5 μm in diameter further into the diagnostic frequency range.

It is also possible to produce contrast effects by altering other acoustic properties of the tissue, such as the speed of sound or the attenuation. However, as no functional ultrasound images of such parameters are currently in clinical use, no further details will be given here. Instead we refer to two recent review articles (1, 2).

Clinical applications

The first report on the use of an ultrasound contrast agent (in the aortic root) appeared over 25 years ago. Since then, considerable efforts have been made to produce agents capable of increasing echogenicity and Doppler signal intensities for both cardiac and noncardiac applications. The ideal agent would be 1/ nontoxic; 2/ injectable intravenously; 3/ capable of traversing the pulmonary, cardiac and capillary circulations; and 4/ stable for recirculation. It is only within the last decade that pharmaceutical companies and researchers have approached this goal. Ultrasound contrast agents are often grouped according to their target area; vascular agents versus organ or tumor-specific agents. Moreover, the vascular agents are subdivided depending on how closely they match the ideal agent; so called first and second generation agents.

Organ or tumor-specific agents

Aqueous solutions, emulsions and suspensions have all been used as organ or tumor-specific agents. However, the amounts of solutions and emulsions required to produce enhancement is often very large. Hence, their usefulness have been limited. Colloidal suspensions, on the other hand, have demonstrated some success in increasing the backscattering from soft tissue as well as blood. Work with iodipamide ethyl esther (IDE) has demonstrated enhancement of the liver after an intravenous injection (5). These particles are less than 1 μm in size and can, therefore, easily pass through the capillary circulation. They appear to be taken up by the reticuloendothelial system in the liver and spleen (the Kupffer cells). IDE seems to enhance normal liver tissue rather than abnormal.

The most extensive investigations, and currently the most promising, have been those using perfluorochemicals. They have been shown to increase backscattering from tissue, as well as blood (6) due to their high density (1.9 g/ml) and low speed of sound (600 m/s), which creates differences in acoustic impedance of 30 % between the perfluorocarbon and the adjacent tissue. Like IDE particles perfluorocarbon increases the echogenicity of normal liver tissue; this improves the detection of tumors, which have destroyed normal liver cells (Figure 1). Most work so far has been in animal experiments, but human studies of one particular perfluorocarbon based agent (Imagent™, Alliance Pharmaceuticals Corp., San Diego, CA) are ongoing.

First generation microbubble agents

Almost any solution which is agitated and then injected into a blood vessel will produce echoes. However, such bubbles are often too unstable for practical use and too large to traverse the capillaries. Alternatively, contrast agents based on sonicated solutions, such as Renografin -76, have smaller, more uniform, and stable bubbles. These agents have been used to enhance Doppler signals from the heart and peripheral vessels. One particularly successful contrast agent is sonicated human serum albumin (Albunex™; Molecular Biosystems, Inc., San Diego, CA). The albumin coating of the microbubbles stabilizes them sufficiently to circulate beyond the right side of the heart and lungs, increasing the reflectivity of blood within the left atrium and ventricle, as well as in different systemic arteries (7). The half-life of this contrast agent in blood has been shown to be less than 1 minute. After three minutes, more than 80 % of the Albumin was found in the liver.

Investigations using naturally occurring hepatocellular tumors in woodchucks have shown that intravenous injections of Albunex produced immediate Doppler signal enhancement within the inferior vena cava, followed by enhancement within the abdominal aorta, hepatic artery and its branches. While the B-mode images

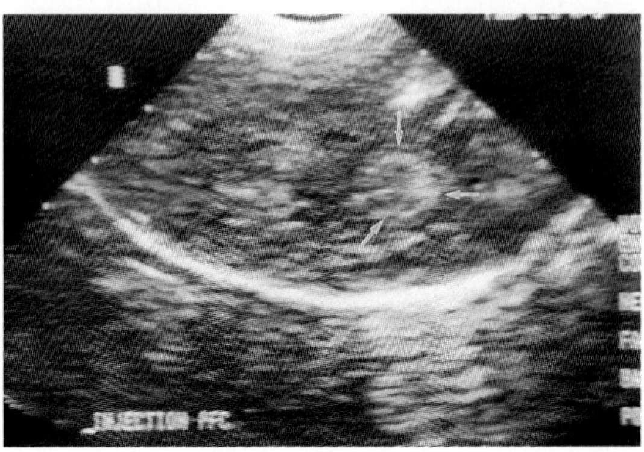

Figure 1 *Woodchuck liver 24 hours post injection of a perfluorochemical; a rim (arrows) of increased liver tumor echogenicity is seen. Reproduced with permission from ref. 2.*

showed no perceivable change in tissue echogenicity with Doppler (both spectral and color) there was clear signal enhancement in normal, as well as tumor vessels. In the larger tumors the greatest increase in Doppler signal intensity occurred at the tumor periphery; the central portion tended to be less vascular and, in some cases, was even necrotic (Figure 2).

Albunex when injected intraarterially has also been used to quantify myocardial perfusion with echocardiography. Studies have been able to assess collateral flow to determine tissue viability after myocardial infarction and to confirm the success of graft placement after coronary artery bypass surgery (8). Intravenous injections in humans have been effective in filling the right and left chambers of the heart but not in producing myocardial enhancement. Based on these results Albunex has been approved for clinical use as an echocardiographic contrast agent in Japan and the USA. However, studies by de Jong et al. have shown that quantitative analysis of the contrast effect in the left side of the heart after an intravenous injection of Albunex had limitations due to the instability of the microspheres and the filtering action of the lung capillaries (9).

An attempt to answer these problems was the development of soluble saccharide (galactose) microparticles containing microbubbles of gas (Echovist™, Schering AG, Berlin, Germany). The microbubbles have a mean diameter of 3.5 μm with 99 % smaller than 12 μm. Trials have been carried out in both animals and humans in which contrast injected intravenously was imaged in the right atrium and ventricle. However, since the bubble sizes in suspension range from 5 to 15 μm they cannot easily pass from the right to the left side of the heart. Echovist is approved for clinical use as a right heart agent in Europe. Essentially, Echovist is (like Albunex) a one-pass only agent, which constitutes the major limitation of first generation vascular contrast agents.

Second generation microbubble agents

Based on experiments with first generation agents new contrast media have been developed, so called second generation contrast agents, that persist for longer in the blood stream (typically 3 to 6 minutes). One such agent is Levovist™ (Schering AG, Berlin, Germany),

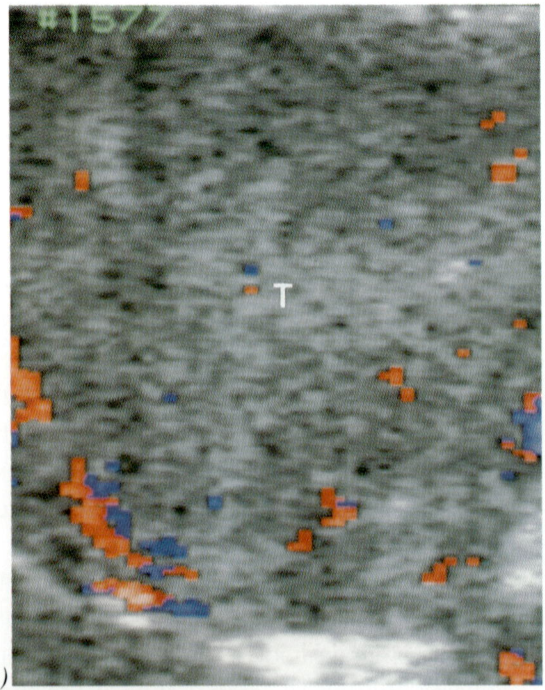

(a)

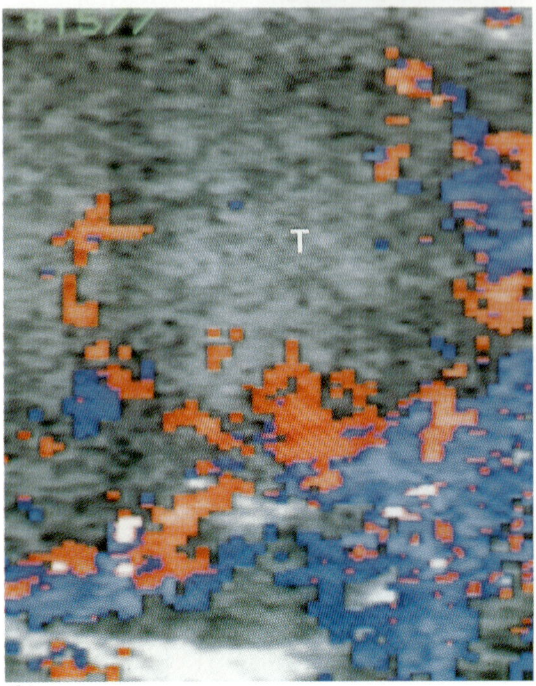

(b)

Figure 2 *Hepatoma (T) in woodchuck. a. pre injection b. post injection of 1.0 cc of Albunex. Marked blood flow enhancement is seen around the periphery of the tumor. Reproduced with permission from ref. 7.*

which like Echovist is made from galactose but is provided with a slight change in its chemical composition to produce smaller, more stable and uniform bubble sizes ranging from 2 to 8 μm in diameter. This agent has been used successfully to visualize not only the right but also the left side of the heart. Levovist appears to be useful in delineating the circumference of the chambers of the heart, as well as assisting in the calculation of the ventricular ejection fraction.

In animal studies, peripheral intravenous injections of Levovist have resulted in enhancement of the Doppler signals throughout the body lasting in excess of three to five minutes. Of more interest is its ability to enhance Doppler signals in the portal circulation, which means that this contrast agent has passed through two capillary beds and still maintains a significant contrast effect. However, no parenchymal enhancement has been reported. Re-

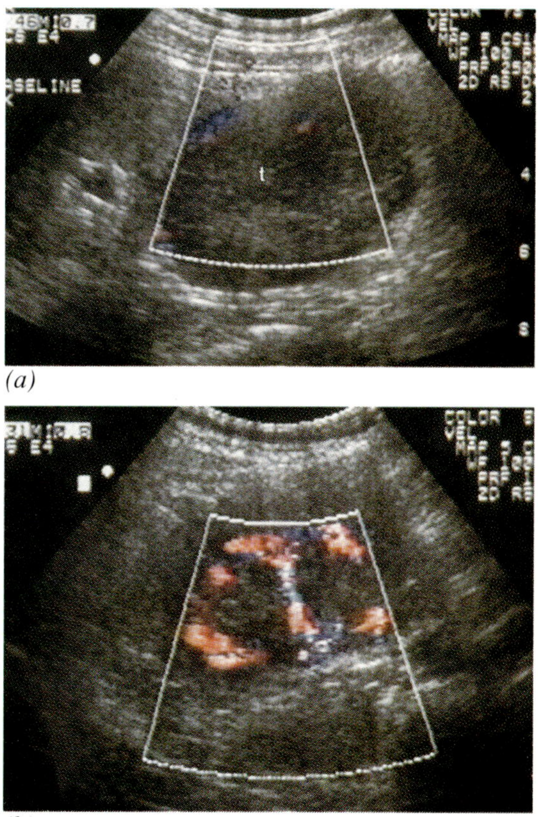

(a)

(b)

Figure 3
Color Doppler imaging of a patient with a renal tumor (T).
a. pre injection
b. post injection of 16 cc of Levovist, tumor blood flow enhancement is demonstrated.
Reproduced with permission from ref. 2.

search with naturally-occurring hepatocellular carcinomas in woodchucks has confirmed Levovist's ability to increase the reflectivity of small vessels not only within the normal portions of the liver, but also within tumors. There was an increasing effect (up to approximately 14 dB) with increasing dose. In large animal models (dog and sheep) this agent produced enhancement of the Doppler signals in the vessels of the retina of the eye, as well as the gallbladder, urinary bladder, and bowel walls.

Clinical trials in humans using Levovist have been carried out for the evaluation of normal and tumor vascularity. Enhancement of both color and spectral Doppler signals within normal and tumor vessels was demonstrated in the liver, kidney, ovary, pancreas and breast (Figure 3). Color Doppler enhancement proved useful for localizing sample volume placement for spectral analysis. Levovist was able to improve the spectral Doppler signal quality and added additional information in assessment of tumor vascularity and vessel displacement. In the examination of a wide variety of vessels, the agent was able to improve the reliability of vascular diagnosis by better demonstrating the presence or absence of high velocity jets, by better demonstrating collateral or runoff vessels, by showing longer segments of vessels or by showing flow through regions with pre-contrast absent or weak Doppler signals.

Microbubble based agents containing gases other than air (e.g., nitrogen or carbon dioxide) are also under investigation. One such newly developed contrast agent is called EchoGen™ (Sonus Pharmaceuticals, Bothell, WA). It has the ability to change from an emulsion of a water-immiscible liquid, dodecafluoropentane (DDFP), and surfactants to echogenic DDFP gas bubbles (diameter 1–5 µm) upon injection into the blood stream. This is due to the boiling point of DDFP being 28–30°C. Echocardiograhic studies following intravenous administration of this agent in monkeys and dogs demonstrated cardiac chamber opacification and myocardial wall enhancement. Further animal studies in woodchucks and rabbits (with VX2 tumors) demonstrated enhancement (of up to 19 dB) in spectral as well as color Doppler imaging (CDI) modes lasting approximately 3 minutes. Grey-scale enhancement of abdominal organs, such as liver and kidney, was observed for over 20 minutes (Figure 4). Smaller hepatomas (< 6 mm) became

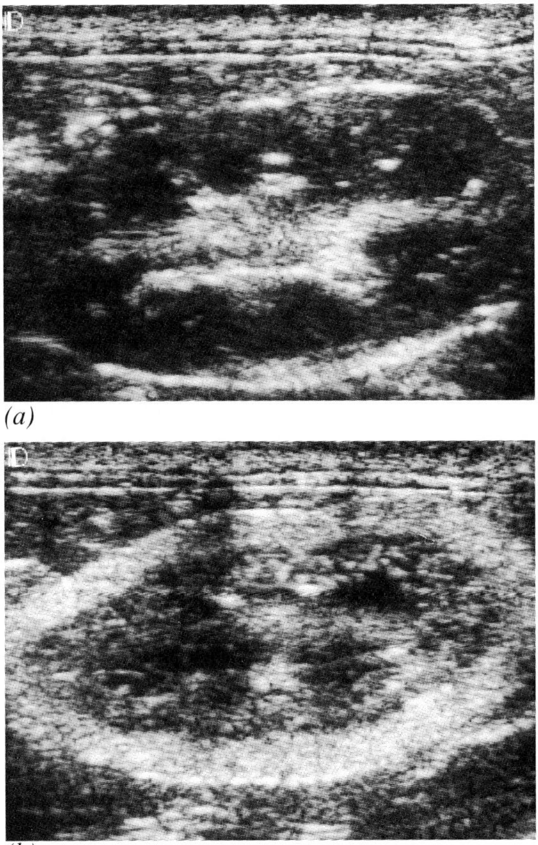

(a)

(b)

Figure 4
Gray-scale enhancement in rabbit kidney.
a. pre injection
b. post injection of 0.4 ml/kg of EchoGen: a significant increase in cortical reflectivity is seen.

more echogenic centrally, while larger tumors only showed an increase in Doppler signals from peripheral vessels (due to central necrosis). Phase I clinical trials in humans have been completed and Phase II trials are in progress.

Recently, two new agents developed from experiences with Albunex have appeared: FS069 (Molecular Biosystems, Inc., San Diego, CA, USA) and NUS (Nycomed Imaging, Oslo, Norway). The former consists of proteinaceous microspheres, while the latter is based on stabilized microbubbles. Both agents have mean sizes in the 3 to 6 μm range, and are capable of recirculating over 4 to 6 minutes. Preliminary animal studies have shown excellent contrast effects (Figure 5).

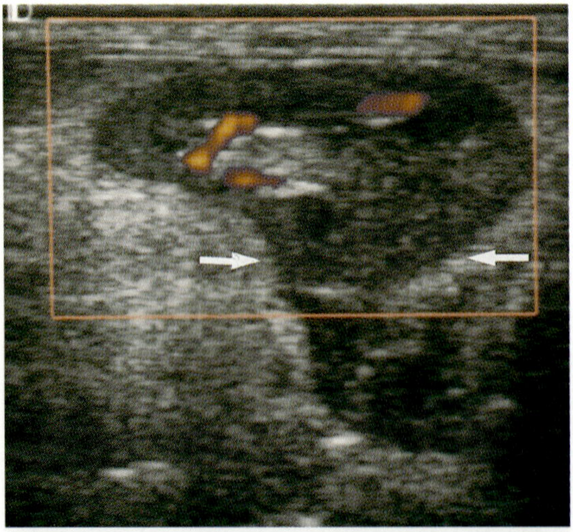

(a)

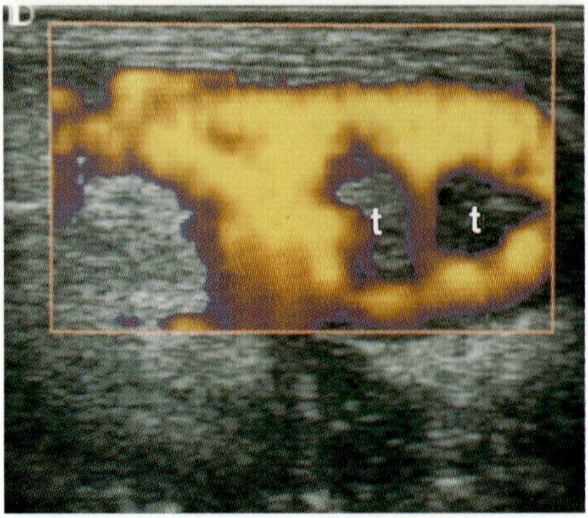

(b)

Figure 5
Rabbit kidney with induced VX-2 tumors.
a. pre injection, the shape of the kidney is distorted (bulge; arrows) but the tumor outline is not well defined.
b. post injection of 0.1 ml/kg of NUS two VX-2 tumors (T) are clearly delineated.

Evaluating contrast effects

By displaying only the power or amplitude of the Doppler signal, so called color amplitude imaging (CAI), it is possible to increase the display dynamic range by up to 10 dB; without administrating a contrast agent. This increase is achieved by sacrificing velocity and direction related information (10). As ultrasound contrast increases the intensity of Doppler signals combining the two (contrast and CAI) allows better delineation of small, deep vessels as in the renal cortex (Figure 6). It is also possible to follow the course of blood vessels for longer. Thus, this technique improves the evaluation of vascular contrast agents. The only major drawback is the susceptibility of CAI to motion artifacts (10).

Another possibility for evaluation of ultrasound contrast agents is to measure the contrast uptake and washout times via videodensitometry. Work on breast masses using Levovist indicate that it might be possible to separate benign from malignant lesions (11). Tumors tend to enhance quickly and washout early probably due to tumor AV-shunts. Further studies are underway to confirm these initial reports and evaluate their potential in other areas of the body.

Figure 6
Color amplitude images of a dog kidney.
a. pre injection
b. post injection of 0.5 cc of FS069, the outline of the kidney is well defined.

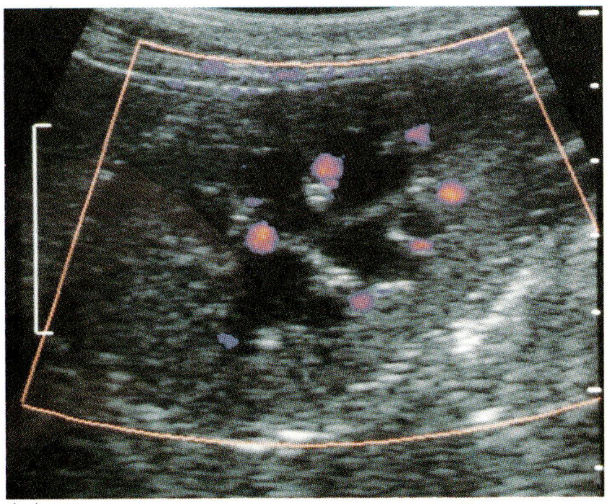

(a)

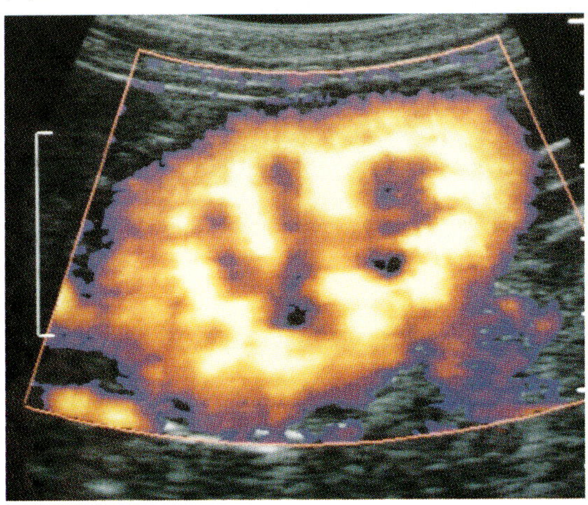

(b)

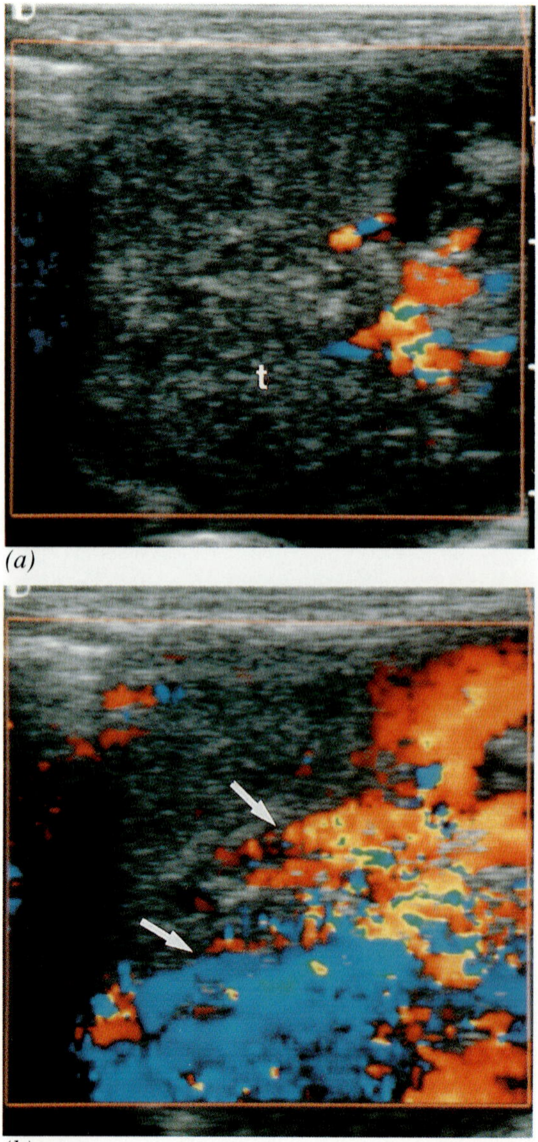

(a)

(b)

Figure 7
Example of color blooming in a rabbit kidney with an avascular VX-2 tumor (T).
a. pre injection
b. after injection. The avascular lesion is completely obscured by color pixels (arrows).

Artifacts and contrast agents

The specific artifacts associated with ultrasonic contrast agent studies are color blooming, spectral bubble noise and increaseed maximum Doppler shifts (12). Color blooming occurs immediately after the bolus injection of contrast media arrives at the imaging location.

This artifact is seen as gray-scale pixels changing to color display in regions where blood flow is not possible (Figure 7). It is caused by the increase in Doppler signal intensity, induced by the contrast, which effectively lowers the threshold below which weak flow signals are excluded from display (the so called color reject threshold). Hence, the amount of color in the image increases. Color blooming can be eliminated either by reducing the overall color gain, or by waiting for the peak enhancement to pass, or by employing a continuous infusion of contrast agent instead of a bolus injection. Spectral bubble noise is seen as very large excursions in the spectral display (Figure 8) and is always associated with a loud "crackling" noise in the audio output. The latter is due to the limited dynamic range of the audio circuitry, while the former is caused either by the breakdown of bubbles within the Doppler sample volume or by large individual bubbles traversing the sample volume. Both bubble noise and color blooming are easy to identify in practice. Consequently, these artifacts are of limited clinical significance.

The increase in maximum Doppler shifts is more troublesome. Increases in peak Doppler frequency shifts ranging from 20 to 45 % have been observed (Figure 9) (12). This change is mostly artifactual and arises from the limited dynamic range of the spectral display. As the Doppler signal power is enhanced the highest frequency

Figure 8 *Spectral bubble noise obtained from a woodchuck liver tumor.*

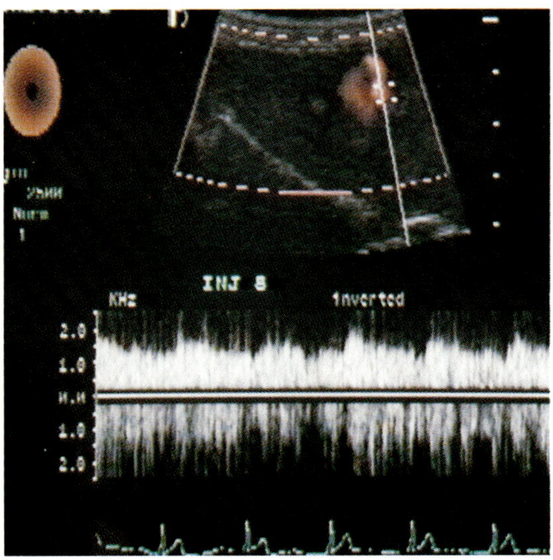

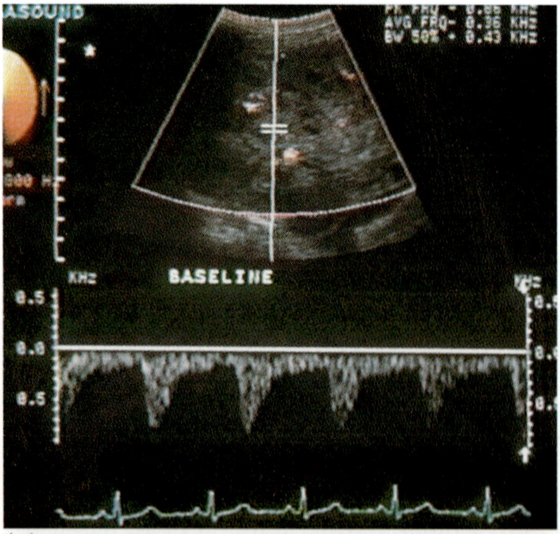

(a)

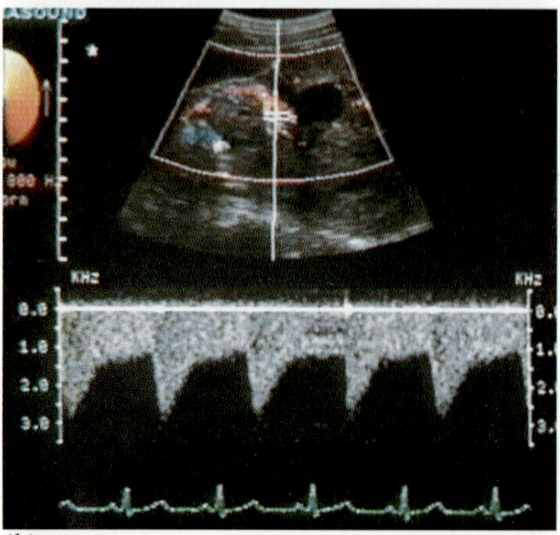

(b)

Figure 9 *Increased peak Doppler shifts obtained from human abdominal mass.*
a. pre injection, the peak Doppler shift is approximately 0.8 kHz.
b. post injection, the peak Doppler shift increases to around 3 kHz.

shown also increases. This artifact affects all indices derived from the maximum Doppler shift, such as the pulsatility index (PI), in a nonlinear fashion due to the nonlinear scanner compression curves. Hence, spectral parameters obtained pre- and post contrast injection cannot be compared. Eliminating this problem will either require scanners with a larger dynamic range than currently available or new spectral indices, which are unaffected by the increase in Doppler signal intensity (e.g., based on the bandwidth of the spectrum).

Harmonic imaging

In principle no modifications of existing ultrasound scanners are required to perform contrast enhanced imaging. Nonetheless, a recent development in scanner technology, called Harmonic Imaging, appear well suited for the evaluation of contrast agents (13, 14). This technique is unique by requiring the presence of a contrast agent, and it opens up the possibility of measuring blood perfusion or capillary blood flow; a clinically important task. Harmonic Imaging utilizes the nonlinear properties of ultrasound bubble contrast agents by transmitting at the fundamental transducer frequency but receiving at the second harmonic (twice the fundamental). Because a free air bubble can act as a harmonic oscillator, contrast enhanced echo signals will contain significant energy components at not only the resonance (fundamental) frequency, but also at higher and lower harmonics.

The advantage of the processing scheme described above is due to the difference in backscattering for tissue and contrast agent at the two frequencies. The magnitude of the backscattered contrast enhanced signal was measured by Schrope and co-workers who found that, in water, the harmonic component was 5 dB down from the fundamental (13). Even though the harmonic signal is weaker than the fundamental the theoretical analysis found the blood-to-tissue intensity ratio (the signal-to-noise ratio; SNR) enhancement achievable is over 1000. Attenuation will be higher at the harmonic frequency than at the fundamental. Nonetheless, further in vitro experiments (in an excised sheep kidney) demonstrated harmonic enhancement of 26 dB compared to 29 dB at the fundamental frequency. Preliminary in-vivo measurements in rabbits ears, recorded an SNR for the backscattered harmonic signal of 5–10, while data acquired at the fundamental frequency had a negative SNR (14). In other words, the nonlinearity of the contrast agent produced a "signature" which could be separated from tissue echoes and large vessel blood flow allowing capillary blood flow (i.e., perfusion) to be calculated.

The first reports on the use of real-time in-vivo harmonic images, both in B-mode and Doppler, have appeared in the literature (15, 16). An example of tumor blood flow visualization using

Harmonic Imaging is given in Figure 10. These early results suggest that it should be possible to achieve real-time blood pool imaging (i.e., perfusion imaging) by subtracting conventional ultrasound images from simultaneously acquired harmonic images. Furthermore, very recently color amplitude imaging (also known as "power Doppler") and Harmonic Imaging have been combined (17). As Harmonic Imaging suppresses tissue echoes this combination reduces the flash artifact, which otherwise can be a substantial problem in color amplitude imaging.

Oral ultrasound contrast agents

Evaluation of the upper gastrointestinal tract with ultrasound can be difficult due to the presence of the airfilled stomach and bowel gas in general. Water is used to displace the air, but often it is not successful. As an alternative, investigators have evaluated cellulose-based suspensions as an oral ultrasound contrast agent. One

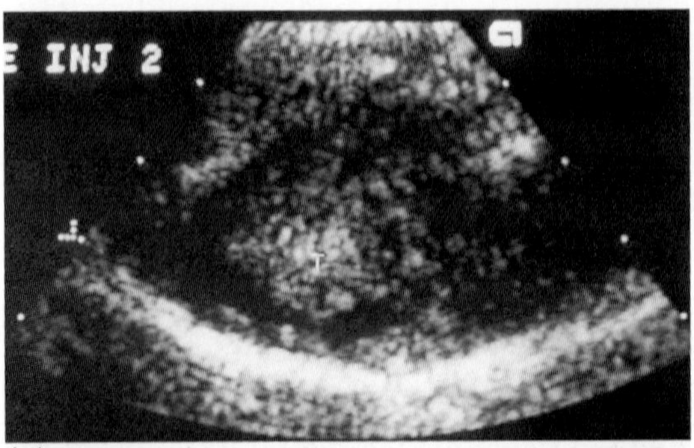

(a)

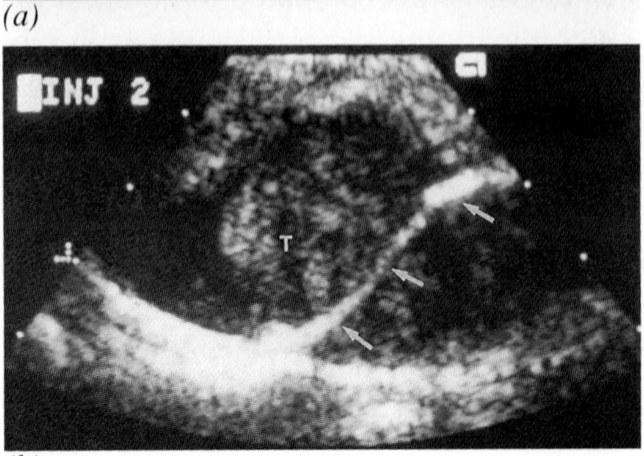

(b)

Figure 10 *Woodchuck hepatoma (T) imaged in gray-scale Harmonic Imaging (2.5 MHz/5.0 MHz transmit/receive frequencies).*
a. pre injection
b. post injection of 2.0 cc of FS069. Notice the excellent contrast between the contrast material and the tissue (arrows).

such agent is SonoRX™ (Bracco, Milan, Italy) which consists of Simethicone-coated cellulose and has been employed in doses of 200–1000 cc. Preliminary results in humans demonstrated improved visualization of the stomach, duodenum and pancreas (Figure 11) (18). Tumors of the upper GI tract were also easier to detect with SonoRX. Several different oral contrast agents are under development.

Figure 11
Stomach (S).
a. pre injection
b. post administration of 800 ml of SonoRX. Notice the improved visualization of the stomach wall (small arrows) and the pancreatic tail (large arrows).

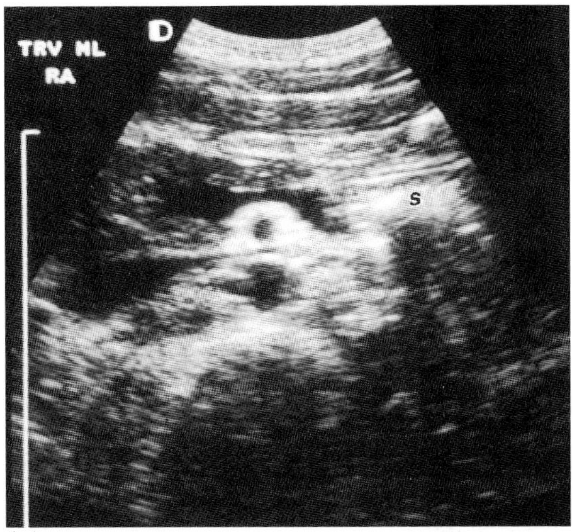

(a)

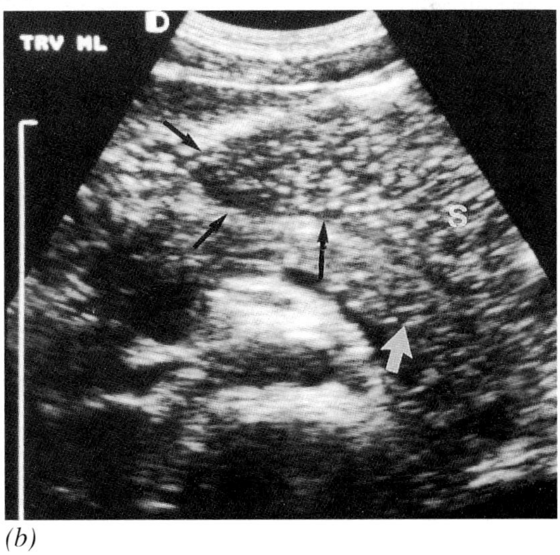

(b)

3D ULTRASOUND

3D reconstruction techniques

Ultrasound presents a special challenge to 3D imaging, since the images are processed in real time and the transducer is moved freely in space acquiring images in any desired plane. The former limits the time available for processing and display, while the latter requires precise localization of the image geometry being acquired to avoid introducing erroneous distortions. Conversely, ultrasound also presents special advantages to 3D imaging: the images are tomographic and can be gated to correspond to other physiological events (e.g., the heart rate). Furthermore, it is typically possible to acquire a total 3D volume in a single breath-hold (thus, reducing motion artifacts) and also to investigate flow conditions using Doppler ultrasound. Producing an accurate 3D ultrasound image relies critically on the data acquisition technique, and on exact definition of the acoustic 3D volume.

Localizing the 3D volume

In a static image collection modality with fixed slice thickness, such as CT or MRI, the geometry of the 3D volume is given. In ultrasound a different approach has to be taken to specify the 3D data set: mechanical tracking, dedicated 3D probes or remote sensing have been used. The only exception in sonography occurs when the anatomy defines the 3D volume; for example in intravascular ultrasound using catheter based miniature transducers inside blood vessels or in endorectal scanning.

The simplest way of defining the 3D volume is to mount a conventional transducer in a mechanical arm and either monitor the probe movements in space (similar to a static B scanner) or move the probe under automatic motor control. The latter approach is often limited to movement along a single axis. Mechanical tracking can be difficult to carry out on curved surfaces such as the female breast or the third trimester abdomen. Instead a dedicated 3D transducer can be utilized. Typically this consists of a conventional transducer (mechanical or more often phased array) mounted with a stepping motor in a hand held assembly. The motor either translates or rotates the transducer around an axis, which defines the 3D volume. Image acquisition lasts from 10 seconds and up to 1 minute (with cardiac gating) during which the probe is held motionless. Due to the need for additional motors 3D probes are often more bulky and, hence, more cumbersome to use than conventional transducers. However, not to a degree where this constitutes a major problem.

Finally, the 3D volume can be specified by placing sensors on a conventional transducer and then tracking its location in space via remote localizers. Acoustic, optical and magnetic positioning devices have been utilized. All these approaches offer great flexibility of movement, but require additional sensor equipment to be placed near the patient (e.g., microphones or a magnetic field generator). Hence the current trend on commercial 3D scanners is to have dedicated 3D probes. Particularly promising are two-dimensional electronic arrays, capable of acquiring a 3D data set directly in real-time. Such arrays are currently under development, but none have yet made the transition to clinical use.

Surface and volume rendering

Once the 3D volume is defined and a set of 2D ultrasound images have been acquired (and digitized for computer manipulations) the 3D data set needs to be displayed. Two main ways for viewing 3D data exist; one is termed surface rendering and the other is called volume rendering (Figure 12).

As the name indicates, surface rendering techniques create a display of the boundaries within the 3D volume. Early attempts in echocardiography applied simple thresholding to the original 3D volume, thus creating a binary data set. This in turn was used (via boundary detection) to produce wireframe 3D displays. This allows the geometric features (i.e., the anatomy) within the region of interest to be assessed, but makes an evaluation of disease morphology more difficult to perform. Later efforts took a voxel oriented approach, which does not rely in extracting any specific information but uses the entire 3D volumetric data set. Voxels are volume elements which expand the traditional digital picture element (or pixel) into 3D space. These algorithms have improved the accuracy of 3D displays. A data set of voxels can be created by segmentation of the digitized 2D images (Figure 12). Segmentation refers to the process by which structures of interest within the gray-scale 2D images are identified and assigned voxels. Next a surface tracking algorithm can be used to create a shaded surface display. Voxel based surface displays are superior to wireframe (i.e., binary) types, because the morphology of the tissue in question can be studied. For example, in intravascular images the arterial wall rather than just the lumen can be visualized.

It is also possible from a voxel data set to produce a volume display. The main feature of such a method is the display of data directly from the gray scale volume, which allows both surface visualization and volume manipulation, e.g. the "peeling" away of layers. One very important function is to display several imaging planes simultaneously. Such a multiplanar display typically shows three orthogonal planes; the acquisition plane, the transverse plane and the so called C-plane (orthogonal to the transducer) (3). Certain methods also allow for oblique cuts of the 3D volume. As the C plane can never be visualized with a conventional 2D scanner,

Figure 12 *Overview of 3D reconstruction techniques.*

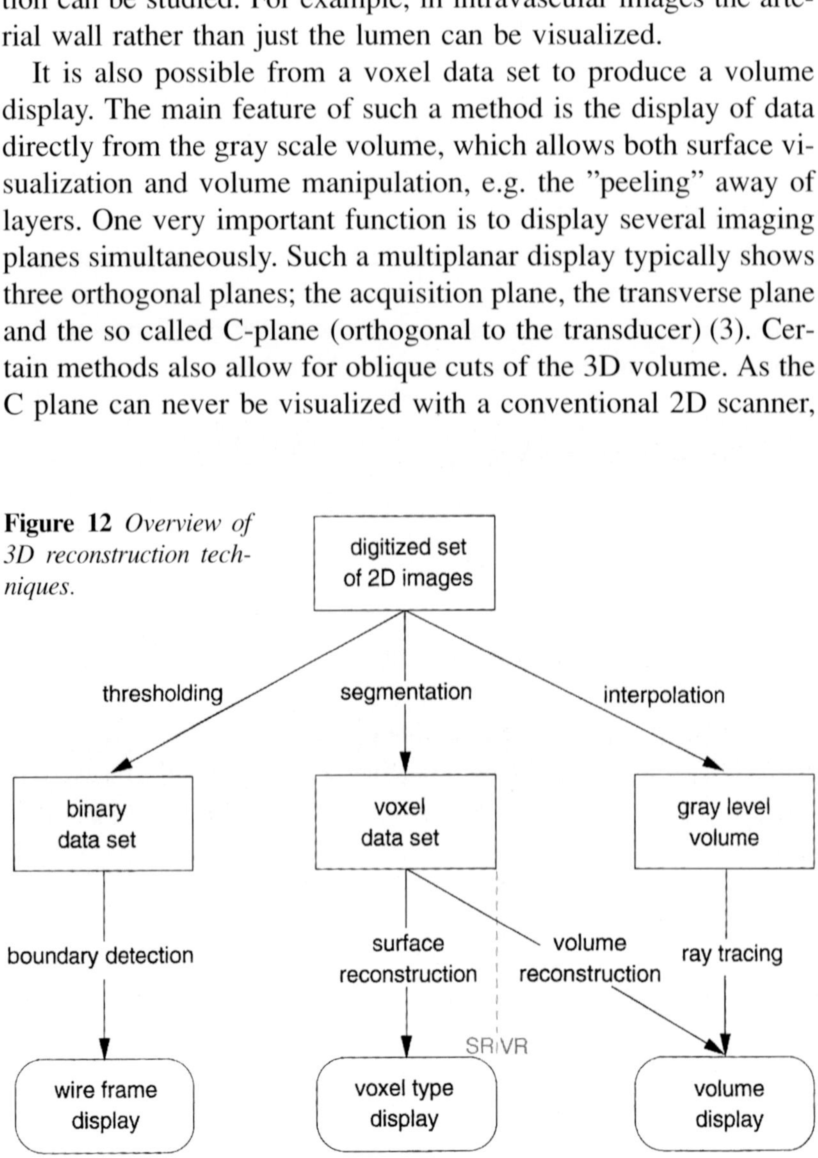

there are hopes that the multiplanar display format in itself will be a valuable adjunct to 2D imaging (Figure 13).

Volume rendering techniques can also be applied to the interpolated 2D gray scale images directly. Interpolation refers to the process required to correctly link individual pixels in separate slices. Linear interpolation is often sufficient, provided the slice separation is not too great. The method used to produce the volume display is called ray tracing, since it tracks a computer simulated ray of light from a source through the object to a viewing screen (the display). Further technical details can be found elsewhere (19). Ray tracing is currently the most sophisticated, and general method for displaying 3D data. Consequently, it is also the most computationally intensive.

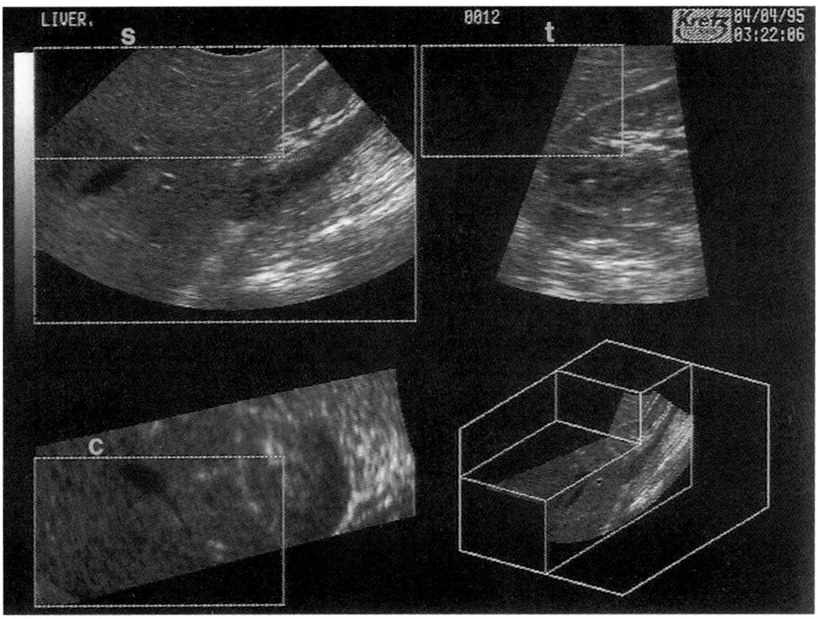

Figure 13 *Multiplanar display of human liver and kidney. Top left to bottom right are the sagittal (S), transverse (T), and coronal (C) planes, as well as the 3D volume.*

Clinical use of 3D ultrasound

3D ultrasound images will suffer from the same limitations imposed by the physics of acoustics as conventional images (lack of penetration of air, bone, etc.). Hence, 3D ultrasound will most likely become an adjunct to standard ultrasound imaging in areas where specific anatomical information or more precise volume calculations are required.

Gray-scale 3D imaging

By far, the most common approach to 3D ultrasound is based on digitizing the B-mode video signal directly to produce gray-scale 3D images. One area which has received a lot of interest is the fetus. Surface rendering techniques have been used to visualize the fetus in general and the fetal face in particular (20). While many fetal abnormalities are relatively easy to detect with conventional 2D ultrasound some facial abnormalities, such as cleft palate and lips, can have very subtle presentations. 3D ultrasound should be able to increase the diagnostic confidence in many cases, and in some cases may even detect abnormalities which were otherwise not observed. Furthermore, some structures (e.g., the fetal spine) can be difficult to visualize in completeness. There the ability of 3D imaging to display planes otherwise not seen (e.g., orthogonal to the transducer) should prove advantageous. Growth retardation is today determined via volume measurements and, here too, 3D ultrasound might have a role to play by increasing the accuracy of volume determinations. Finally the total exposure time for the fetus could be reduced by acquiring all data needed in a single 3D volume, which would then be available for viewing at different angles, planes, etc. An example of surface rendering of a fetal face is presented in Figure 14.

However, 3D imaging of the fetus is technically challenging. Fetal movement is a major problem, which ideally requires data acquisition times of less than 5 seconds. Furthermore, the 3D volume to be interrogated can be very large; especially later in pregnancy. The third trimester may also present some types of mechanical arms with localization problems due to the curvature of the abdomen.

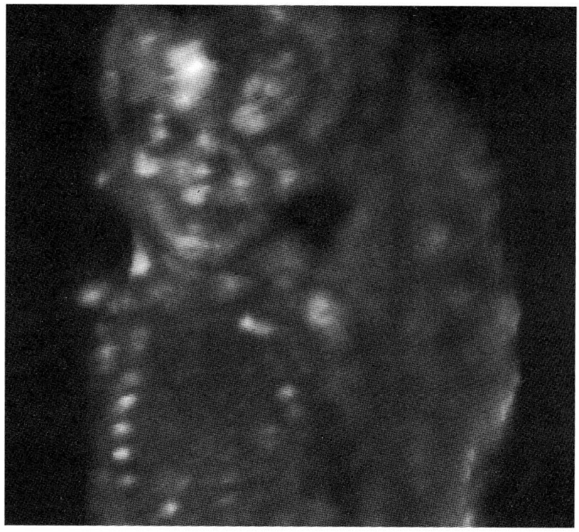

Figure 14 *Surface rendering of fetal face.*

Areas where localization is not a problem include catheterized vessels (as in intravascular ultrasound) and the prostate. Cancer of the prostate is the second largest cause of death for men, and the volume of the prostate, as well as of the tumor itself can be of importance. Since the transducer is positioned in the rectum, simple timed pull-back at a constant velocity will suffice to define the 3D volume. This should also help to shorten the procedure. Timed pull-back can also be applied to 3D intravascular imaging. High frequency, miniature, catheter-based transducers provide circumferential images of the vascular lumen, plaque and adjacent structures beyond the vessel walls. 3D images of plaque morphology, as well as lesion size determination (for staging) appear to be promising areas of clinical utility.

The eye and orbit has been described as an area ideally suited for 3D ultrasound or because of the limited depth and the specific anatomy involved (20). Direct evaluation of some orbital diseases, as well as assisting in the surgical planning are areas where 3D ultrasound imaging might have a role to play. Even though it is more difficult to provide clinical reasons for performing 3D examinations of abdominal organs, such as the liver and kidneys, some preliminary work has been reported. It is feasible to construct 3D reconstructions of hepatic structures, but more research in this area will be required to establish usefulness.

The heart, on the other hand, offer many clinical uses for 3D ultrasound imaging. The spatial relationship between different cardiac structures is of interest, as is visualization of abnormalities such as arterial septal defects. Furthermore, calculation of ventricular volumes and masses are important and should be improved with 3D. Data acquisition must be cardiac gated and is either performed transthoracically or transesophagally; the former is often limited by rib interference, while the latter approach often does not visualize the left ventricular apex well. However, the transesophageal approach does provide improved spatial resolution due to the higher frequencies (≥5 MHz) employed when in close proximity to the heart. Wire frame displays have been used with success in 3D cardiac imaging, since volume calculations are easy to perform.

Color 3D imaging

The ability of ultrasound to perform real-time studies of blood flow (without the use of ionizing contrast) is very important. Thus, it is not surprising that the prospect of combining color Doppler imaging with 3D displays has aroused interest; in spite of the considerable demand on computer resources.

The technically most advanced system for color Doppler imaging was developed by Picot and co-workers (21). They used a 5

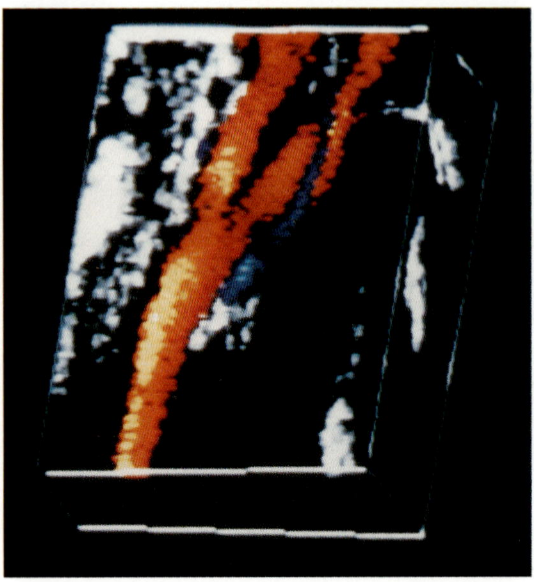

Figure 15 *3D color flow image of the carotid artery. Reproduced with permission from ref. 21.*

MHz linear array transducer mounted in a motor-driven, handheld translation assembly to image flow in the carotid artery (Figure 15). The duration from scanning to 3D display is approximately 10 minutes. The angle between the translation axis and the imaging plane of the transducer is adjustable (66° was used for the carotid study). The velocity estimates were found to be accurate to within 1.3 % with a precision of 11 % and not particularly sensitive to ECG timing problems. The system is also capable of acquiring multiple images at several points during the cardiac cycle to form a set of 3D reconstructions, which can then be viewed in a cine-loop fashion. This ability is sometimes referred to as 4D ultrasound imaging.

The clinical applications of color 3D imaging include the visualization of cardiac jets due to valve defects, which can be difficult to see in conventional ultrasound, as well as the display of the vasculature in an area suspected of containing a mass. The 3D display should make it easier to detect any abnormal changes in the relationship between closely spaced vessels, thus, revealing the location of the lesion. Other areas where color 3D imaging has been attempted are the prostate and the brain (20). The former research centers around attempts to monitor tumor flow after radiation therapy, while the latter attempts to overcome the difficulties of transcranial Doppler to globally evaluate the major brain arteries. The benefit is being able to localize a functional abnormality relative to the underlying anatomy.

Preliminary work has begun on improving color 3D ultrasound imaging. The easiest way to increase the quality of the 3D display is to acquire color amplitude instead of color Doppler images. CAI has, as mentioned, the ability to display smaller vessels as well as showing vessels over longer length than has conventional CDI. This increase in display dynamic range is achieved by sacrificing directional and velocity information, which makes vessels in CAI appear more like those of x-ray angiograms. The added completeness of the depiction of the vasculature will also result in more complete 3D color images. Another approach is to combine 3D imaging with ultrasound contrast agents. Given the large enhancement of Doppler signals produced by the contrast quite spectacular 3D color images should be feasible. The problem of the limited duration of the contrast effects could be overcome through continuous infusion, instead of bolus injection, of the agent. Both of the concepts described above are actively being pursued by a number of researchers and it is only a question of time before the first results appear in the literature.

SUMMARY

A large variety of ultrasound contrast agents have been, or are, under development. The majority utilize gas-based microbubbles to enhance Doppler, as well as B-mode signals; other types e.g., aimed at specific organs also exist. There appear to be numerous potential clinical applications ranging from straightforward improved vessel visualization to measurements of myocardial perfusion. The possibility of contrast-specific imaging is being developed. Some first generation agents are already commercially available and others are expected to follow suit in the not too distant future.

Due to the advances in computer processing and display powers 3D ultrasound imaging is quickly becoming an available clinical tool. To date, only a rather limited number of specific clinical applications have been identified. However, given the research efforts devoted to 3D ultrasound and considering the impact 3D displays have had in other imaging modalities, there will undoubtedly be areas where 3D ultrasound imaging will emerge as a viable adjunct to conventional 2D imaging.

REFERENCES

1. Ophir J, Parker KJ. Contrast agents in diagnostic ultrasound. Ultrasound Med Biol 1989;15:319–333.
2. Goldberg BB, Liu JB, Forsberg F. Ultrasound contrast agents: a review. Ultrasound Med Biol 1994;20:319–333.
3. Hamper UM, Trapanotto V, Sheth S et al. Three-dimensional US: preliminary clinical experience. Radiology 1994;191:397–401.
4. Tickner EG, Rasor NS. An instrument for the noninvasive assessment of pulmonary hypertension. Adv Bioengin ASNE 1978;101–103.
5. Parker KJ, Baggs RB, Lerner RM et al. Ultrasound contrast for hepatic tumors using IDE particles. Invest Radiol 1990;25:1135–1139.

6. Andre MP, Steinbach G, Mattrey RF. Enhancement of the echogenicity of flowing blood by the contrast agent perfusion. Invest Radiol 1993;28:502–506.
7. Goldberg BB, Hilpert PL, Burns PN et al. Hepatic tumors: signal enhancement of Doppler US after intravenous injection of a contrast agent. Radiology 1990;177:713–717.
8. Winkelmann JW, Kenner MD, Dave R et al. Contrast echocardiography. Ultrasound Med Biol 1994;20:507–515.
9. de Jong N, ten Cate FJ, Vletter WB, Roelandt JRTC. Quantifacation of transpulmonary echocontrast effects. Ultrasound Med Biol 1993;19:279–288.
10. Rubin JM, Bude RO, Carson PL et al. Power Doppler US: a potential useful alternative to mean frequency-based color Doppler US. Radiology 1994;190:853–856.
11. Duda VF, Rode G, Schlief R. Echo contrast enhanced color flow imaging of the breast. Ultrasound Obstet Gynecol 1993;3:191–194.
12. Forsberg F, Liu JB, Burns PN et al. Artifacts in ultrasonic contrast agent studies. J Ultrasound Med 1994;13:357–365.
13. Schrope B, Newhouse VL, Uhlendorf V. Simulated capillary blood flow measurement using a nonlinear ultrasonic contrast agent. Ultrasonic Imaging 1992;14:134–158.
14. Schrope BA, Newhouse VL. Second harmonic ultrasonic blood perfusion measurement. Ultrasound Med Biol 1993;19:567–579.
15. Burns PN, Powers JE, Fritsch T. Harmonic imaging: new imaging and Doppler method for contrast-enhanced ultrasound. Radiology 1992;182(P):142 (abstract).
16. Forsberg F, Newhouse VL, Liu JB et al. In-vivo application of contrast-enhanced harmonic imaging. Radiology 1993;189(P):285 (abstract).
17. Burns PN, Powers JE, Hope-Simpson D et al. Power Doppler imaging combined with contrast-enhancing harmonic Doppler: a new method for small-vessel imaging. Radiology 1994;193(p):366 (abstract).
18. Lev-Toaff AS, Merton DA, Dumsha J, Goldberg BB. Evaluation of an oral contrast agent to improve ultrasonic visualization of abdominal anatomy: a phase I trial. J Ultrasound Med 1994;13:S8 (abstract).
19. Barillot C. Surface and volume rendering techniques to display 3D data. IEEE Eng Med Biol Mag 1993;12:101–119.
20. Rankin RN, Fenster A, Downey DB et al. Three-dimensional sonographic reconstruction techniques and diagnostic applications. AJR 1993;161:695–702.
21. Picot PA, Rickey DW, Mitchell R et al. Three-dimensional colour Doppler imaging. Ultrasound Med Biol 1993;19:95–104.

Index

B

C

I

J

K

L

M

N

W

X

Y